From Conventional to Innovative Approaches for Pain Treatment

Edited by Marco Cascella

Published in London, United Kingdom

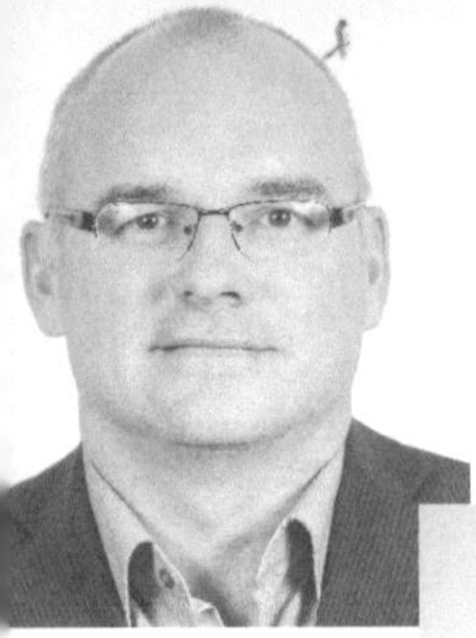
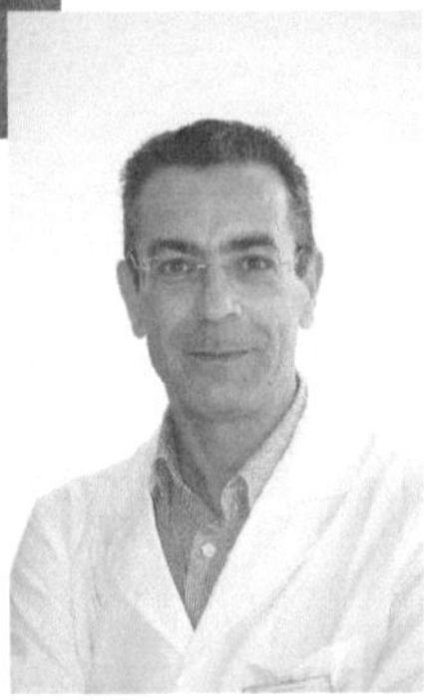
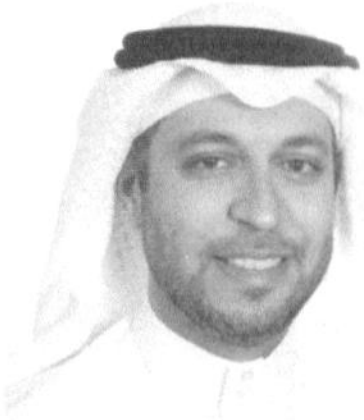
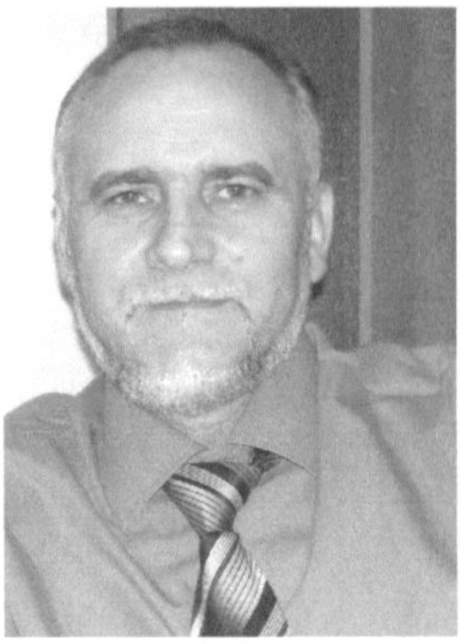
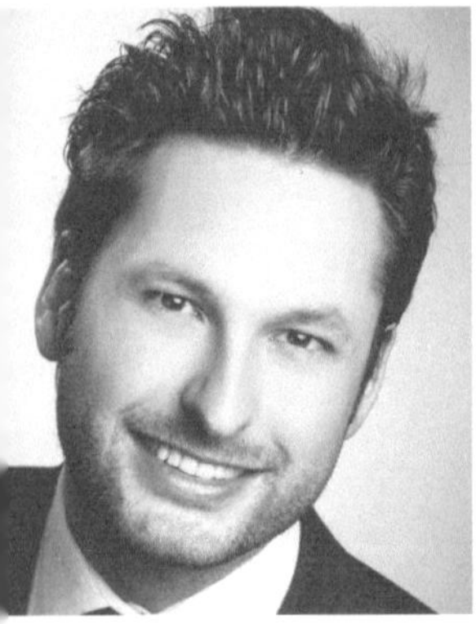
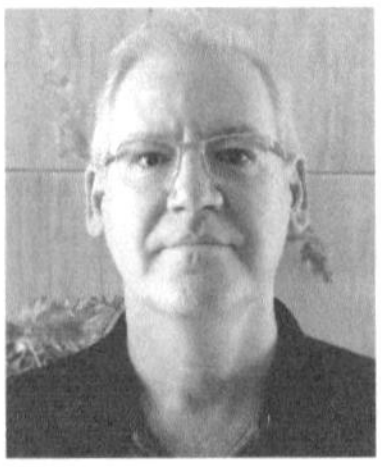
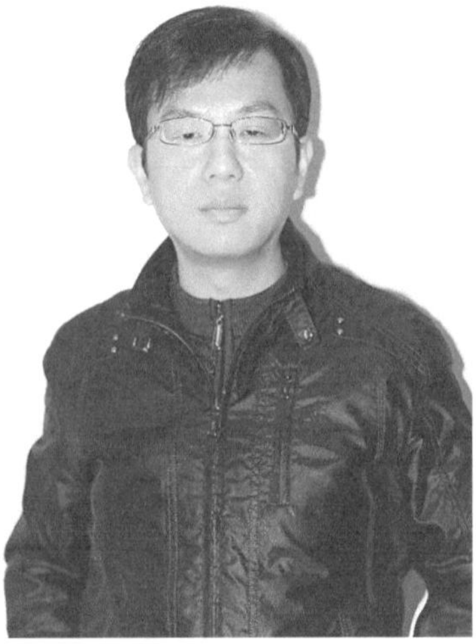

IntechOpen

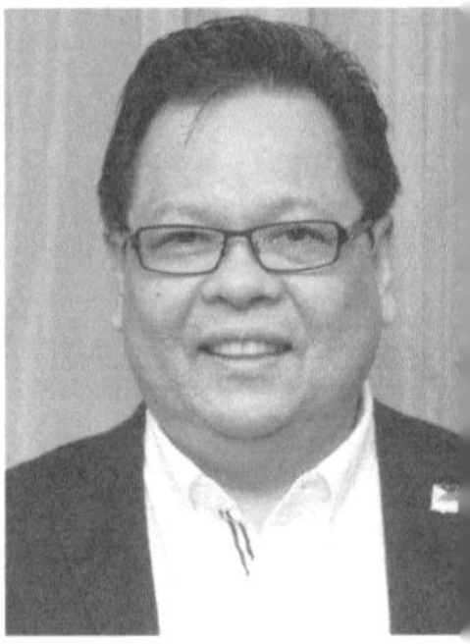
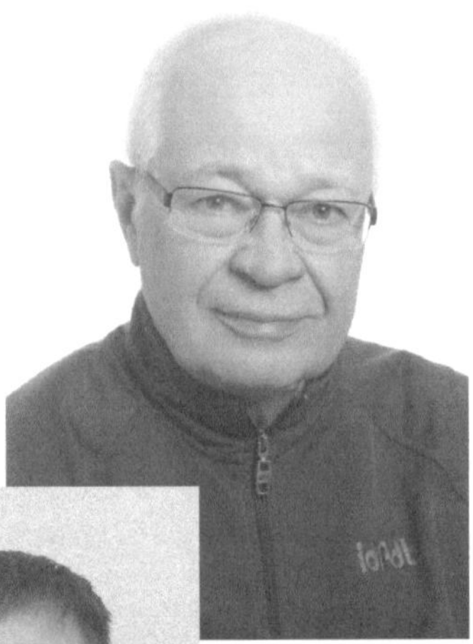
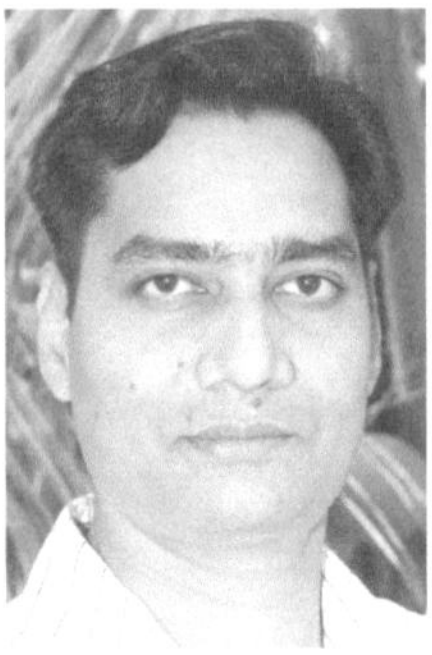
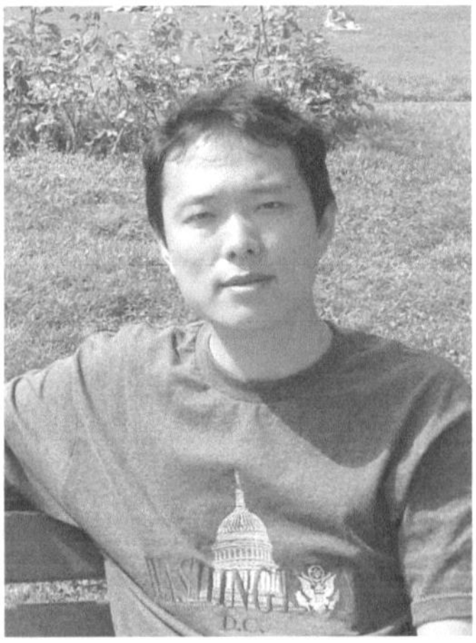
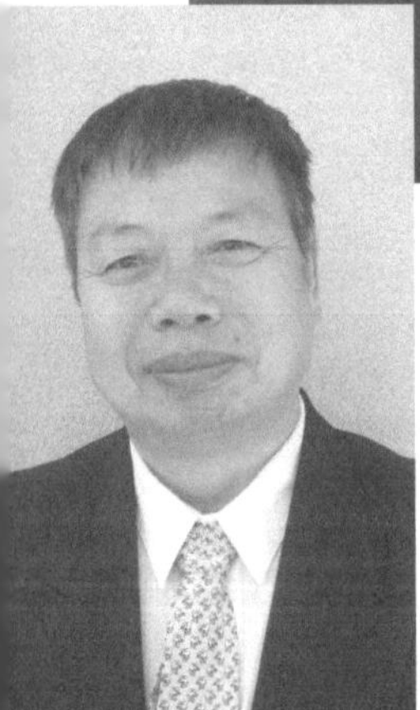
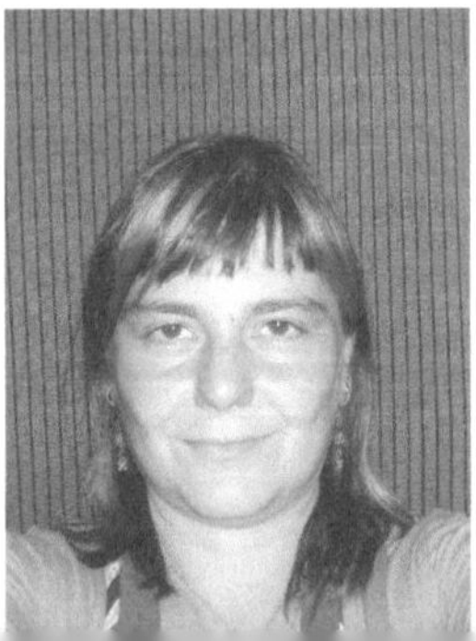

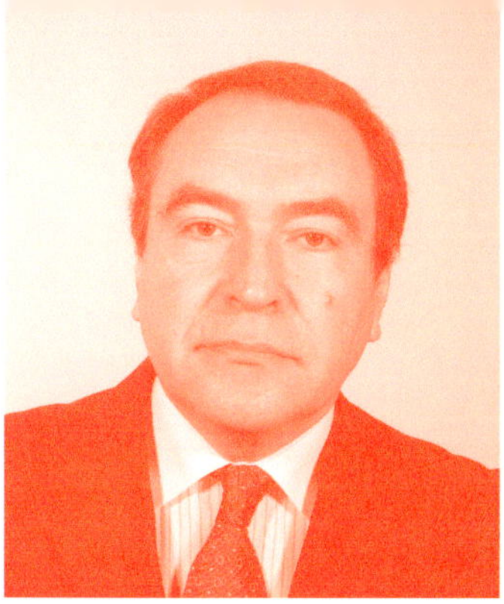

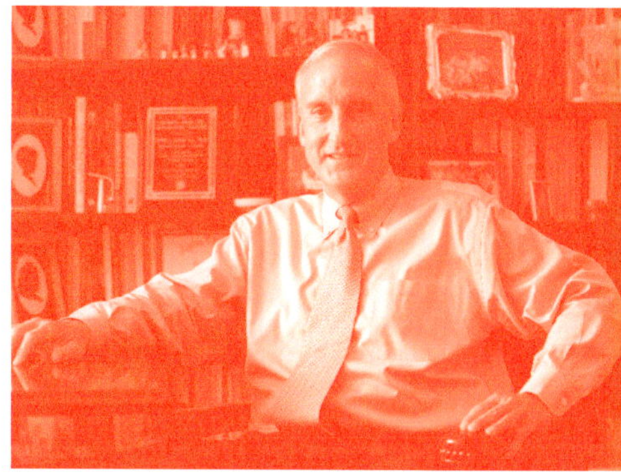

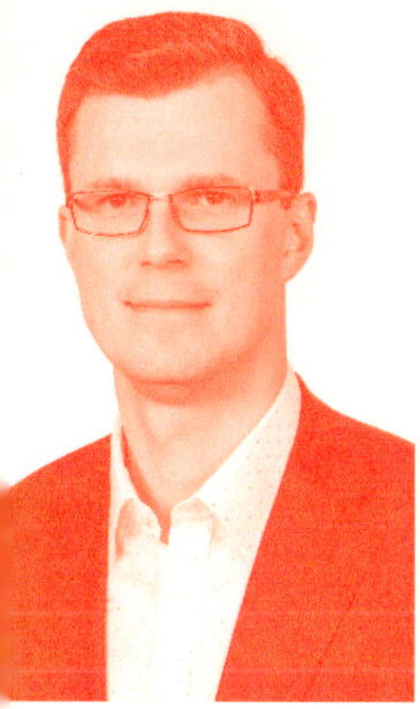

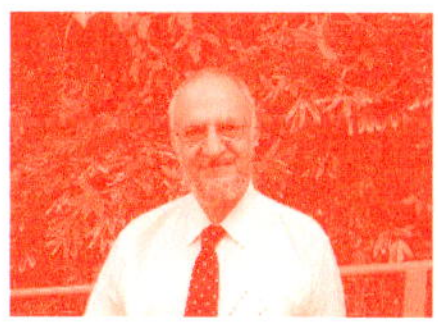

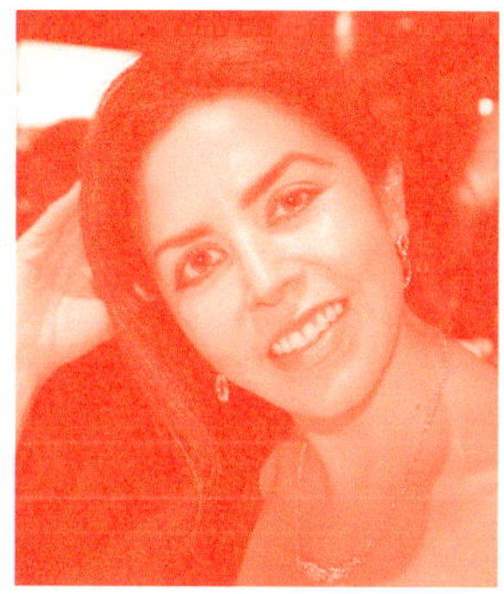

Supporting open minds since 2005

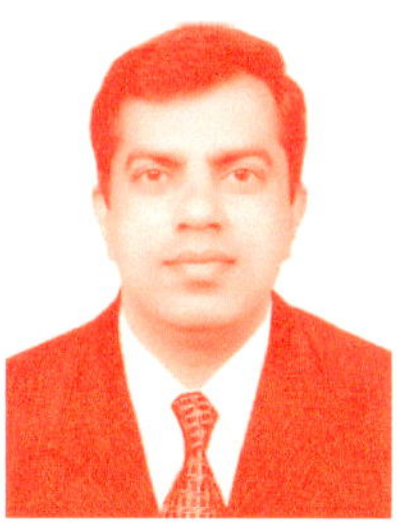

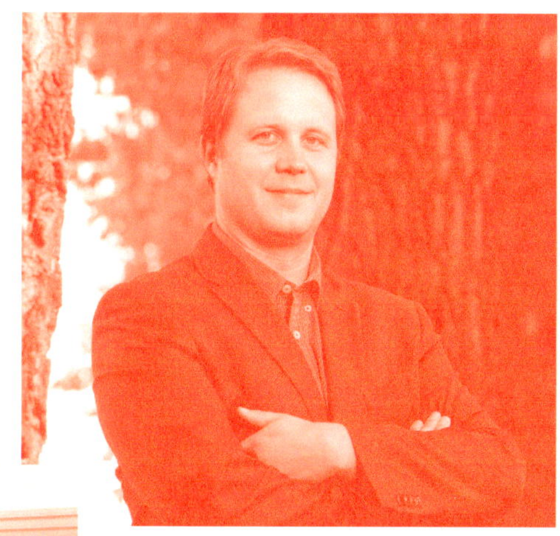

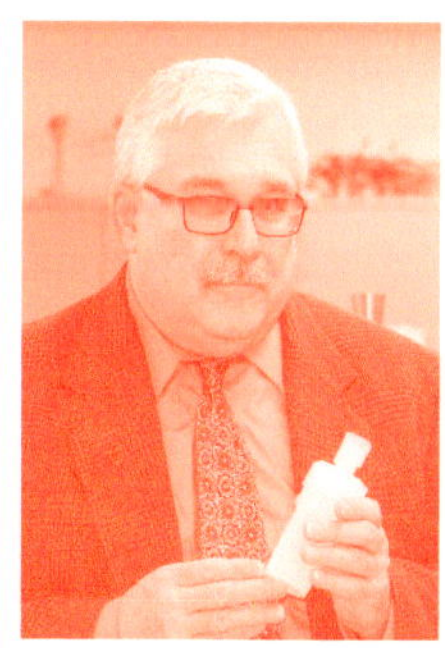

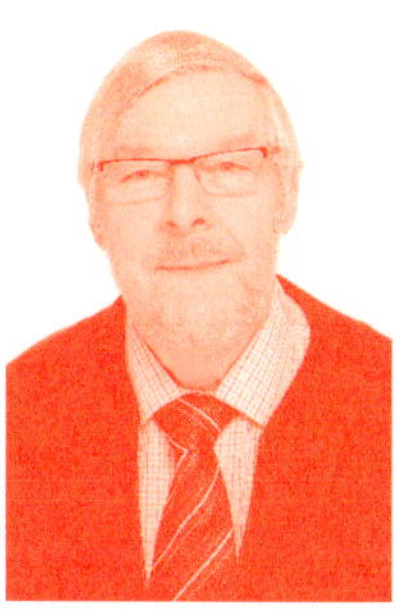

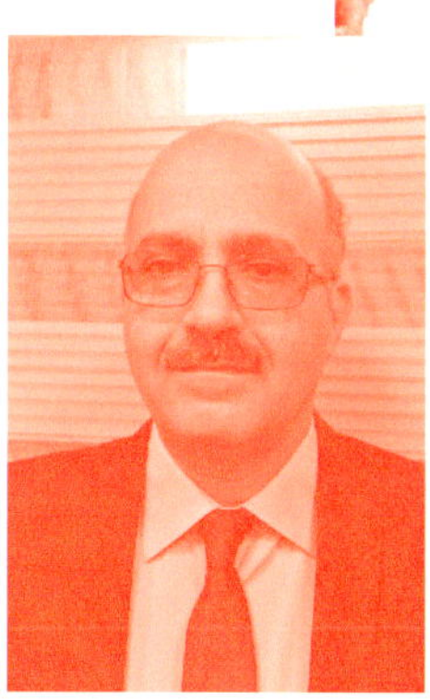

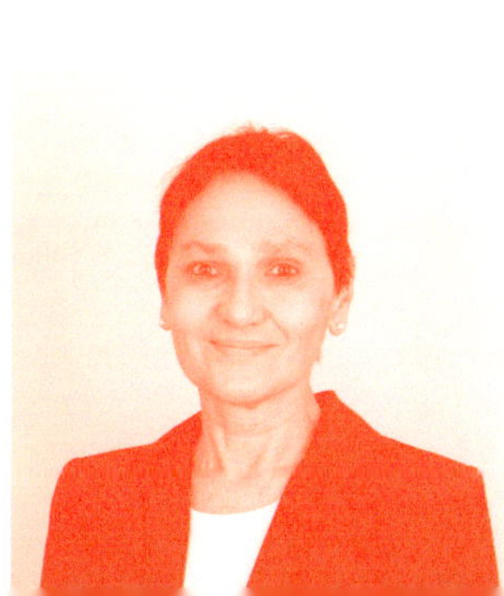

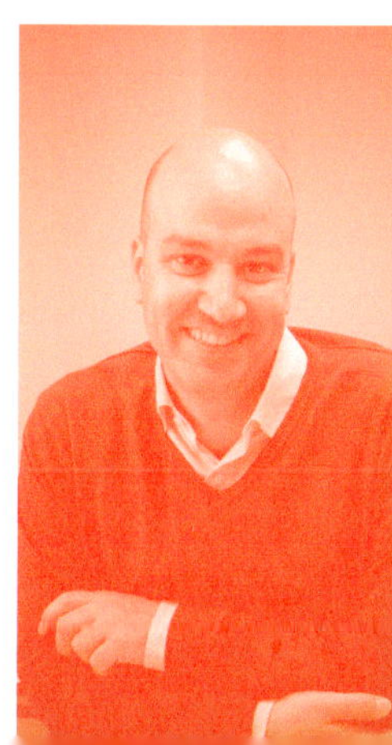

From Conventional to Innovative Approaches for Pain Treatment
http://dx.doi.org/10.5772/intechopen.77716
Edited by Marco Cascella

Contributors
Sameer Shaikh, Xue-Bin Yan, Nicholas West, Gillian R. Lauder, Greg Siren, Özlem Aytekin, Sevda Arısoy, Işık Çoban, Arunas Sciupokas, Liuda Brogienė, Dalia Skorupskienė, Laura Perryman, Hollis Krug, Linda Papa, Mark Bender, Nicholas Yim, Fereydoun Don Parsa, Ilker Solmaz, Aydan Orscelik, Marco Cascella

First published in London, United Kingdom, 2019 by IntechOpen
IntechOpen is the global imprint of INTECHOPEN LIMITED, registered in England and Wales, registration number: 11086078, The Shard, 25th floor, 32 London Bridge Street
London, SE19SG – United Kingdom
Printed in Croatia

British Library Cataloguing-in-Publication Data
A catalogue record for this book is available from the British Library

Additional hard and PDF copies can be obtained from orders@intechopen.com

From Conventional to Innovative Approaches for Pain Treatment
Edited by Marco Cascella
p. cm.
Print ISBN 978-1-78984-163-3
Online ISBN 978-1-78984-164-0
eBook (PDF) ISBN 978-1-83962-197-0

Meet the editor

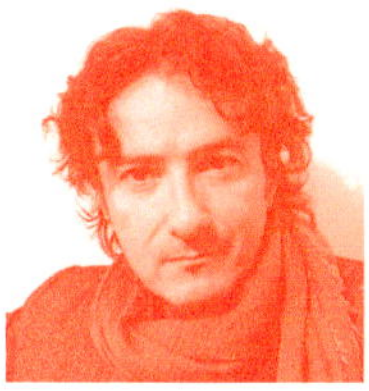

Marco Cascella, MD, works in the Department of Anesthesia Pain Medicine and Supportive Care at the National Cancer Institute, Istituto Nazionale Tumori IRCCS "Fondazione G. Pascale" (INT – Pascale), Naples, Italy, where he conducts clinical and preclinical research projects in anesthesia and pain medicine. He is also a professor of Physiology in Biomedical Laboratory Techniques at the Faculty of Medicine, University of Naples Federico II, and a professor of Anesthesia and Pneumology in the School of Nursing at the same university. Dr. Cascella graduated in Medicine and Surgery with honors in 1997 from the Second University of Naples. He undertook postgraduate studies in anesthesia and intensive care, earning his doctorate in 2001. He is a member of the expert committee in cancer pain and palliative care of the Italian Society of Anesthesia, Analgesia, Reanimation and Intensive Care (SIAARTI). He is a research editor for the Italian Ministry of Health and an editorial board member of several medical journals. He has spoken at numerous conferences and conventions and is the author of about 100 scientific publications, books, and book chapters in the fields of anesthesia, pathophysiology, pain treatment, oncology, and palliative care.

Contents

Preface

Non est vivere, sed valere vita est
Marcus Valerius Martialis
Epigrammaton Liber VI, Carmen 70, 15

In recent decades, notable advances have been carried out in pain medicine due to enhanced knowledge of the pathophysiology of acute and chronic pain, the newest pharmacological options, the significant role of nonpharmacological strategies, and the development of minimally invasive approaches. In particular, individualized, dynamic, and multicomponent paths (multimodal therapy) represent a real revolution in this field of medicine.

Nevertheless, to date, pain relief often remains an unmet need. For instance, up to 80% of postsurgical patients experience pain, which is described as severe in 10–20% of cases. Furthermore, primary and secondary chronic painful conditions are often managed by focusing only on pain intensity instead of considering the multiple aspects related to disease and disability. This poses a great challenge because pain as a symptom and pain as a disease are leading causes of suffering and disability. Furthermore, undertreated pain leads to serious problems such as increased opioid prescription and use, which can result in opioid addiction.

This book analyzes several important aspects of pain treatment, from acute pain in surgical settings to chronic pain in cancer and other diseases, from opioids research to interventional procedures, and from optimization of conventional strategies to innovative therapeutic approaches. Coverage of these topics augmented with attractive iconography and up-to-date references. This volume is an important source for specialized pain therapists, owing to the comprehensive coverage of the topics and the scientific value of each chapter. Furthermore, for nonspecialized physicians, it is a very useful guide for managing different types of pain.

I would like to express thanks to all the internationally recognized experts in the treatment of pain who collaborated in producing this volume. Finally, I am especially grateful to Mr. Luka Cvjetkovic, author service manager at IntechOpen publishing. This book offered me the opportunity to collaborate with a qualified professional and it is my sincere belief that this significant partnership will be further strengthened in the years to come.

Marco Cascella
Division of Anesthesia and Pain Medicine,
Istituto Nazionale Tumori – IRCCS – Fondazione 'G. Pascale',
Naples, Italy

Section 1

Acute Pain

Chapter 1

Introductory Chapter: The Rationale for a Multimodal Approach to Pain Treatment

Marco Cascella

1. Common issues in acute and chronic pain management

The symptom pain is a perception affected by complex interconnections of biological, psychological, and social factors. Analgesic monotherapy can often provide pain relief in clinical conditions featuring non-severe pain. In other circumstances, such as those characterized by intractable cancer pain, or concerning acute/chronic non-cancer neuropathic pain, the intensity and quality of the pain require individualized multidrug approaches, with different analgesics and adjuvants used in combination according to clinical practice guidelines published by international and regional professional associations [1]. Moreover, because pharmacological strategies may not be able to successfully treat all patients with acute or chronic pain, nonpharmacological strategies should be included in the analgesic program, supporting and strengthening drug therapy [2]. Again, especially, chronic pain represents a dynamic experience, profoundly changeable in a spatial-temporal manner; thus, standardized and fixed protocols are not universally applicable for pain therapy. From these premises, the individualized, dynamic, and multicomponent pathway is summarized by the concept of the multimodal approach to pain management and represents a real revolution in this field of medicine. This optimization strategy can allow managing the pain by treating this symptom in its variegated clinical expressions through multiple interventions. According to the concept of multimodal therapy, the objective of pain relief is possible by targeting different sites of the nociceptive pathway [3] and by managing the galaxy of pain-related conditions through pharmacologic and nonpharmacologic modalities [4]. However, several considerations should be addressed in order to better understand its rational application for both acute (e.g., postoperative) and chronic pain management.

1.1 The unmet need of postoperative pain relief

According to the Lancet's data, more than 230 million people undergo surgery each year worldwide and this huge number tends to increase year over year [5]. Postoperative pain is a typical example of acute pain and, probably, it represents the classic example of unmet need in surgery as up to 80% of postsurgical patients experience pain which in 10–20% of cases is described as severe [6]. This topic is of paramount importance, as inadequately controlled pain impairs quality of life (QoL) and functional recovery, increases the risk of postsurgical complications, and lengthens the time of hospitalization. Increased morbidity and prolonged opioid use during and after hospitalization are serious problems which call for effective preventive interventions. Furthermore, treating chronic pain induced by ineffective acute pain management increases the cost of care, enormously [7]. From these data, it is clear that the commonly used strategies to address postoperative pain are very often inadequate.

1.2 The issue of pain chronitization

Undertreated acute postoperative pain is the main cause determining the development of postsurgical chronic pain (PSCP), which is difficult to treat and often invalidating in form. The pain chronitization is the final stage of a complex pathogenetic cascade. Summarizing, these mechanisms involve the activation of peripheral and central sensitization pathways. Data from a wide number of preclinical investigations demonstrated that activation and sensitization of peripheral nociceptors, spinal dorsal horn neurons, and central nervous system (CNS) brain areas may occur [8]. The role of specific peripheral mechanisms contributing to pain after surgical incision and manipulation has been investigated as well. The literature on the topic encompasses an incredible number of studies on nociceptors, molecular mechanisms, fiber sensitization processes, inflammatory cytokines, and so on [9–13]. While according to a classical point of view, the CNS involvement is strictly related to the mechanisms of chronic pain; however, it may result in difficulty to identify the borderline between acute and chronic pain. There are many good reasons to believe that many gaps such as the role of the environment (i.e., epigenetic) and genetics are not still well explained. Again, no clear criteria for diagnosing central sensitization have been recognized. The chronicity of pain is the effect of changes in pain processing through transcription and transduction processes. Preclinical studies suggested that alterations in the mRNA expression occur within the first 42–48 hours after surgery [14]. These sensitization processes seem to be quite rapid, at least in the experimental field. Thus, postoperative pain is a convoluted process engaging both the peripheral nervous system (PNS) and the CNS and, in turn, the exact distinction between acute and chronic postoperative pain is not always easy to establish.

1.3 Toward an early and combined strategy

Rather than dissecting the precise pathophysiology of acute and chronic pain, our knowledge on the matter must be translated in the most effective way to limit acute pain and to prevent mechanisms of sensitization. For these aims, all our "analgesic arsenal" must be defused as soon as possible, and before that surgery may trigger the first fuse. For instance, it has been demonstrated that tailored preoperative educational programs reduced postoperative opioid requirement and shortened the length of stay [15]. Furthermore, several self-management programs focused on patient's education and training may reduce risk factors (e.g., lifestyle-related), enhance protective factors, and, finally, prevent pain chronitization [16]. As a consequence, individualized programs for perioperative pain management can be performed by acting simultaneously on different targets or implementing different strategies according to the timing.

1.4 The opioid crisis

Ineffective management of perioperative pain and poorly controlled postoperative pain may induce development of PSCP, increased opioid prescription and use, until opioid addiction. Because the opioids epidemic in the United States and Canada is a dramatic phenomenon which has been responsible for up to 70,000 drug overdose deaths, in 2017 [17], the time has come to look at more effective solutions and less harmful approaches capable of inducing optimal pain relief combined with lessening opioid use, opioid prescriptions, and reduced opioid-related complications. Controlled investigations and evidence-based analysis demonstrated that multimodal approaches to postoperative pain improved analgesia and lowered opioid consumption is several clinical settings such as those underwent orthopedic [18] or colorectal surgery [19].

1.5 Chronic pain

These problems, linked to a lack of efficacy and to a criticality due to the use of opioids, do not only concern the postoperative pain chapter but also involve the management of chronic pain in its two sides of the coin, chronic cancer pain and chronic non-cancer pain. To understand the numerical terms of the matter, chronic pain is among the most common reasons for seeking medical care because it is reported by up 50% of patients seen in primary care [20]. Of note, chronic pain with neuropathic features, which often represents a hard task for clinicians, seems to be more common in the general population than earlier reported [21]. Because in cancer patients, pain has a multifactorial etiology and is quite a dynamic process, its management should be conducted through a careful combination of pharmacological agents with nonpharmacological strategies. This dynamical approach should be based on pain intensity and the complexity of symptoms, pain pathophysiology, and presence of comorbidities.

2. Features of the multimodal approaches to pain management

The concept of "multimodal" analgesia was introduced by Kehlet and Dahl, in 1993 [22]. This approach is based on the use of two or more distinct methods or drugs to treat pain rather than using opioids, or other strategies, alone. The rationale is that by combining medications and techniques with different mechanisms and sites of action, better pain relief can be achieved, with reduced side effects [23]. Different combinations of analgesic medications, adjuvants, and procedures can act on different sites and pathways in an additive or synergistic fashion. Clinicians may choose among a wide range of options included in several categories: pharmacologic, physical medicine, education and behavioral approaches, interventional, and surgical modalities. In the surgical setting, anesthesiologists may combine regional anesthetics, and/or nonopioid analgesics, such as nonsteroidal anti-inflammatory drugs (NSAIDs), cyclooxygenase-2 (COX2) inhibitors, NMDA-receptor antagonists, and antiepileptic, and antidepressant medications with or without conventional opioids. On the other hand, chronic cancer and non-cancer pain chronic cancer treatment often requires the involvement of a multidisciplinary team which combines resources based on the patient's needs, obtaining an individually tailored program.

2.1 Surgical settings

Multimodal approaches to pain management can be included among more complex systematic processes adopted for managing the whole perioperative course. The Enhanced Recovery After Surgery (ERAS) pathway, for instance, is a multidisciplinary model of care born with the aim of guaranteeing optimal recovery and an early and safe return to daily activities after surgery. The pathway is a patient-tailored process provided by a team of surgeons, anesthesiologists, nurses, nutritionists, and physical therapists. In this scenario, the perioperative pain management is a keystone of the whole pathway [24]. Indeed, reduced need for opioids through regional anesthetic block used in addition to general anesthesia during surgery, or other minimally invasive approaches, may be effective for both pain relief and enhanced recovery target [25]. Apart from the ERAS strategy, another recent approach to perioperative pain management is the so-called opioid-free anesthesia (OFA) [26]. This term refers to a fascinating option for anesthesia administration that maximizes the patient's comfort (including pain relief) while eliminating the unwanted side effects of opioids. Through this model, no intraoperative systemic, neuraxial, or intracavitary opioid is administered during the anesthetic course. The rationale of the OFA model is the avoidance of the opioid-induced hyperalgesia phenomenon, a paradoxical effect in which opioid therapy enhances or aggravates preexisting pain [27], the reduced occurrence of postoperative delirium, and postoperative cognitive dysfunction in elderly [28, 29] and in high-risk patients [30]. Furthermore, the OFA technique seems to be appropriate for minimizing respiratory depression in patients that have impaired respiratory function (e.g., due to sleep apnea, or obesity), for reducing postoperative nausea and vomiting, and for treating patients who have chronic pain conditions, or are on chronic opioid therapy, or opioid addiction [31, 32]. Although the effect of opioids on cancer recurrence or progression remains an open issue [33], the OFA approach can be considered as a protective strategy against cancer progression [34]. In the surgical setting, it is possible to obtain a multimodal strategy without completely avoiding opioids. Low-dose opioids can be combined with one or more additional pain management methods (e.g., peripheral nerve blocks and neuraxial analgesia) and/or medications such as acetaminophen, steroids, gabapentin/pregabalin, NSAIDs, dexmedetomidine, intravenous lidocaine, COX-2 inhibitors, or ketamine. Recently, Cozowicz et al. [35] demonstrated that this approach was correlated with a reduction in opioid use, postoperative complications, and less resource utilization. Again, multimodal analgesia may reduce the occurrence of PSCP, even when expressed as postsurgery pain syndrome [36], although the link between perioperative analgesic modes and the postoperative chronitization of pain should be better investigated [37]. The challenge of the OFA or the opioid-sparing regimens remains the choice of medication pathway in terms of number, the timing of use, and doses useful in different patient subgroups. While the use of a single drug (e.g., intravenous acetaminophen or methylprednisolone) was not associated with decreased opioids consumption [38], complex regimens featuring numerous medications may only increase drug-related side effects without improving outcomes.

2.2 Chronic cancer pain: beyond the analgesic ladder

In 1986, the World Health Organization (WHO) developed the classic three-step ladder model based on the use of analgesics for pain management in accordance with pain intensity in a linear movement directed toward the high or low steps of the ladder [39]. Subsequently, it was proposed a further step concerning interventional methods such as neurosurgical procedures (e.g., neuromodulation, nerve blocks, brain stimulators, and nerve lysis) robustly recommended for managing persistent pain even following the use of strong opioids. This revised four-step path can be adopted in a bidirectional way on the basis of the type of pain and its intensity [40]. Other attempts to modify the ladder strategy have also been proposed. According to the neuromatrix theory, chronic pain represents a multidimensional experience induced by the activation of a neural network ("neurosignature patterns") extensively distributed in the CNS [41]. From these premises, Leung hypothetically revised the original analgesic WHO ladder into a new analgesic path illustrated as a platform [42]. In this model, pain management followed a three-dimensional perspective including different areas of expertise that, in a multimodal fashion, can be combined with classical analgesics, on the basis of the pain condition. Despite its novelty, Leung's system seems to be lacking in completeness because it does not consider the dynamic perspective. The Cuomo et al. [43] "trolley analgesic model" is focused on individualized tailored therapies with dynamic multimodal approaches which are modulated according to the pain intensity, the physiopathology of pain, the multiplicity of symptoms, the presence of comorbidities, and psychological status and the patient's social context. The pharmacological agents and the nonpharmacological methods are included in different drawers of the trolley. It is possible to draw on one, or more, drawers of the trolley, and to choose within the contents of each drawer the most useful therapeutic method. According to the patient's needs, therapists can close or open different drawers, in a dynamic fashion.

2.3 Chronic non-cancer pain: toward a winning strategy

Chronic non-cancer pain conditions such as low back pain (LBP), osteoarthritis, headache, and neuropathic pain represent a significant problem in terms of psychosocial and socioeconomic consequences [44]. Due to the complexity of clinical features and multiple underlying mechanisms, this issue requires a multimodal approach. Since the 1980s, Kohles et al. [45] proposed a combined (multimodal) strategy focused on medical, behavioral, physical, and educational programs. Through this approach, defined as "functional restoration," the restoring of physical and psychological performances was obtained by the involvement of a multidisciplinary team composed of clinicians from a variety of medical disciplines (e.g., pain therapists, neurologists, orthopedics, rheumatologists), psychologists and psychiatrists, nurses, physical, and occupational therapists [46]. More recently, a task force of the German International Association for the Study of Pain (IASP) chapter has defined the principles of this approach, in terms of resources and operating methods [47]. Currently, the multimodal path has been widely recognized as winning strategy for addressing several chronic non-cancer pain conditions such as LBP, headache, and fibromyalgia although several obstacles still limit its routinely clinical application [48].

3. Conclusion

Multimodal approaches through the combined use of multiple modalities in analgesic protocols have the potential to offer a significant improvement in pain management for different acute, or chronic, clinical settings. Concerning perioperative pain management, included or not among ERAS or OFA pathways, multimodal modes can allow reducing opioid use, opioid prescriptions, and common opioid-related side effects, improving, in turn, outcomes. It seems that multimodal pain management may be able to prevent the development of chronic postsurgical pain conditions. Moreover, different attempts to better frame chronic pain in its many components, and for an effective treatment through a holistic approach, are being made to address the matter. Thus, the combined use of multiple modalities in analgesic protocols is worldwide encouraged. However, further research is needed to evaluate optimal multimodal regimens in terms of medications, doses, and timing (including the duration) of the administration, as well as to offer data useful for evidence-based practice. Finally, because lack of training (e.g., for invasive techniques or new techniques in regional anesthesia) and poor sources are huge obstacles for a routine application of multimodal approaches, identification of key barriers for their implementation seems to be a research priority.

Author details

Marco Cascella
Department of Anesthesia and Pain Medicine, Istituto Nazionale Tumori, IRCCS—Fondazione G. Pascale, Naples, Italy

*Address all correspondence to: m.cascella@istitutotumori.na.it

References

[1] Cruccu G, Truini A. A review of neuropathic pain: From guidelines to clinical practice. Pain and therapy. 2017;**6**(Suppl 1):35-42

[2] Cascella M, Thompson NS, Muzio MR, Forte CA, Cuomo A. The underestimated role of psychological and rehabilitation approaches for management of cancer pain. A brief commentary. Recenti Progressi in Medicina. 2016;**107**(8):418-421

[3] Manworren RC. Multimodal pain management and the future of a personalized medicine approach to pain. AORN Journal. 2015;**101**(3):308-314

[4] Bonakdar RA. Integrative pain management. The Medical Clinics of North America. 2017;**101**(5):987-1004

[5] Weiser TG, Regenbogen SE, Thompson KD, Haynes AB, Lipsitz SR, Berry WR, et al. An estimation of the global volume of surgery: A modeling strategy based on available data. Lancet. 2008;**372**(9633):139-144

[6] Apfelbaum JL, Chen C, Mehta SS, Gan TJ. Postoperative pain experience: Results from a national survey suggest postoperative pain continues to be undermanaged. Anesthesia and Analgesia. 2003;**97**:534-540

[7] Gan TJ. Poorly controlled postoperative pain: Prevalence, consequences, and prevention. Journal of Pain Research. 2017;**10**:2287-2298

[8] Pogatzki-Zahn EM, Segelcke D, Schug SA. Postoperative pain-from mechanisms to treatment. Pain Reports. 2017;**2**(2):e588. DOI: 10.1097/PR9.0000000000000588

[9] Pace MC, Passavanti MB, De Nardis L, Bosco F, Sansone P, Pota V, et al. Nociceptor plasticity: A closer look. Journal of Cellular Physiology. 2018;**233**(4):2824-2838

[10] Pasquinucci L, Turnaturi R, Montenegro L, Caraci F, Chiechio S, Parenti C. Simultaneous targeting of MOR/DOR: A useful strategy for inflammatory pain modulation. European Journal of Pharmacology. 2019;**847**:97-102

[11] Tsuda M. Modulation of pain and itch by spinal glia. Neuroscience Bulletin. 2018;**34**(1):178-185

[12] Zhang L, Terrando N, Xu ZZ, Bang S, Jordt SE, Maixner W, et al. Distinct analgesic actions of DHA and DHA-derived specialized pro-resolving mediators on post-operative pain after bone fracture in mice. Frontiers in Pharmacology. 2018;**9**:412. DOI: 10.3389/fphar.2018.00412. eCollection 2018

[13] Lueptow LM, Fakira AK, Bobeck EN. The contribution of the descending pain modulatory pathway in opioid tolerance. Frontiers in Neuroscience. 2018;**12**:886. DOI: 10.3389/fnins.2018.00886

[14] Spofford CM, Brennan TJ. Gene expression in skin, muscle, and dorsal root ganglion after plantar incision in the rat. Anesthesiology. 2012;**117**(1):161-172

[15] Chou R, Gordon DB, de Leon-Casasola OA, Rosenberg JM, Bickler S, Brennan T, et al. Management of postoperative pain: A clinical practice guideline from the American Pain Society, the American Society of Regional Anesthesia and Pain Medicine, and the American Society of Anesthesiologists' Committee on Regional Anesthesia, Executive Committee, and Administrative Council. The Journal of Pain. 2016;**17**(2):131-157

[16] Institute of Medicine. Relieving Pain in America: A Blueprint for Transforming Prevention, Care, Education, and Research. Washington, DC: National Academies Press; 2011

[17] National Institute on Drug Abuse. Overdose Death Rates. Available at: https://www.drugabuse.gov/related-topics/trends-statistics/overdose-death-rates [Accessed: 28-01-2019]

[18] Halawi MJ, Grant SA, Bolognesi MP. Multimodal analgesia for total joint arthroplasty. Orthopedics. 2015;**38**(7):e616-e625

[19] Wick EC, MC2 G, Wu CL. Postoperative multimodal analgesia pain management with nonopioid analgesics and techniques: A review. JAMA Surgery. 2017;**152**(7):691-697

[20] Elliott AM, Smith BH, Penny KI, Smith WC, Chambers WA. The epidemiology of chronic pain in the community. Lancet. 1999;**354**(9186):1248

[21] Torrance N, Smith BH, Bennett MI, Lee AJ. The epidemiology of chronic pain of predominantly neuropathic origin. Results from a general population survey. The Journal of Pain. 2006;**7**(4):281-289

[22] Kehlet H, Dahl JB. The value of "multimodal" or "balanced analgesia" in postoperative pain treatment. Anesthesia and Analgesia. 1993;**77**(5):1048-1056

[23] Clarke H, Poon M, Weinrib A, Katznelson R, Wentlandt K, Katz J. Preventive analgesia and novel strategies for the prevention of chronic post-surgical pain. Drugs. 2015;**75**(4):339-351

[24] Simpson JC, Bao X, Agarwala A. Pain management in enhanced recovery after surgery (ERAS) protocols. Clinics in Colon and Rectal Surgery. 2019;**32**(2):121-128

[25] Beverly A, Kaye AD, Ljungqvist O, Urman RD. Essential elements of multimodal analgesia in enhanced recovery after surgery (ERAS) guidelines. Anesthesiology Clinics. 2017;**35**(2):e115-e143

[26] Harkouk H, Fletcher D, Beloeil H. Opioid free anaesthesia: Myth or reality? Anaesthesia Critical Care & Pain Medicine. 2019;**38**(2):111-112. DOI: 10.1016/j.accpm.2019.01.005

[27] Tompkins DA, Campbell CM. Opioid-induced hyperalgesia: Clinically relevant or extraneous research phenomenon? Current Pain and Headache Reports. 2011;**15**(2):129-136

[28] Cascella M, Bimonte S. The role of general anesthetics and the mechanisms of hippocampal and extra-hippocampal dysfunctions in the genesis of postoperative cognitive dysfunction. Neural Regeneration Research. 2017;**12**(11):1780-1785

[29] Cascella M, Muzio MR, Bimonte S, Cuomo A, Jakobsson JG. Postoperative delirium and postoperative cognitive dysfunction: Updates in pathophysiology, potential translational approaches to clinical practice and further research perspectives. Minerva Anestesiologica. 2018;**84**(2):246-260

[30] Cascella M, Di Napoli R, Carbone D, Cuomo GF, Bimonte S, Muzio MR. Chemotherapy-related cognitive impairment: Mechanisms, clinical features and research perspectives. Recenti Progressi in Medicina. 2018;**109**(11):523-530

[31] Miceli L, Bednarova R, Vetrugno L, Cascella M, Cuomo A. Is the limit of 60mg of oral morphine equivalent daily dose still actual for the access to rapid onset opioids therapy? Current Problems in Cancer. 2018;**42**(3):367-368

[32] Miceli L, Bednarova R, Rizzardo A, Cuomo A, Riccardi I, Vetrugno L, et al. Opioids prescriptions in pain therapy

and risk of addiction: A one-year survey in Italy. Analysis of national opioids database. Annali dell'Istituto Superiore di Sanità. 2018;**54**(4):370-374

[33] Bimonte S, Barbieri A, Cascella M, Rea D, Palma G, Del Vecchio V, et al. The effects of naloxone on human breast cancer progression: In vitro and in vivo studies on MDA.MB231 cells. OncoTargets and Therapy. 2018;**11**: 185-191. DOI: 10.2147/OTT.S145780. eCollection 2018

[34] Clarke H, Soneji N, Ko DT, Yun L, Wijeysundera DN. Rates and risk factors for prolonged opioid use after major surgery: Population based cohort study. BMJ. 2014;**348**:g1251. DOI: 10.1136/bmj.g1251

[35] Cozowicz C, Poeran J, Zubizarreta N, Liu J, Weinstein SM, Pichler L, et al. Non-opioid analgesic modes of pain management are associated with reduced postoperative complications and resource utilisation: A retrospective study of obstructive sleep apnoea patients undergoing elective joint arthroplasty. British Journal of Anaesthesia. 2019;**122**(1):131-140

[36] Cascella M, Cuomo A, Viscardi D. Pain syndromes associated with cancer therapy. In: Cascella M, Cuomo A, Viscardi D, editors. Features and Management of the Pelvic Cancer Pain. Springer: Verlag; 2016. pp. 25-62. DOI: 10.1007/978-3-319-33587-2_3

[37] Jian W, Rejaei D, Shihab A, Alston TA, Wang J. The role of multimodal analgesia in preventing the development of chronic postsurgical pain and reducing postoperative opioid use. Journal of Opioid Management. 2018;**14**(6):453-461

[38] Wasserman I, Poeran J, Zubizarreta N, Babby J, Serban S, Goldberg AT, et al. Impact of intravenous acetaminophen on perioperative opioid utilization and outcomes in open colectomies: A claims database analysis. Anesthesiology. 2018;**129**(1):77-88

[39] Ventafridda V, Saita L, Ripamonti C, De Conno F. WHO guidelines for the use of analgesics in cancer pain. International Journal of Tissue Reactions. 1985;**7**(1):93-96

[40] Vargas-Schaffer G. Is the WHO analgesic ladder still valid? Twenty-four years of experience. Canadian Family Physician. 2010;**56**(6):514-517

[41] Melzack R. Evolution of the neuromatrix theory of pain. The Prithvi Raj Lecture: Presented at the Third World Congress of World Institute of Pain, Barcelona 2004. Pain Practice. 2005;**5**(2):85-94

[42] Leung L. From ladder to platform: A new concept for pain management. Journal of Primary Health Care. 2012;**4**(3):254-258

[43] Cuomo A, Bimonte S, Forte CA, Botti G, Cascella M. Multimodal approaches and tailored therapies for pain management: The trolley analgesic model. Journal of Pain Research. 2019;**12**:711-714. DOI: 10.2147/JPR.S178910. eCollection 2019

[44] Cheatle MD. Biopsychosocial approach to assessing and managing patients with chronic pain. Medical Clinics of North America. 2016;**100**:43-53

[45] Kohles S, Barnes D, Gatchel RJ, Mayer TG. Improved physical performance outcomes after functional restoration treatment in patients with chronic low-back pain. Early versus recent training results. Spine. 1990;**15**(12):1321-1324

[46] Cascella M, Cuomo A, Viscardi D. Pain management team and palliative care setting. In: Cascella M, Cuomo A, Viscardi D, editors. Features and Management of the Pelvic Cancer Pain.

Springer: Verlag; 2016. pp. 151-157. DOI: 10.1007/978-3-319-33587-2_11

[47] Arnold B, Brinkschmidt T, Casser HR, Gralow I, Irnich D, Klimczyk K, et al. Multimodal pain therapy: Principles and indications [in German]. Schmerz. 2009;**23**:112-120

[48] Kaiser U, Treede RD, Sabatowski R. Multimodal pain therapy in chronic noncancer pain-gold standard or need for further clarification? Pain. 2017;**158**(10):1853-1859

Chapter 2

Management of Odontogenic and Nonodontogenic Oral Pain

Sameer Shaikh

Abstract

Pain in the orofacial region is by far the commonest reason for patients to seek treatment. Tooth and intraoral structures are often the main sources of orofacial pain. Odontogenic pain, also commonly known as tooth pain, originates from dental structures, pulpal or periodontal. Nonodontogenic oral pain can originate from intraoral structures such as gingiva and buccal mucosa. Arriving at a correct and definitive diagnosis is of paramount importance to institute an appropriate treatment. Obtaining a detailed history from the patient including the location, duration, frequency, periodicity, character, and quality of pain assists in differentiating odontogenic from nonodontogenic causes. Wide varieties of pharmacological agents, along with invasive and noninvasive procedures, are available to manage odontogenic and nonodontogenic pain. While managing orofacial pain, clinical and pharmacological judgment should encompass a systematic and objective assessment in compliance with the strongest evidence available. In this chapter, there will be a discussion of various choices and options available to manage a few of the orofacial pain complaints.

Keywords: orofacial pain, odontogenic pain, nonodontogenic oral pain, pain management, pulpitis, periapical periodontitis, traumatic periodontitis, cracked tooth syndrome, noninfectious and nonmalignant oral ulcers, burning mouth syndrome, oral mucositis

1. Introduction

Odontogenic pain, a common malady globally and the most prevalent type of orofacial pain, originates from dental structures, pulpal or periodontal [1]. Differential diagnosis for odontogenic pain is outlined in **Table 1**. Oral pain of nonodontogenic origin can originate from the intraoral structures, such as buccal mucosa, gingival tissues, and alveolar bone. Some of the main causes for nonodontogenic pain of oral origin are shown in **Table 2**. The complexity of the orofacial region makes the management of odontogenic and nonodontogenic pain of oral origin a challenging task for the clinicians. For an effective diagnosis and treatment, the clinician should have a thorough knowledge of the various pain complaints pertaining to the orofacial region and the different options available for their optimal management [2, 3].

For managing odontogenic pain, The “3-D’s” principle—diagnosis, dental treatment, and drugs—should be used. The first and foremost step is to determine the condition causing the pain and then to discover that what caused that condition. Removal of the cause usually leads to rapid recovery and should be done by an appropriate dental treatment. Medications should only be used to complement the dental treatment [4].

Origin	Possible causes
Pulpal pain	Dentine hypersensitivity Reversible pulpitis Irreversible pulpitis Cracked tooth syndrome
Periodontal pain	Periapical periodontitis • Periapical abscess • Periapical granuloma and cyst Traumatic periodontitis Periodontal (lateral) abscess Perio-endo, endo-perio, and combined lesions

Table 1.
Differential diagnosis for odontogenic pain.

• Noninfectious and nonmalignant oral ulcers
• Acute pericoronitis
• Acute alveolar osteitis (dry socket)
• Burning mouth syndrome (BMS)
• Oral mucositis (OM)
• Acute necrotizing ulcerative gingivitis (ANUG)
• Desquamative gingivitis (DG)

Table 2.
Causes of nonodontogenic pain of oral origin.

For managing nonodontogenic pain particularly in complex cases, a multidisciplinary pain management approach should be adopted encompassing both nonpharmacological and pharmacological modalities [5].

2. Odontogenic pain

2.1 Pulpal pain

2.1.1 Dentine hypersensitivity

Dissolution of the dental enamel results in development of dental caries. If caries goes unchecked, it may involve the dentin and the pulp, resulting in pain. In the initial stages, caries penetrates and exposes the dentin leading to dentine hypersensitivity. The pain due to dentin exposure is of a sharp and shooting nature with a shorter duration and is classically stimulated by exposure to heat, cold, sweet drinks/food, and mechanical trauma such as tooth brushing. Apart from caries, there exist other predisposing factors for dentine hypersensitivity. These include anatomical defects, gingival recession, erosion, abrasion, and attrition. The diagnosis of dentine hypersensitivity is based upon detection of dentin exposure or tooth wear. Therapies for managing dentinal hypersensitivity are aimed at: sealing the exposed dentinal tubules (composite resin application), reducing dentinal neuron activity (application of desensitizing agents such as potassium nitrate and strontium chloride), and making the enamel and dentin more resistant to demineralization (application of fluoride-containing medicaments) [6, 7].

2.1.2 Reversible and irreversible pulpitis

The extension of caries to pulp leads to pulpal inflammation known as pulpitis. Other cause of pulpitis can be operative dental procedures. The chemicals, heat, and friction involved in such procedures may trigger pulpal inflammation. Pulpitis has two clinical forms: acute (reversible) and chronic (irreversible). Acute pulpitis represents mild inflammation and is characteristically associated with sharp and shooting pain of a shorter duration. On the other hand, inflammation in irreversible pulpitis is severe enough to undermine the pulp. It is characterized by spontaneous and dull pain that persists even after the removal of a stimulus such as cold or heat [6–8].

Diagnosis of pulpitis is based mainly on clinical evaluation and pulp vitality tests. Radiographs can be helpful in cases where carious lesions are not clinically visible [8, 9].

The management strategies are determined based on the type of pulpitis and presence of infection involving the periapical area. In reversible pulpitis, pulp vitality can be maintained if the tooth is treated, usually by removing the caries, and then restored [10]. In irreversible pulpitis, management options include endodontic (root canal) therapy or tooth extraction. In root canal treatment, an opening is made in the tooth and the pulp is extirpated. The root canal system is thoroughly cleaned, shaped, and then obturated with gutta-percha points. Following root canal therapy, adequate healing is manifested clinically by resolution of symptoms and radiographically by bone filling in the radiolucent area at the root apex over a period of months. If symptoms persist or worsen, root canal therapy is usually repeated in case a root canal was missed [11, 12].

2.1.3 Cracked tooth or cracked cusp syndrome

Cracked tooth syndrome occurs when a crack has occurred in the enamel or dentine and reaches the pulp chamber. The crack is usually not visible to the naked eye. Application of excessive force on a normal tooth or physiologic forces applied to a weakened tooth can lead to cracks. The diagnosis of cracked tooth is often tricky. Radiography is not helpful in detection of fractures, as cracks occur in a mesiodistal direction, parallel to that of the plane of the film. Simple test is to have patient bite on a cotton roll that evokes a sharp pain. Pain due to cracked tooth is sharp and shooting in nature, and is usually associated with biting and chewing. Hot and cold stimuli also evoke the pain. Restorable teeth should be treated endodontically, followed by a full-coverage restoration of tooth. However, tooth with large cracks may require extraction [7, 13].

2.2 Periodontal pain

2.2.1 Periapical periodontitis (periapical abscess, granuloma, and cyst)

Pulpitis, if untreated, is followed by death of the pulp. The necrotic pulp is infected and leads to spread of infection through the apical foramina into the periapical tissues. This in turn causes inflammation and destruction of the periradicular tissues known as periapical periodontitis. It includes acute/chronic nonsuppurative inflammation and suppurative inflammation. Periapical granuloma forms due to chronic inflammation without pus, while periapical abscess is the result of inflammation involving pus. The other likely cause of periapical periodontitis can be chemical irritation. This irritation can be due to the escape of antiseptics used for root canal sterilization through the root apex into the surrounding periapical area [11, 12].

Acute periapical abscesses characteristically present with severe pain in the area of the nonvital tooth particularly on percussion, inflammation, or complaint of pus drainage (with its associated foul taste). Pain also typically interferes with sleep. Treatment includes drainage through an opening in the tooth itself or through the soft tissue surrounding the jaw, if cellulitis has developed. If patients with abscess have systemic signs of infection (e.g., fever), an oral antimicrobial is prescribed (amoxicillin 500 mg every 8 hours; for patients allergic to penicillin, clindamycin 150 or 300 mg every 6 hours). On resolution of the abscess, the patient should undergo root canal therapy or extraction [8, 10, 11, 14].

Periapical granulomas or cysts usually follow acute pulpal infection that remains unresolved due to inadequate drainage. Tooth with periapical granulomas may present with a dull pain or may be asymptomatic. Radiographically, abscesses, granulomas, or cysts have the same features and microscopic examination should be done for distinction. Teeth with periapical granulomas are nonvital and needs root canal treatment or removal. Root canal treatment done competently leads to healing even if cystic phase has started. Persistence of periapical radiolucency after 6–12 months may be due to technical faults associated with root canal treatment. In such a case, apical curettage with apicoectomy may be indicated [6, 8, 14, 15].

2.2.2 Traumatic periodontitis

Traumatic periodontitis is a painful condition that arises because of injury to the periodontium. This injury is caused by the trauma from excessive occlusal forces. The occlusal trauma affecting periodontium can be primary, secondary, or combined. Tooth or teeth with normal periodontal support enduring increased occlusal loads may undergo primary occlusal trauma. The causes may include bruxism, overextended margins of restorations, excessive loading during orthodontic movements, and recent fitting of a new partial denture. Tooth or teeth with inadequate periodontal support if subjected to normal occlusal forces may undergo secondary occlusal trauma. Excessive occlusal force on a diseased periodontium may lead to combined occlusal trauma. The excessive occlusal forces are generally from parafunctional movements such as bruxism. The clinical features of traumatic periodontitis include pain on chewing/biting or percussion, progressive tooth mobility, and nonphysiological movement of tooth during function (fremitus). Additionally, there can be gingival inflammation with pocket formation in combined occlusal trauma.

Radiographic features include evidence of circumferential and furcal bone loss, in combination with widening of the periodontal ligament space.

The goal of management of traumatic periodontitis is the removal of excessive occlusal forces and brings the dentition in occlusal harmony. Primary occlusal trauma can be managed with analysis and correction of occlusion. One or more of the following steps can do occlusal adjustments: tooth movements, tooth removal, dental restorations, coronoplasty, etc. Progressive tooth mobility due to secondary occlusal trauma may be reduced by occlusal adjustment. Pain occurring due to hypermobility can be managed by splinting of teeth. The aim of splinting is to increase the resistance of dentition to the occlusal forces through stabilization. It involves joining of two or more teeth [16, 17]. Managing the periodontal inflammation is of primary importance in cases of combined occlusal trauma. Premature occlusal contacts usually contribute to the progression of periodontitis. This can be tackled by simple correction of the occlusion that may eradicate the premature occlusal contacts [16, 17].

2.2.3 Periodontal (lateral) abscess

A periodontal abscess arises because of acute infection of a periodontal pocket. Unlike a periapical abscess, periodontal abscess is associated with a vital tooth.

Varieties of reasons are implicated in causation of periodontal abscess. Primarily incomplete calculus removal can be a causative factor. Occasionally, it may occur following root planing, as the trauma to pocket lining implants bacteria into the periodontal tissues. Other contributing factors can be food packing down between teeth with poor contact points or foreign body (e.g., fish bone) driven through the floor of a pocket. Poorly controlled diabetes mellitus can also be a predisposing factor for periodontal abscess formation.

Periodontal abscess has a rapid onset. The gingival swelling and inflammatory edema prevent drainage through the pocket orifice. The initial gingival tenderness progresses to throbbing pain that is well localized. The affected tooth is tender to percussion or biting. There is tooth mobility with its elevation in the socket. Pus exudation may occur from the pocket; however, a deep abscess has a sinus tract that points on the alveolar mucosa. Fever and regional lymphadenopathy can be occasional clinical features. The vitality of the tooth, deep pocketing, and less severe tenderness helps to differentiate between a periodontal and pulpal abscess.

Periodontal abscess should be ideally drained through pocket or occasionally by an incision through the gingiva. If the abscess is too large and drainage cannot be done, subgingival scaling and root planing or deferring the surgical access until the major clinical signs have subsided. Before initiating the treatment of acute periodontal abscess, the evaluation of patient's medical history, dental history, and systemic conditions is crucial to determine the need for antibiotics. The indications for antimicrobial therapy in patients with acute abscess are fever, lymphadenopathy, evidence of spreading of infection (cellulitis), deep periodontal pocketing, and immunosuppression. Administration of antibiotics alone without the local drainage of the abscess is contraindicated. The drainage is mandatory in order to eliminate the etiologic factors. Extraction of the affected tooth can be considered as a last resort to treat the periodontal abscess, if there is poor response to therapy, horizontal tooth mobility exceeding 1 mm, pocketing exceeding 8 mm, and more than 40% alveolar bone resorption [6, 18, 19].

2.2.4 Perio-endo, endo-perio, and combined lesions

In perio-endo lesions, microorganisms from the periodontal pockets can reach the pulp through accessory canals, thereby leading to pulpal inflammation and necrosis.

In endo-perio lesions, pulpal necrosis leads to involvement and destruction of the periodontal ligament and adjacent alveolar bone. Clinically endo-perio lesions present as deep periodontal probing depth extending to the apex of the tooth.

In managing the lesions of pulpal or periodontal origin, making an accurate diagnosis as to the source of infection is a critical determinant of the treatment outcome. Sequence of the disease process can be an important factor in determining the exact nature of lesions: perio-endo and endo-perio lesions. Conventional root canal therapy (RCT) alone leads to a complete resolution of the periodontal defects arising from primary pulpal infection. However, pulpal infections resulting from primary periodontal infections require both endodontic and periodontal treatments for achieving complete healing [18].

3. Nonodontogenic pain of oral origin

Oral ulcers are a broad entity that encompasses a variety of causes, such as infections (bacterial, viral, and fungal), neoplasia, immunological disturbances, drug reactions, etc.

3.1 Noninfectious and nonmalignant oral ulcers

A detailed clinical history and examination, and laboratory investigations including biopsy, culture, and immunochemistry tests are essential for ruling out the neoplastic, infectious, and immunological causes of oral ulcerations. The causative factors for noninfectious and nonmalignant oral ulcers usually include mechanical trauma (self-induced trauma such as on chewing and biting, aggressive tooth brushing, and iatrogenic causes particularly due to dental treatment) and chemicals (aspirin, acetylsalicylic acid, acid etchants, etc.)

Superficial ulcers usually lead to soreness; severe pain and discomfort are the features of deep ulcers.

On elimination of cause, acute forms of traumatic- and chemical-induced ulcers usually heal in 7–10 days. They develop chronicity if subjected to continuous trauma or irritation. The considerations in management of such type of ulcers are as follows:

1. Maintenance of oral hygiene. In the presence of an ulcer, tooth brushing particularly near to the ulcerative area can be detrimental. In such as case, an antiseptic mouthwash (e.g., 0.2% chlorhexidine solution) can be of considerable help. Chlorhexidine mouth rinse is recommended to be used three times daily after meals and held in the mouth for at least 1 minute. Oral rinsing with chlorhexidine has been found to lessen down the discomfort and duration of aphthous stomatitis.

2. Avoidance of irritation or injury to the area of ulceration. Covering agents, e.g., carboxymethylcellulose paste (Orabase®) and carmellose sodium can be helpful in safeguarding the ulcers from the effects of friction or injury. When correctly applied, these covering agents absorb moisture and form an adhesive gel, which can remain in place for several hours.

3. For management of pain, over-the-counter anesthetic agent (an example is Orobase® with 20% benzocaine). Topical application of weak potency corticosteroids (hydrocortisone hemisuccinate) and medium potency steroids (triamcinolone acetonide) also assist in reducing the associated pain and inflammation; however, they are unlikely to expedite the healing of ulcers. Hydrocortisone hemisuccinate 2.5 mg pellets allowed to be dissolved in the mouth close to ulcers, three times a day. Triamcinolone 0.1% in Orabase applied to ulcer three times daily. However, long-term and/or repeated topical application of such corticosteroids has a downside in the form of adrenal suppression. This concern can be addressed by using the topical corticosteroids at the lowest possible concentration and frequency. The problem of adrenal suppression is not evidenced with 0.05% fluocinonide in adhesive paste and betamethasone-17-valerate mouth rinse.

Tetracycline (e.g., doxycycline), or tetracycline plus nicotinamide in rinse form may provide significant pain relief and reduce ulcer duration, particularly in aphthous ulcers. However, usage of tetracycline should be avoided in children below 12 years of age due to the risk of tooth staining. For oral rinsing, a tetracycline capsule (250 mg) is crushed and stirred in a little water and held in the mouth for 2–3 minutes, three times daily.

Tetracycline mouth rinses can also reduce the frequency of aphthous ulcers on regular usage for 3 days each week.

Salicylates based on their anti-inflammatory role can be helpful in reducing the discomfort of oral ulcers. Over the counter, preparation of choline salicylate in gel form is recommended for application to ulcers, 3–5 times daily [6, 20, 21].

3.2 Acute pericoronitis

It is the inflammation of the flap of tissues (operculum) around an erupting tooth, and most commonly associated with impacted mandibular third molars. The chief complaints in this condition are severe pain that can radiate to surrounding areas and swelling of the pericoronal tissues. The hyperplastic-inflamed flap of tissue can become a hotbed for bacteria, as it readily holds food particles and debris. This scenario leads to bacterial infection with clinical manifestations of discharge of pus, trismus, fever, regional lymphadenopathy, and in some cases spread of the infection to adjacent tissue spaces.

If the pain and inflammation are limited to the tooth, local measures, such as debridement of food debris and plaque, irrigation with normal saline or hydrogen peroxide, and avoidance of occlusal trauma are recommended.

Antimicrobial therapy is indicated for patients presenting with fever, trismus, and pus exudation. Metronidazole 400 mg three times a day for 5 days is to be prescribed in combination with phenoxymethylpenicillin 500 mg four times a day for 5 days.

If it is envisaged that the tooth can be useful for chewing and patient also has the desire to retain the tooth, hyperplastic pericoronal tissue should be excised out through a minor oral surgery procedure known as operculectomy. This will allow better access to properly clean the area and prevent the accumulation of bacteria and food debris. In some unfortunate instances, the gum tissue may grow back and create the same problem.

Since impacted teeth frequently are unfavorably aligned and do not erupt completely, extraction of such tooth is commonly performed. This method eliminates any chance of recurrence of pericoronitis.

The risks and benefits of removal of impacted molars are mired in controversy, as extraction can lead to inferior alveolar nerve damage; retention can precipitate serious, even life-threatening infection [14, 22].

3.3 Acute alveolar osteitis (dry socket)

This painful condition is a complication that may occur following dental extraction. It presents with a severe throbbing pain caused by bone exposure at the site of extraction. Following the extraction, a blood clot forms within the extraction socket to safeguard the bone. If a blood clot forms inadequately in the socket or it is dislodged, the bone and nerves are exposed, leading to pain. Smoking, excessive extraction trauma, difficult disimpactions of third molars, vasoconstrictor in local anesthetic, and oral contraceptives are some of the predisposing factors to alveolar osteitis. Alveolar osteitis can strike 3–5 days after an extraction and may persist for a week. The exposed bone is acutely tender to touch; hence, mechanical stimulation by tongue movement and food particles results in frequent acute pain. On clinical examination, the socket appears empty with visible bony lamina dura.

Minimization of trauma related to the extraction procedure can be an important factor in prevention of dry socket. Since removal of the debris from the socket expedites healing, irrigation with warmed saline or chlorhexidine is suggestive. Use of intra-alveolar dressing materials such as bismuth iodoform paraffin paste and lidocaine gel on ribbon gauze can protect the socket from painful stimuli and collection of food debris. These dressing materials also impart a soothing sensation of warmth in the painful area. Usually after one or two dressings, significant pain relief is achieved. It is better to be on the lookout for signs of infection, such as pus in the socket, localized swelling, and lymphadenopathy. Antibiotics should be prescribed if these signs are there. It is crucial that the reason for infection is determined such as retained root or bony fragments. A radiograph can be helpful. Surgical extraction is indicated for removal of root tip or bone sequestrum [6, 13, 23].

3.4 Burning mouth syndrome (BMS)

Burning mouth syndrome (BMS) is a complex painful disorder that is characterized by warm, burning, or tingling sensation in the oral mucosa, tongue, or lips. The pain may be associated with a feeling of intermittent numbness. Other associated features may include metallic taste and dryness in the mouth. Interestingly, a variety of names has been associated with this condition such as oral dysesthesia, stomatodynia, glossodynia, stomatopyrosis, glossopyrosis, sore mouth, and sore tongue. BMS is a reasonably common chronic complaint to affect middle age or elderly patients, especially females. Diagnosis of BMS is challenging, because usually no clear-cut dental or medical cause is evident and laboratory findings does not reveal any abnormality.

BMS can be classified into two clinical variants, namely, primary and secondary BMS. If no underlying medical or dental problem becomes evident on investigations, the diagnosis is primary or idiopathic BMS. Probably, the damage to the nerves that control pain and taste leads to primary BMS. Secondary BMS is caused by local, systemic, or psychological factors. A few common causes of secondary BMS include, dry mouth, acid reflux, deficiency of iron or vitamin B, hormonal disturbances (such as from thyroid problem or diabetes), etc. Because burning mouth syndrome can be associated with a wide array of local, systemic, or psychological conditions, an ambitious diagnostic approach is warranted. This approach should be based on a detailed history, clinical examination, laboratory tests, and exclusion of all other possible oral and systemic problems.

If no organic cause can be found and diagnosis suggests psychological factors such as anxiety, stress, and depression, it is advisable to make the patient aware by explaining that depression and other emotional disturbances are just as much illnesses and cause as much suffering as physical diseases. Apart from psychogenic medications, cognitive behavioral therapy is indicated in BMS.

Depending on the causative factors, medications used for BMS include antidepressants, analgesics, antiepileptic, antifungal, antibacterial, sialagogues, antihistamines, anxiolytics, antipsychotics, and vitamin, mineral, and hormonal replacements.

The topical application of clonazepam (by sucking a tablet of 1 mg), three times a day for 14 days can reduce the burning symptoms. *Aloe vera* gel also helps to reduce the burning sensation and pain in the sore areas of the tongue. Symptoms of secondary BMS go away when the underlying medical condition, such as diabetes or acid reflux, is treated [24, 25].

Overall, successful management of BMS is dependent on a holistic diagnostic workup and collaborative management involving dental practitioners, psychologist, and physician.

3.5 Specific anticancer treatment painful oral complications: oral mucositis (OM)

This grossly painful disorder usually occurs as a complication of chemo- and radiotherapy. An allergic reaction to certain medications, dental materials, or infections may also lead to nonspecific mucositis. Oral mucosal injury is the hallmark of OM that occurs due to the interference of chemotherapy and/or radiation therapy with normal turnover of oral mucosal cells.

Chemotherapy-induced and/or radiation therapy-induced OM clinically manifests as the painful swelling, atrophy, and ulceration of the oral mucosa. *Candida* and streptococcal infections may also occur due to the disintegration of the oral mucosa.OM-affecting pharynx and other areas of alimentary canal can lead to complications, including dysphagia, electrolyte disturbances, systemic infection, malnutrition, and even death [20, 26].

Oral mucosal injury tends to be acute in cases where chemotherapy is administered over a short span of time. Chemotherapy-induced mucosal damage usually develops within a week after the start of therapy and peaks within 2 weeks. Radiotherapy-induced mucositis has a slower onset since it is most often administered in small fractions given over weeks. Radiation-induced mucositis typically starts in 1–2 weeks of starting the radiotherapy at cumulative doses of about 15 Gy (gray, a unit of absorbed radiation). At doses greater than 30 Gy, OM attains full severity and may last for weeks or even months.

Factors related to treatment and patient characteristic can influence the development of OM. Treatment factors that influence the severity and presence of mucositis include the class, dose, and administration frequency of systemic chemotherapeutic agents, radiation dose and field, and use of adjuvant chemotherapy and radiation. The majority of patients treated for head and neck cancers or those receiving high-dose chemotherapy develop severe OM. Usually the healing within lesions of OM is evidenced within 2–4 weeks after stoppage of either therapy.

So much so, the OM is a painful and agonizing condition that it has a drastic impact on oral hygiene maintenance, nutritional intake, and quality of life. Current clinical management of OM is largely supportive and aimed at maintaining oral hygiene, pain relief, and nutritional support. A majority of patients with mucositis pain has difficulty in food intake through mouth and a nasogastric tube or gastrostomy tube helps to achieve nutrition. Diet modifications in the form of liquid and soft diet are suggested to facilitate the food intake during the cancer therapy [27].

Maintenance of oral hygiene has an important contribution in the prevention and management of OM; however, it remains a neglected habit. Moreover, a good oral care helps to prevent secondary infection and sepsis in the lesions of OM. Oral hygiene measure such as tooth brushing, flossing, rinsing with sterile water, and using mouth moisturizers helps control pain and bleeding and prevent infections of the oral soft tissue. However, at the same time, caution must be exercised that tooth brushing and flossing do not traumatize the oral mucosa. In case, a patient with OM is unable to tolerate the use of a tooth brush, oral sponges and foam brushes can be used instead.

Simple analgesia, e.g., paracetamol (1 g four times a day) in soluble form used as a mouth rinse will be adequate to control the mild-to-moderate pain of OM. For controlling severe pain, opioid analgesics (e.g., hydromorphone or morphine) can be used. Use of opioids is both logical and appropriate to alleviate the intolerable pain of OM, and strong opioids can be helpful in this direction.

When swallowing pills can be problematic in patients with severe OM, the use of parenteral administration of opioid analgesics is required. For seeking short-term relief in pain of OM, oral rinsing with 2% viscous lidocaine (topical anesthetic) in combination with diphenhydramine and magnesium aluminum hydroxide may allow the patient to eat and maintain oral hygiene. Mucosal-coating agents such as sucralfate, Gelclair®, and Caphosol® by adhering to oral mucosa form a protective coating. This coating aids in patient comfort by shielding the exposed and overstimulated nerve endings [20].

Prevention of OM is also an important aspect to be considered and has involved multiple medications. The updated clinical practice guidelines for the prevention and treatment of mucositis have suggested the use of chemo-preventative agents to prevent and/or reduce severity of OM. The most commonly prescribed preventative agents for OM are ice chips (given 30 minutes prior to chemotherapy) or amifostine (a thiol drug) and keratinocyte growth factor-1 (palifermin). Moreover, the Multinational Association of Supportive Care in Cancer (MASCC) and the International Society for Oral Oncology (ISOO) guidelines for treatment of oral recommends the use of benzydamine for prevention of radiation-induced OM. Benzydamine hydrochloride (HCl) is a cytoprotectant with analgesic, anti-inflammatory, and antimicrobial activity. On being used as an oral rinse, it significantly reduced OM-related erythema and ulceration [20].

3.6 Acute necrotizing ulcerative gingivitis (ANUG)

Acute necrotizing ulcerative gingivitis (ANUG) is an acute infection of the gingiva and is characterized by pain, bleeding, fetid breath, and gingival necrosis. Fever, malaise, and regional lymphadenopathy may be accompanying features. Oral functions including speaking and swallowing become difficult due to intense gingival pain.

Destructive pattern in the form of gingival ulcerations, necrosis, and 'punched-out' ulcerated papillae makes ANUG unique when compared with other periodontal diseases. Initially cratered ulcers affect the tips of interdental papilla, later on spreading along gingival margins. ANUG most commonly affects smokers and stressful immunocompromised individuals. Other risk factors are neglected oral hygiene, sleep deprivation, and malnutrition. ANUG is an opportunistic bacterial infection that is caused by a complex of *fusiforms* and *spirochaetes*.

Maintenance of oral hygiene through self-care and gentle debridement by the dentist is the stepping stone to the successful management of ANUG. Patients may be advised to use mouth rinses, such as warm normal saline or 1.5% hydrogen peroxide or 0.12% chlorhexidine at hourly intervals for the first few days. Analgesics may help to ward off the intense pain associated with ANUG. In order to prevent recurrence of ANUG, the patient must be educated to maintain high personal oral hygiene, to have adequate nutrition, and to get sufficient rest. Antibiotics are indicated in case of systemic involvement. The recommended antibiotics are amoxicillin 500 mg, three times daily for 10 days plus metronidazole 250 mg, three times daily for 10 days. The healed gingival craters can act as stagnation areas where plaque can accumulate and ANUG may reoccur. For correction of superficial craters, gingivectomy and/or gingivoplasty procedures may be helpful. For rehabilitation of deep craters, periodontal flap surgery or regenerative surgery may be considered [28–30].

3.7 Desquamative gingivitis (DG)

Desquamative gingivitis (DG) is a specific clinical presentation of unknown etiology in which the attached gingiva appears fiery red, glazed, and friable. Desquamative gingivitis may be a clinical manifestation of various mucocutaneous disorders—erythema multiforme, erosive lichen planus, pemphigus, pemphigoid, and psoriasis. DG is characterized by gingival soreness and burning sensation, which worsens on eating spicy and acidic food. The typical clinical feature in severe cases is of desquamation of gingival epithelium. The treatment of DG is aimed at minimizing the gingival injury and irritation. Therefore, the patient should avoid spicy or acidic foods. Oral hygiene maintenance can be helpful in removal of exacerbating factors, particularly dental plaque. However, in order to avoid injury to the friable gingiva, tooth brushing should be done gently with a soft tooth brush or toothette. Use of an anesthetic mouthwash, e.g., benzydamine hydrochloride can be helpful in tackling the pain. Topical therapies are the mainstay of treatment for DG. High potency corticosteroid gels are commonly used as first-line topical therapy. Clobetasole-17-propionate or fluocinonide 0.05% in gel form can be prescribed. Ease of gel application can be facilitated via the use of custom fabricated trays. Furthermore, 0.1% triamcinolone orabase can also be used. For complete resolution of DG, it is important that the underlying disease leading to DG is diagnosed and treated appropriately by specific therapies [31, 32].

4. Conclusion

Odontogenic and nonodontogenic pain may occur due to a variety of factors and causes. A differential diagnosis of orofacial pain, distinguishing between odontogenic pathologies and nonodontogenic painful etiologies, is a requisite before taking any clinical or pharmacological decision for pain management. Exactness of differential diagnosis is dependent on a thorough medical and dental history, comprehensive clinical examination, and appropriate investigations. Any decision on pain management should encompass a treatment regimen (e.g. palliative, dental, pharmacological, and psychological) that can adequately address the clinical problem of pain. For the successful accomplishment of a durable pain management, the treatment decisions should be based upon the best-available evidence, consideration of cost-effectiveness, and patient's expectation. Specialist referral is warranted, if the conventional clinical and pharmacological measures fail to control the odontogenic or non-odontogenic oral pain [1].

Conflict of interest

The author declares no potential conflicts of interest with respect to the authorship and/or publication of this chapter.

Author details

Sameer Shaikh
Department of Oral Diagnosis and Oral Medicine, University of Ha'il, Ha'il, Saudi Arabia

*Address all correspondence to: smrshaikh@gmail.com

References

[1] Odontogenic pain management. International Dental Journal. 2018;**68**:20-21. DOI: 10.1111/idj.12375. https://onlinelibrary.wiley.com/doi/pdf/10.1111/idj.12375

[2] Romero-Reyes M, Uyanik JM. Orofacial pain management: Current perspectives. Journal of Pain Research. 2014;7:99-115. DOI: 10.2147/JPR.S37593

[3] Clark GT. Chapter 1: The 30 most prevalent chronic painful diseases, disorders, and dysfunctions that occur in the orofacial region. In: Clark GT, Dionne RA, editors. Orofacial Pain: A Guide to Medications and Management. Oxford , England: Wiley-Blackwell; 2012

[4] Hargreaves K, Abbott PV. Drugs for pain management in dentistry. Australian Dental Journal. 2005;**50**(4 Suppl 2):S14-S22

[5] Clark GT. Chapter 2: Top 60 most important medications used in an orofacial pain treatment center. In: Clark GT, Dionne RA, editors. Orofacial Pain: A Guide to Medications and Management. Oxford, England: Wiley-Blackwell; 2012

[6] Cawson RA, Odell EW, Porter S. Cawson's Essentials of Oral Pathology and Oral Medicine. 8th ed. Edinburgh: Churchill Livingstone; 2008

[7] Shephard MK, Macgregor EA, Zakrzewska JM. Orofacial pain: A guide for the headache physician. Headache. 2014;**54**(1):22-39. DOI: 10.1111/head.12272

[8] Regezi JA, Sciubba JJ, Jordan RCK. Oral Pathology: Clinical Pathologic Considerations. 6th ed. St. Louis, Missouri: Saunders; 2012

[9] Dabuleanu M. Pulpitis (reversible/irreversible). Journal of the Canadian Dental Association. 2013;**79**:d90

[10] Ubertalli JT. Pulpitis [Internet]. 2018. Available from: http://www.msdmanuals.com/professional/dental-disorders/common-dental-disorders/pulpitis [Accessed: November 15, 2018]

[11] Marchick M. Chapter 4: Sore throat, dental pain, and other oral issues. In: Desai B, Desai A, editors. Primary Care for Emergency Physicians. Cham: Springer; 2017

[12] Rosenberg PA. Chapter 2: Odontogenic and non-odontogenic pain. In: Rosenberg PA, editor. Endodontic Pain: Diagnosis, Causes, Prevention and Treatment. 1st ed . (Endodontic Topics). Heidelberg, Germany: Springer Publishing; 2014. DOI: 10.1007/978-3-642-54701-0

[13] Greenwood M, Corbett I. Dental Emergencies. Chichester, West Sussex: Blackwell Publishing Ltd; 2012. DOI: 10.1002/9781118702895

[14] Eversole LR. Clinical Outline of Oral Pathology: Diagnosis and Treatment. 4th ed. USA: People's Medical Publishing House; 2011

[15] Graunaite I, Lodiene G, Maciulskiene V. Pathogenesis of apical periodontitis: A literature review. Journal of Oral & Maxillofacial Research. 2011;**2**(4):e1

[16] Patel B. Chapter 1: Pain of odontogenic and non-odontogenic origin. In: Patel B, editor. Endodontic Diagnosis, Pathology and Treatment Planning. Switzerland: Springer International Publishing. p. 2015. DOI: 10.1007/978-3-319-15591-3

[17] Barzilay I. Splinting teeth—A review of methodology and clinical case reports. Journal of the Canadian Dental Association. 2000;**66**(8):440-443

[18] Newman MG, Takei HH, Klokkevold PR, Carranza FA. Carranza's Clinical Periodontology. 11th ed. St. Louis, Missouri: Saunders; 2012

[19] Patel PV, Sheela Kumar G, Patel A. Periodontal abscess: A review. Journal of Clinical and Diagnostic Research. 2011;**5**(2):404-409

[20] Kumar S, Teruel A, Clark GT. Chapter 12: Treatment for oral mucositis and noninfectious, non-neoplastic oral ulcerations. In: Clark GT, Dionne RA, editors. Orofacial Pain: A Guide to Medications and Management. Oxford, England: Wiley-Blackwell; 2012

[21] Scully C, Felix DH. Oral medicine—Update for the dental practitioner. Aphthous and other common ulcers. British Dental Journal. 2005;**199**(5):259-264

[22] Moloney J, Stassen LF. Pericoronitis: Treatment and a clinical dilemma. Journal of the Irish Dental Association. 2009;**55**(4):190-192

[23] Mamoun J. Dry Socket etiology, diagnosis, and clinical treatment techniques. Journal of the Korean Association of Oral and Maxillofacial Surgeons. 2018;**44**:52-58

[24] Zakrzewska J, Buchanan JAG. Burning mouth syndrome. BMJ Clinical Evidence. 2016;**2016**:1301

[25] Jimson S, Rajesh E, Krupaa RJ, Kasthuri M. Burning mouth syndrome. Journal of Pharmacy & Bioallied Sciences. 2015;**7**(Suppl 1):S194-S196

[26] Naidu MU, Ramana GV, Rani PU, Mohan IK, Suman A, Roy P. Chemotherapy-induced and/or radiation therapy-induced oral mucositis—Complicating the treatment of cancer. Neoplasia. 2004;**6**(5):423-431

[27] Raber-Durlacher JE, Elad S, Barasch A. Oral mucositis. Oral Oncology. 2010;**46**:452-460

[28] Malek R, Gharibi A, Khlil N, Kissa J. Necrotizing ulcerative gingivitis. Contemporary Clinical Dentistry. 2017;**8**(3):496-500

[29] Dufty J, Gkranias N, Donos N. Necrotising ulcerative gingivitis: A literature review. Oral Health & Preventive Dentistry. 2017;**15**(4):321-327

[30] Ubertalli JT. Acute Necrotizing Ulcerative Gingivitis (ANUG) (Fusospirochetosis; Trench Mouth; Vincent Infection or Vincent Angina) [Internet]. 2018. Available from: https://www.msdmanuals.com/professional/dental-disorders/periodontal-disorders/acute-necrotizing-ulcerative-gingivitis-anug [Accessed: November 15, 2018]

[31] Karagoz G, Bektas-Kayhan K, Unur M. Desquamative gingivitis: A review. Journal of Istanbul University Faculty of Dentistry. 2016;**50**(2):54-60

[32] Maderal AD, Lee Salisbury P, Jorizzo JL. Desquamative gingivitis: Diagnosis and treatment. Journal of the American Academy of Dermatology;**2018**(5):78, 851-861

Chapter 3

From the Origins of the Opioid Use (and Misuse) to the Challenge of Opioid-Free Pain Management in Surgery

Nicholas Yim and Fereydoun Don Parsa

Abstract

Pain is a physiologic mechanism of the human body. Early cultures believed pain to have demonic and spiritual origins. In the early nineteenth century, morphine was first isolated by the German pharmacist Friedrich Wilhelm Adam Ferdinand Serturner. Since then, synthetic opioids and other derivatives of morphine have been developed for a wide variety of purposes, including pain relief during surgery. Opioids mainly act through the stimulation of μ-receptors, which has inhibitory effects on the propagation of pain signals to the brain. However, opioids also have unwanted side effects like nausea, vomiting, constipation, postoperative sedation, dizziness, and addiction, and are associated with significant morbidity, prolong hospital stays, increase use of medications needed to reverse side effects, and decrease patient satisfaction. Furthermore, use and abuse of opioids have contributed to an opioid epidemic, especially in the United States since the beginning of the twenty-first century. Opioid-free anesthesia is an alternative aimed at providing pain relief without the opioid-related adverse effects and to enhance recovery. Non-opioid alternatives and preoperative patient education strategies have been shown to be superior in the management of postoperative pain and opioid requirements. Clinicals have embraced these concepts enthusiastically and have begun to incorporate an opioid-free pain management approach in surgery.

Keywords: opioids, opioid-free anesthesia, opioid-free pain management, surgery

1. Introduction

The perception of pain is an integral part of human existence. Although uncomfortable to the individual, the perception of pain is necessary to protect the body from harm. A painful sensation causes man to seek an explanation for the reason of this discomfort. A brief history of the origins of pain and the development of pain medications is presented, followed by the current understanding of the physiology of pain and modern concern about opioid use. In the second half of the twentieth century, synthetic opioids were introduced to achieve hemodynamic stability during anesthesia. Furthermore, combined with hypnotics and muscle relaxants, the opioids administration is considered a keystone of anesthesia. For instance, a prevalence of 30% of unwanted effects of opioids such as nausea, vomiting, dizziness and constipation has been reported [1].

An increased occurrence of confusion and postoperative delirium [2], respiratory depression, increased postoperative pain and opioids consumption with abuse, immunodepression, hyperalgesia and chronic postoperative pain have also been described. Of note, opioid tolerance to analgesia can occur after a single dose. Thus, the management of pain in surgery is currently moving in the direction of the reduction of opioid use preoperatively, perioperatively, and postoperatively. The modern multimodal anesthesia and analgesia with intraoperative hemodynamic stability, immobility and anticipation of postoperative analgesia can be achieved without opioids. The concept of opioid-free anesthesia (OFA) is based on the idea that hemodynamic stability can be obtained without opioids during anesthesia. In particular, OFA is a fascinating multimodal approach to anesthesia which provides the combination of hypnotics, N-methyl-D-aspartate (NMDA) antagonists, local anesthetics, anti-inflammatory drugs and alpha-2 agonists such as dexmedetomidine, and no intra-operative systemic, neuraxial, or intracavitary opioid is administered during anesthesia and the perioperative course. This strategy is aimed to prevent postoperative opioid-related adverse effects and to enhance recovery after surgery.

2. Pain and pain management from ancient cultures to the nineteenth century

Early theories of the origin of pain, especially from internal diseases, revolved around demonic and religious beliefs. Shamans and sorcerers treated patients with the use of amulets, magic sculptures, talismans, magic ceremonies and rituals to ward off demons and evil spirits. It was believed that spirits and demons should leave the body from the same way it entered, resulting in cultural scarifications to allow bad fluids, spirits and demons to escape. In Egypt, religious ceremonies and prayers were believed to help relieve pain. Incantations to God Horus and other deities were thought to relieve unilateral headaches [3].

Ancient cultures have used leaves of cocoa plant and opium for religious and medical purposes. The earliest anthropological evidence of the use of cocoa leaves was from the pre-Inca culture in Peru, dated to 1300 B.C. The Peruvians used cocoa leaves as a local anesthetic in trepanation operations. Opium was introduced to Egypt around 1500–1300 B.C., and was used as a cream for external application and for the fumigation of toothaches. In India and China, opium was used for the treatment of toothache and joint pain. In these cultures, opium could not be separated from its "recreational" use [3].

In the seventeenth century, physicians began to consider the human body as a machine with different parts in constant motion. The French philosopher Rene Descartes proposed one of the earliest concepts of modern physiology: a movement or touch initiated at the peripheral nerve endings propagated to the brain. This concept, which formed the basis of nineteenth century pain theories, is illustrated by Descartes famous figure [3] of a boy, whose foot is being stimulated by heat from a fire. Several scientific discoveries followed Descartes physiologic concept of pain, including that of Sir Humphrey Davy's reports of pain relief from inhalation of nitrous oxide in 1800 and James Moore's report of opium use for postoperative analgesia in 1784 [3].

3. The era of opioid analgesics and the discovery of anesthesia

With a better understanding of the physiology and pathways of pain, pharmacologic discoveries, particularly of morphine, were made in the beginning of the nineteenth century. The German pharmacist Friedrich Wilhelm Adam Ferdinand

Serturner was the first to isolate morphine from poppy in 1805. He named the substance after Morpheus, the Greek god of sleep. The invention of the hypodermic hollow needles and syringes by Charles Gabriel Pravaz and Alexander Wood in the 1850s allowed the ease of subcutaneous application. While this helped the widespread use of morphine, it also paved way for the use and abuse of morphine that spread rapidly during the American Civil War (1861–1865) and the French-German War (1870–1871). Opioid addiction became known as the "soldier's disease" and spurred research efforts to find substances with a lower risk of abuse [3].

Stemming from the discovery of morphine, scientists began to experiment and develop different forms of morphine. In 1874 Charles Adler Wright synthesized diacetyl-morphine, which in 1898 was registered under the name of heroin. This drug showed stronger cough suppression but lower analgesic effects when compared to morphine in animal models. Toward the beginning of the twentieth century, addiction to heroin became a growing problem in the USA, and in 1914, the government began implementing stricter regulations, limiting the maximum amount of heroin in preparations. These regulations also prohibited opium, morphine, cocaine, and several other substances from non-prescription preparations [3].

The development of new opioid analgesics continued. Derivatives of morphine and codeine such as hydromorphone, dihydrocodeine, hydrocodone, oxymorphone, meperidine, and oxycodone emerged at the beginning of the twentieth century. Methadone was developed during World War II in Germany and was used primarily as a substitution therapy in drug addicts. Methadone is a μ-receptor agonist and a noncompetitive NMDA antagonist. The NMDA receptor is involved in the pathophysiology of neuropathic pain. Fentanyl was developed by Paul A.J. Janssen in 1953 and was proved to be approximately 40 times more active than morphine. Subsequently, similar compounds with stronger potency developed, including carfentanil, sufentanil, and alfentanil [3].

The techniques for pain relief, such as spinal cord analgesia, knee surgeries, and different routes of administration for medications, began to develop after further research suggested opioid receptors in the human brain and the demonstration of endogenous opioids, the endorphins and enkephalins, constituting an internal system of pain modulation. Opioid receptors were found in high density in the substantia gelatinosa of the spinal cord, as well as the limbic system and periaqueductal gray area of the brainstem. This led to the reintroduction of spinal opioid application in clinical medicine. Peripheral opioid receptors were demonstrated in the late 1980s, and Stein and colleagues showed reduced operative pain following arthroscopy of the knee joint following intraarticular injection of morphine. Sustained release formula and transdermal route of administration provided a profound impact on the management of chronic pain. It made pain management much more comfortable for the patients, resulting in an improved quality of life. Morphine was available in the sustained release formula in 1983, while fentanyl was available in the transdermal system. Various opioids in sustained release formula and transdermal systems followed [3].

Surgical anesthesia experimentations in the nineteenth century allowed for major development in pain-free surgeries. One of particular note was the Dr. William Morton's experimentation with ether as a local anesthetic for a surgical neck operation. The dentist Horace Wells previously used gas during teeth extraction procedures. The first surgical ether anesthetized procedure was by the dentist William Thomas Green Morton at Massachusetts General Hospital, Boston, in 1846. Dr. John C. Warren was the senior surgeon operating on a congenital vascular tumor on the neck of a young man, Gilbert Abbott. To the audience's amazement, Abbott did not cry out in pain during the procedure, and this ushered in the era of pain-free surgery [3]. Painters Warren and Lucia Prosperi were commissioned in 2000 to immortalize this milestone in anesthetic surgery with a painting that became known as the Ether Dome painting.

Further significant steps in anesthesia in surgical environments continued. The use of chloroform in the management of childbirth was introduced into the medical world by Sir James Young Simpson in 1847, the same year physiologist Marie Jean Pierre Flourens had discovered the anesthetic properties of chloroform in animals. Chloroform remained the preferred anesthetic until the end of the nineteenth century even though the use of chloroform resulted in significantly more deaths than with ether [3].

Cocaine in local anesthesia marked another milestone in the advancement of pain management in surgery. During the nineteenth century, Albert Niemann, a scientist from Gottingen, isolated cocaine out of the mixture of alkaloids of the cocoa plant. The extracts became popular for conditions such as toothaches, digestive disorders, hysteria, and melancholia, as well as for being an aphrodisiac. Carl Koller experimented with cocaine as a local anesthetic on frog eyes, other animals, his assistants, and even himself. His paper, which demonstrated cocaine's efficacy, was presented at the Heidelberg Ophthalmological Society in 1884 by his colleague Josef Brettauer. The presentation was widely received and others began experimenting with cocaine's surgical applications [3].

After the Heidelberg presentation, scientists began experimenting with cocaine as a nerve block, in advanced cancer patients, and in spinal cord operations. American surgeon William Steward Halsted [4] began experimenting with cocaine as a nerve block, which opened up new possibilities in surgery anesthetics. Halsted and several of his colleagues eventually became addicted to cocaine during their experimentations with the drug. James Leonard Corning used cocaine as a spinal anesthetic in 1885. Dr. Herbert Snow was the first physician to incorporate cocaine into cancer pain treatment. In 1896, he administered cocaine with opium for pain relief to patients with advanced diseases. He later developed the "Brompton Cocktail," a mixture containing morphine, cocaine, and alcohol. German surgeon August Bier and his colleagues published their clinical results of spinal anesthesia, including intrathecal injections on each other. He introduced intravenous regional anesthesia in 1908. Rudolph Matas administered the first morphine anesthetic to the spinal cord in 1909. Most of the nerve blocking techniques during this time period were developed for surgical anesthesia [3].

Further experimentation with cocaine as an analgesic continued during the nineteenth century, resulting in the development of new local anesthetics including synthetic substitutes. Alfred Einhorn synthesized procaine in 1905. Lofgren and Lundqvist synthesized Lignocaine in 1943. Other local anesthetics followed including cinchocaine and amethocaine in the 1920s, mepivacaine, prilocaine, and bupivacaine in the late 1950s, etidocaine in the 1970s, and ropivacaine in the 1980s [3].

The current understanding of the physiology of pain involves the activation of the nervous system. Noxious stimuli, including intense thermal, mechanical, or chemical stimuli, are recognized by nociceptors in the peripheral nervous system. The threshold for pain activation is relatively high, requiring a large stimulus for signal propagation. The signals either travel through Aδ-fibers, Aβ-fibers, or C-fibers. While the Aδ-fibers and Aβ-fibers are myelinated and transmit "acute, well-localized, fast pain," the C-fibers are unmyelinated and transmit "slow" pain, often described as an ache. The signals travel to the dorsal root ganglion, are transmitted through the spinal cord and synapse on the somatosensory cortex and limbic system. The modification of this pathway by medications aims to reduce or eliminate pain [5].

4. The public health issue of prescription opioid abuse

Although opioids have historically been significant medications in the management of pain, opioids have also been the source of significant public health concern because of the addictive and destructive adverse effects of the medication. During the twentieth century, there were positive attitudes for the use of opioids, as a letter written to the New England Journal of Medicine underscored the safety and low addictive potential of opioid use in chronic pain patients, with subsequent letters and reviews supporting this perspective. With the impression that there was very little risk, particularly of addictive potential, in prescribing opioids for chronic pain, the demand for opioid use increased in clinical settings. However, by 2000, attitudes are beginning to shift and a reduction of opioid use is becoming the trend [5].

The detrimental overuse, abuse and addiction of opioids can precipitate from prolonged treatment of opioids. Opioid tolerance occurs when there is a reduction in the analgesic and sedative effects of these medications. Tolerance to the euphoric effects also develop, further increasing the risk of addiction. Opioid dependence results from the overactivation of the somatomotor cortex and autonomic nervous system due to the increased signaling of the cells while on the inhibitory medications. Cessation of opioid use or the administration of opioid receptor antagonists such as naloxone or naltrexone cause the withdrawal symptoms, including diarrhea, vomiting, agitation, hyperalgesia, hyperthermia, and hypertension [5].

In the United States, the opioid abuse has reached epidemic proportions and have become a public health issue. The treatment of opioid dependence is unclear, but there have been significant public health prevention efforts to combat the trends of increased abuse and overdose deaths [5]. On the topic of opioid epidemic, the United States Surgeon General Dr. Jerome Adams supports overdose education and awareness, and suggests co-prescribing naloxone to patients on high morphine milligram equivalent who are at risk [6]. Nearly all the U.S. states have laws supporting naloxone provision to lay persons. Further, the U.S. Department of Health and Human Services highlighted naloxone rescue kit access and emergency overdose as a priority to address the opioid crisis. The benefits of naloxone programming have been demonstrated in San Francisco, as well as in North Carolina, where a 70% decline in prescription opioid-related overdose death rates was observed from 2009 to 2010 [7].

5. Special issues on perioperative opioids administration

The current trend in surgery is in the direction away from general anesthesia that traditionally requires opioids preoperatively, intraoperatively, and postoperatively, and toward a more multi-modal regimen approach with preoperatively patient education, specifically highlighting the interplay between opioids and the human body's natural pain management system.

Currently, many surgical operations have been traditionally performed under general anesthesia with adjunct opioid use. The main mechanism of action of opioids is the stimulation of μ receptors, which has inhibitory effects on the propagation of pain signals to the brain [8]. However, there are a wide variety of associated adverse effects of opioids including nausea, vomiting, constipation, postoperative sedation, dizziness, and addiction [9]. Opioid use also carries significant morbidity, prolong hospital stays, increase use of medications needed to reverse side effects, and decrease patient satisfaction [10, 11]. Further, opioids may also cause paradoxical hyperalgesia due to opioid-induced neural plasticity. This appears to affect both the central and peripheral nervous systems, and may lead to sensitization of the pain pathways [12].

In addition to the wide variety of adverse effects, opioids use may also hamper the effects of the human body's own natural pain killers, endorphins. Opioid administration reduces the production of beta-endorphins and impairs the function of mu-opioid receptors [13]. Beta-endorphins have significant natural analgesic effects and have been proposed to yield 18–33 times greater analgesic potency than morphine. Endorphin release is believed to enhance in response to a stressor, such as sharp pain, and can be quickly utilized to control the pain. The stressor causes the hypothalamus to release corticotrophin-releasing hormone (CRH), a peptide hormone and neurotransmitter, from the periventricular nucleus. CRH stimulates the cleavage of protein proopiomelanocortin (POMC) from basophilic cells, resulting in smaller proteins, one of them being beta-endorphin. In the peripheral nervous system, beta-endorphins bind to the μ receptors on both pre-synaptic and post-synaptic nerve terminals. The binding leads to the release of gamma-aminobutyric acid (GABA), which inhibits the release of substance P, a tachykinin protein involved in the transmission of pain. Endorphins not only have greater analgesic potency than morphine, but also enhances individuals' mood and well-being, due to indirect elevation of dopamine [13]. In the central nervous system, beta-endorphins bind the μ receptors on the pre-synaptic nerve terminals and inhibit release of GABA, which normally inhibits the release of dopamine. The overall effect of beta-endorphins, which is decreased in opioid use, is a decrease in pain and an elevation in wellbeing.

6. The concept of opioid-free anesthesia

Opioid-free anesthesia is an anesthetic technique without intraoperative systemic, neuraxial or intracavitary opioids, and that avoids perioperative opioids. There are a number of therapeutic uses and indications for opioid-free anesthesia including narcotic history (acute and chronic opioid addiction), opioid intolerance, morbidly obese patients with obstructive sleep apnea, hyperalgesia, history of chronic pain, immune deficiency, oncologic surgery, inflammatory disease, chronic obstructive pulmonary disease, and asthma [14].

Postoperative complications, such as respiratory depression, central muscle rigidity, pharyngeal muscle weakness, obstructed breathing, negative inotropism, nausea, vomiting, ileus and constipation, urinary retention, tolerance and addiction, dizziness, and excessive somnolence, can be reduced or prevented. Decrease histamine release (allergy/anaphylaxis), increase patient satisfaction, and enhanced recovery after surgery and anesthesia (ERAS) are other beneficial effects of opioid-free anesthesia [14–16].

Opioid-free anesthesia should be avoided in patients with allergy to any adjuvant drugs, and should be used cautiously in patients with disorders of autonomic failure, cerebrovascular disease, critical coronary stenosis, acute coronary ischemia, heart block, extreme bradycardia, non-stabilized hypovolemic shock or polytrauma patients, controlled hypotension for minimal blood loss, and elderly patients on beta-blockers.

Interest and use of adjuvant modalities, including ketamine, gabapentinoids, intravenous lidocaine, magnesium sulfate, alpha-2 adrenoreceptor agonists, and beta-blockers, is increasing because of enhanced recovery, particularly in specific patient populations like chronic pain and opioid dependent patients [15].

7. Opioid alternatives for postoperative pain control

In light of the serious adverse effects associated with opioids, many clinicians are forgoing prescribing opioids excessively and using opioid alternatives for postoperative pain control. These non-opioid alternatives, including acetaminophen, nonsteroidal anti-inflammatory drugs (NSAIDS)/cyclooxygenase-2 (COX-2) inhibitors, gabapentin, local anesthetic infusion pumps, paravertebral or transverse abdominis plane nerve blocks, long-acting local anesthetics, and botulinum toxins, have been shown to produce analgesic effects and decrease opioid use postoperatively. Combinations of non-opioid alternatives have been shown to be superior in the management of postoperative pain and opioid requirements. In 2008, Parsa demonstrated that gabapentin and celecoxib in combination preoperatively for subpectoral breast augmentation was significantly superior than celecoxib alone in reducing postoperative pain and opioid use [17]. Stephan and Parsa have extensive experience using non-opioid modalities of postoperative pain control, which has resulted in significant reduction in opioid administration postoperatively for patients undergoing various plastic surgery procedures [13].

Several other opioid reduction strategies in a surgical setting have been tested and shown to be effective in managing pain and decreasing opioid use. Preoperative patient education has shown to be effective in reducing the opioid requirement postoperatively. Sugai et al. demonstrated that preoperative oral and written education concerning the body's response to pain reduced preoperative and postoperative opioid prescriptions [18]. When comparing patients that had opioid-free procedures to the patients receiving adjunct opioids, Parsa et al. found statistically significant reduction in time from end of operation to discharge, unplanned postoperative hospital admissions, and opioid use in the post-anesthesia care unit [19].

8. Conclusions

Pain treatment and management has come a long way since ancient cultures. Several innovations during the nineteenth century made significant headway in opioid analgesics, and by the end of the twentieth century, hemodynamic stability during anesthesia was achievable through the application of opioids. However, in an era with significant opioid abuse, limiting opioid requirements in postoperative pain management is of greater importance. Opioids are associated with unwanted side effects, including nausea, vomiting, dizziness, constipation, and hyperalgesia. Not only are there several adverse effects with opioid use, including a high addictive potential, opioids also interfere with beta-endorphins, the human body's potent natural analgesic. Opioid-free anesthesia provides a technique that can achieve intraoperative hemodynamic stability, immobility, and postoperative analgesia without opioids, and therefore, in the absence of the significant associated side effects. Judicious utilization of adjuvants like ketamine, gabapentinoids, intravenous lidocaine, magnesium sulfate, alpha-2 adrenoreceptor agonists, and beta-blockers contribute to enhanced recovery in specific patients with chronic pain and opioid dependence. Opioid-free anesthesia and other opioid-free pain relief strategies are essential in the control of the opioid crisis, are key in effective analgesia without unwanted opioid-related side effects, and are needed for postoperative recovery.

Author details

Nicholas Yim and Fereydoun Don Parsa*
Department of Surgery, John A. Burns School of Medicine, University of Hawaii, USA

*Address all correspondence to: fdparsa@gmail.com

References

[1] Boer HD, Detriche O, Forget P. Opioid-related side effects: Postoperative ileus, urinary retention, nausea and vomiting, and shivering. A review of the literature. Best Practice & Research. Clinical Anaesthesiology. 2017;**31**(4):499-504

[2] Cascella M, Bimonte S. The role of general anesthetics and the mechanisms of hippocampal and extrahippocampal dysfunctions in the genesis of postoperative cognitive dysfunction. Neural Regeneration Research. 2017;**12**(11):1780-1785

[3] Sabatowski R, Schafer D, Kasper SM, Brunsch H, Radbruch L. Pain treatment: A historical overview. Current Pharmaceutical Design. 2004;**10**(7):701-716

[4] Rankin JS, Halsted WS. Annals of Surgery. 2006;**243**(3):418-425

[5] Schaefer CP, Tome ME, Davis TP. The opioid epidemic: A central role for the blood brain barrier in opioid analgesia and abuse. Fluids and Barriers of the CNS. 2017;**14**:32

[6] U.S. Surgeon General Discusses the Opioid Epidemic. https://www.thedoctors.com/articles/u.s.-surgeon-general-discusses-the-opioid-epidemic/

[7] Fairbairn N, Coffin PO, Walley A. Naloxone for heroin, prescription opioid, and illicitly made fentanyl overdoses: Challenges and innovations responding to a dynamic epidemic. The International Journal on Drug Policy. 2017;**46**:172-179

[8] Owusu OA, Hamadeh I, Smith M. Review of opioid pharmacogenetics and considerations for pain management. Pharmacotherapy. 2017;**37**(9):1105-1121

[9] Sturkenboom MC, Stricker BH, Bosch R. Drug-induced urinary retention: Incidence, management and prevention. Drug Safety. 2008;**31**(5):373-388

[10] Oderda GM, Said Q, Evans RS, et al. Opioid-related adverse drug events in surgical hospitalizations: Impact on costs and length of stay. The Annals of Pharmacotherapy. 2007;**41**(3):400-406

[11] Swegle JM, Logemann C. Management of common opioid-induced adverse effects. American Family Physician. 2006;**74**(8):1347-1354

[12] Lee M, Silverman SM, Hansen H, Patel VB, Manchikanti L. A comprehensive review of opioid-induced hyperalgesia. Pain Physician. 2011;**14**(2):145-161

[13] Stephan BC, Parsa FD. Avoiding opioids and their harmful side effects in postoperative patient: Exogenous opioids, endogenous endorphins, wellness, mood, and their relation to postoperative pain. Hawai'i Journal of Medicine & Public Health. 2016;**75**(3):63-67

[14] Sultana A, Torres D, Schumann R. Special indications for Opioid Free Anaesthesia and Analgesia, patient and procedure related: Including obesity, sleep apnoea, chronic obstructive pulmonary disease, complex regional pain syndromes, opioid addiction and cancer surgery. Best Practice & Research. Clinical Anaesthesiology. 2017;**31**(4):547-560

[15] Lavand'homme P, Estebe JP. Opioid-free anesthesia: A different regard to anesthesia practice. Current Opinion in Anaesthesiology. 2018;**31**(5):556-561

[16] Lavand-Homme P, Steyaert A. Opioid-free anesthesia opioid side effects: Tolerance and hyperalgesia. Best Practice & Research. Clinical Anaesthesiology. 2017;**31**(4):487-498

[17] Parsa AA, Sprouse-Blum AS, Jackowe DJ, Lee M, Oyama J, Parsa D. Combined preoperative use of celecoxib and gabapentin in the management of postoperative pain. Aesthetic Plastic Surgery. 2009;**33**:98-103

[18] Sugai DY, Deptula PL, Parsa AA, Parsa FD. The importance of communication in management of postoperative pain. Hawai'i Journal of Medicine & Public Health. 2013;**72**(6):180-184

[19] Parsa FD, Cheng J, Stephan B, Castel N, Kim L, Murariu D, et al. Bilateral breast reduction without opioid analgesics: A comparative study. Aesthetic Surgery Journal. 2017;**37**(8):892-899

Chapter 4

The Utility of Patient-Controlled Analgesia for Managing Acute Pain in the Emergency Department

Mark Bender and Linda Papa

Abstract

There is a growing expectation of physicians to treat acute pain more aggressively in the emergency department (ED). This has contributed to an increase in opiate prescribing practices that has resulted in a crisis of medication abuse and misuse. The resultant backlash against physicians has created a void within the realm of acute pain management, as physicians search for a means to treat their patients in a way that is both empathetic and responsible. In an effort to combat this growing epidemic, alternative means of pain control are being explored. Patient-controlled analgesia devices (PCADs) have been used extensively in multiple fields of medicine and have demonstrated significant clinical utility for treating pain postoperatively; however there is a dearth of evidence to support their use within the acute care setting. Due to this lack of evidence, PCADs have not been widely implemented in the ED. Recent studies have shown that the use of PCADs may improve objective pain scores and increase both patient and nurse satisfaction while reducing the likelihood of developing chronic pain. The economic feasibility of this undertaking remains unclear; however there is strong evidence for the clinical utility of this modality to treat acute pain in this population.

Keywords: pain, emergency department, treatment, patient-controlled analgesia, patients-controlled analgesia devices, oligoanalgesia, patient satisfaction, patient autonomy

1. Introduction

Although there are discrepancies in prevalence among different emergency departments (ED), pain is the primary presenting complaint in 45–75% of all ED visits [1]. To put this in perspective, it is important to note just how significantly the landscape of the ED has changed over the last 20 years. Between 1996 and 2015 there was a 46% increase in the utilization of emergency services in the United States with 136 million people seeking emergency care in 2015. This equates to over 100 million patients presenting to the ED in acute pain [2]. As emergency room visits continue to grow every year, so does the need to find effective treatments for patients experiencing such episodes. Currently, the standard of care in most EDs includes the use of intravenous (IV) opiates which are titrated subjectively according to patient complaints; however this is often significantly impacted by outside forces including nursing availability and patient census. Unfortunately, in many cases a baseline pain score is not adequately established which leads to substantial variations in treatment, with the end result being that patients experience increased pain and less satisfaction with their care. Inadequate pain relief, otherwise known as oligoanalgesia, can lead to a myriad of psychological and physiologic consequences which can extend far beyond the initial injury. Thus, early intervention to treat acute pain is integral to effective patient care.

Current guidelines established by the American Academy of Emergency Medicine Physicians suggest that "parenteral opioids should be titrated regardless of the initial dosing regimen (i.e., weight-based, fixed, or nurse-initiated) at 20–30 minutes intervals until pain is relieved to acceptable levels with frequent re-assessment and evaluation for development of opioid-related adverse effects." [3] Although this schedule may appear ideal, re-dosing of medication at this frequency requires significant time from nursing staff and physicians and may prove difficult given the demanding pace characteristic of most emergency departments. This is problematic from both a practice and administrative standpoint, as increasing patient volumes are taxing our already overburdened EDs. From a clinical perspective this translates into substantial delays in achieving adequate analgesia and prolonged wait times between doses for patients in acute pain. In light of these issues, it is clear that physicians and ED staff must reconsider their current approach to pain management and explore novel methods to improve treatment efficiency without sacrificing quality.

Within the last 20 years, there have been increasing demands placed on ED physicians and staff to aggressively treat acute pain in an effort to improve patient satisfaction, improve outcomes and meet core measures. Consequently, the "Emergency Department Measure Set" was developed by the Centers for Medicare and Medicaid Services (CMS) and has been adopted by The Joint Commission's ORYX program in order to maintain alignment with CMS reporting requirements [4]. These, and many additional factors, have contributed to an increase in opiate prescriptions which has resulted in a crisis of medication abuse and misuse which continues to plague EDs all over the country. The resultant backlash against both physicians and pharmaceutical companies has created a void within the realm of acute pain management, as physicians search for a means to treat their patients in a way that is both empathetic and responsible. Patient-controlled analgesia, which has long been accepted as an appropriate form of pain management in post-surgical care, has shown promising results in its application in the acute care setting and may prove to be an invaluable tool which may be used for effective multimodal pain control.

Patient-controlled analgesia offers multiple benefits to patients in acute pain. The devices themselves are relatively easy to set up, they reduce delays and treatment variability, and provide patients with increased control of their analgesic needs. Delivery of medication via this method also avoids the peaks and troughs in blood levels associated with irregular bolus dosing and allows for a steady-state concentration within the plasma [5]. By controlling both the frequency and quantity of medication being delivered, patients are able to achieve improved levels of analgesia while minimizing the risk of adverse events. Dynamic systems such as this allow for increased patient autonomy and improved personalization of care without the requirement of additional supervision by staff.

2. The risks of undertreating pain

Although many patients achieve full resolution of pain after an acute episode, it has been demonstrated that pain may persist in up to 21% of patients being discharged from the ED [6, 7]. The precise mechanism for the transition from acute to chronic pain is poorly understood, however, the practical implications of this issue are becoming increasingly apparent as the number of patients experiencing chronic pain has reached epic proportions. Patients experiencing traumatic pain and acute abdominal pain are especially at risk for developing chronic pain and these populations make up a significant amount of ED admissions. In addition to the mechanism of injury there is also a myriad of different symptoms which can predispose individuals to developing persistent pain including age, gender, genetics, pain trajectory and pre-existing anxiety/depression [7]. Although many of these cannot be adequately controlled for in an acute setting, pain trajectory is one of the main factors that can be actively affected by emergency physicians and PCADs have shown increasing effectiveness in this regard. A recent study conducted by Rockett et al., demonstrated that utilization of PCADs in the emergency room significantly decreased the number of patients experiencing persistent pain from non-traumatic abdominal injuries, 6 months post-injury. "The study findings suggest that it may be possible to reduce persistent pain (at least in patients with abdominal pain) by delivering better acute pain management" [7]. Consequently, it appears that increased utilization of patient-controlled analgesia may be a viable alternative to our current practice model which can provide increased comfort to both provider and patient while diminishing the number of patients developing persistent pain.

3. Background on patient-controlled analgesia devices

Patient-controlled analgesia devices were first developed in the 1960s in an effort to allow patients to control their pain without the requirement of frequent nursing intervention [8]. The device itself has gone through significant changes with regards to technology, however its basic purpose remains the same. PCADs generally consist of a volumetric pump which contains opiate medications that may be delivered intravenously once a patient presses the button controlling outflow. The device often contains additional control measures including anti-siphon and anti-reflux valves which allow for precision in the quantity of dosing while minimizing the risk of inadvertent medication administration [9]. Physicians may control several variables including the loading dose, demand/bolus dose, lock-out interval and quantity required for continuous infusions [5]. In the initial stage of treatment a bolus or loading dose is commonly administered to establish a baseline degree of analgesia. Afterwards there is a lock-out period during which the pump does not release any additional medication. Patients may continue to press the release trigger during this period of time but no additional doses are released. A number of demand requests are logged by the device and can help guide physicians when attempting to determine an optimal dosing strategy for each individual patient.

Dosing parameters are generally set by the physician and should reflect the level of pain being experienced by the patient as well as the patient's expected length of stay in the ED, body habitus, and previous use and tolerance to analgesics. An optimal dosing strategy is one that would allow for maximum analgesia while minimizing potential side effects. With traditional dosing methods this is difficult to achieve. To remedy this, several protocols have been developed for use in patient-controlled analgesia which have been demonstrated to be effective in most patients. For instance, a common protocol used in both the US and UK includes a loading dose of 1 mg of morphine followed by a 5 minutes lockout period and subsequent bolus dosing of 1 mg [10]. Lock-out times are an important safety concern among physicians for obvious reasons, however studies show that increments between 5 and 10 minutes are generally considered safe regardless of the type of medication being used [5]. These parameters can be altered in real time in response to patient feedback. This allows for more dynamic analgesic control which has clear benefits for patients presenting to the ED with acute pain.

It is important to note that there are distinct differences between machine programming parameters for postoperative patients versus those in an emergency setting. A prime example of this is the use of background/continuous infusions. Utilization of this setting allows for increased baseline plasma levels of medication and may improve pain control in certain populations [5]. Although the literature supports this type of treatment in post-operative patients, it may not be ideal for the ED as it requires close maintenance by nursing staff. Additionally, research shows that it does not improve pain control significantly in this patient population and may actually lead to increased incidence of adverse events including respiratory depression and sedation [5]. In another study which specifically examined the use of background infusions in the ED it was also found that manipulation of this setting led to an increased rate of pump programming errors. Although the patients involved in this study did not sustain any long-term side effects, there was an increase in the rate of sedation which further supports that this setting is of limited use in the ED [11].

4. General principles in acute pain management

The use of opiate medication in acute pain management has been a staple in most busy emergency departments. They work via blockade of μ-opioid receptor-channels which inhibit the transmission of pain in the central nervous system. In general, pure μ agonists have a high degree of variation in terms of dose-response relationships among individuals and require close monitoring by medical staff [1]. Side effects of medications which target μ-opioid receptors include respiratory depression, sedation, nausea, vomiting and pruritus. The frequency of adverse events associated with opiate administration in an acute care setting is difficult to predict and often, a trial of medication is necessary before sensitivities can be established. The disparities among these patients in regard to appropriate analgesic control is multifactorial and includes differences in opiate tolerance, pain severity, previous opiate use, body habitus, height and weight, dosing quantity and the frequency of administration. Many of these factors are difficult to control in a fast-paced environment such as the emergency room. However, utilization of patient-controlled analgesia may help offset these issues by allowing patients to take a more active role in the management of their pain.

Common opiates used in this setting include morphine, hydromorphone, and fentanyl. They are widely available and physicians are familiar with their general dose-response relationships and safety profiles. Although studies have shown that usage of specific opiates does not necessarily correlate with significant differences in pain scores among patients using PCADs, this does not obfuscate the need for appropriate medication selection [5]. Thus, it is important to take an individualized approach when selecting which medication a patient will receive.

4.1 Opiate selection

4.1.1 Morphine

Morphine is the most commonly used opiate in EDs which is likely due to its intermediate half-life, moderate strength and familiarity among hospital staff.

The average half-life of morphine is 1.5–2 hours with peak intensity usually being established in approximately 90 minutes [12, 13]. This makes it an effective medication for pain control as its effects wear off in a reasonable amount of time and it is generally well tolerated. Analgesic dosing is usually 0.5–3 mg per bolus, with a lockout period of 5–20 minutes [5]. Due to morphine's longer onset of action it could accumulate in the plasma and could result in analgesic stacking if the lockout times are not calibrated appropriately. Although this could theoretically lead to a significant increase in adverse events; it is very rarely seen clinically when administering conventional PCAD level dosages [5]. Additionally, it is important to recall that morphine has a higher degree of histamine release than other opiates in its class. This may preclude it from use in patients that have a history or pruritus or flushing after morphine use. This is, however, only a relative contraindication and may not manifest as readily due to the decreased quantity of medication administered in each dose.

4.1.2 Hydromorphone (Dilaudid)

Hydromorphone is a medication that is both incredibly effective but also increasingly maligned by emergency physicians. It has gained notoriety due to its strength and efficacy in acute pain management and it is widely available in most EDs. Unfortunately, these attributes have also made it a popular drug of abuse among pain seekers and physicians remain wary of regular use. It is seven times more potent than morphine and is broken down into a biologically inactive metabolite which makes it an excellent candidate for patients requiring repeat dosing of opioid medications. It also has an improved side effect profile, including diminished histamine release, which results in less pruritus. The time to peak analgesic effect for hydromorphone is approximately 20 minutes and its dose equivalent when compared to morphine ranges from 4–8 to 1 which can make precise conversions difficult [13]. Although hydromorphone is considerably more potent than morphine studies have demonstrated that PCADs utilizing hydromorphone are equally effective in comparison to morphine PCADs when dosing toward equianalgesia [13]. Typical dosing for hydromorphone is 0.1–0.5 mg followed by a 5–15 minutes lockout interval [5]. A recent study comparing the efficacy of morphine and hydromorphone concluded that the side effect profile is similar between morphine and hydromorphone in terms of opiate-related side effects [13]. Additionally, pain control and patient satisfaction were also equivalent. Thus it appears that prioritization of one medication over another should likely be guided by patient history as each drug has a unique side effect profile which may preclude it from usage in certain groups. Unfortunately, due to the past history of hydromorphone misuse in the ED it will likely remain as a secondary agent.

4.1.3 Fentanyl

Fentanyl has long been a preferred drug in ED for patients in severe acute pain as it reaches peak concentrations quickly within 1–2 minutes and has a short half-life (6 minutes) [14]. This makes it an excellent candidate for patients that require timely analgesia without a lengthy period of sedation. Fentanyl is well suited for use with PCADs as repetitive dosing at appropriate lockout intervals has not been shown to lead to excessive accumulation in the plasma and thus, does not result in analgesic stacking [15]. Intravenous dosing of Fentanyl usually consists of 15–50 μg followed by a 3–10 minutes lockout period. Although intravenous administration of this medication remains popular, novel delivery methods have recently been explored which show promising results. Transdermal Fentanyl is becoming increasingly popular in the realm of patient-controlled analgesia, as it has been demonstrated to have increased ease of use (i.e. improved confidence/comfort with the device, dosing, and knowledge/understanding) and less technical issues associated with autonomous administration. Although the transdermal route of delivery has been notorious for inconsistencies in medication delivery/absorption it appears as though transdermal Fentanyl produces results in terms of pain control and patient satisfaction which are on par with morphine [16]. Additionally, studies have also demonstrated that it has an improved side effect profile and has less frequent adverse events associated with its use, including hypotension, hypoventilation, nausea, vomiting, pruritus and tachycardia [17]. As such, it may be a viable alternative for patients who have sensitivities to more traditional medications like morphine.

4.1.4 Meperidine (Demerol)

Meperidine is another common opiate that has been studied as an alternative to morphine for use in patient-controlled analgesia, however it has limited utility in the ED. Meperidine has numerous disadvantages, including a short duration of action, a very poor analgesic effect at common doses (25–50 mg), abuse potential, and concerning drug interactions. Meperidine has serotonergic and noradrenergic properties and has the potential to induce serotonin syndrome in patients taking selective serotonin reuptake inhibitors and monoamine oxidase inhibitors [18].

A head-to-head comparison was recently done which evaluated meperidine versus morphine use in patients utilizing patient-controlled analgesia who were chronic opiate users presenting to the emergency room in acute pain. Levels of analgesia among the two groups were similar; however, patients using meperidine had a greater likelihood of experiencing withdrawal symptoms afterwards which was reflected in increased COWS scores [19]. Additionally, meperidine has a less favorable side effect profile when compared to morphine as it is broken down into the biologically active metabolite, normeperidine, which is a neurotoxin that can accumulate in the plasma and increases the risk of seizures, delirium, tremors, myoclonus and restlessness [5, 20]. It is important that patients be closely monitored when receiving this medication. Increased need for staff supervision would likely negate many of the benefits which PCADs provide in an acute care setting. For these reasons, meperidine is a poor choice for acute pain and should be used with caution in the ED [5, 21].

4.2 Additional modes of administration

There are numerous alternative modes of medication administration in patient-controlled analgesia including oral/sublingual, transdermal, intranasal, inhalational, and epidural preparations [22]. Intravenous delivery has remained the most popular route of administration, however, studies have shown promising results for several of these alternatives. Oral/sublingual medication, in particular, may have increased utility in the ED as it has the added benefit of being less invasive than standard IV therapy and may be preferable for some patients who are not candidates for inpatient admission. A meta-analysis of 13 studies demonstrated that sublingual medication administration had less side effects and a statistically significant improvement in global assessment scores (defined as "good" or "excellent") as well as trends which indicated improvements in VAS when compared to both morphine and transdermal Fentanyl [23].

In light of this information, a novel, non-invasive delivery system has recently been developed for the newly FDA approved medication, sufentanil.

This sublingual delivery device has been specifically designed for use in patient-controlled analgesia and has demonstrated excellent titratability and a rapid onset of action which makes it attractive for use in the ED [24]. Phase 3 trials have demonstrated that sublingual Sufentanil has greater efficacy for the treatment of pain than IV medications and has less incidence of oxygen desaturation in the populations being studied [24]. Additionally, a recently conducted prospective, randomized double-blind study has shown that patients receiving sublingual Sufentanil have a higher summed pain intensity difference and improved global assessment scores in comparison to placebo [25]. Although this initial data appears promising, further studies must be done in an acute care setting before this device can be recommended specifically for use in the emergency department.

In additional to oral preparations there may be increased utility for medication delivery via the intranasal or inhalation route as these may also decrease the need for IV insertion and reduce overall cost. Unfortunately there are still significant barriers which must be overcome before these devices become commonplace. Inhalational medication, in particular, offers clear benefits as it is non-invasive, has a rapid onset of action and improved bioavailability [8, 26]. It has not been embraced in its current form; however, due to technical issues with regard to medication delivery, and improper patient compliance. Intranasal administration has been plagued by similar issues; however this may change in the future as technology improves and devices are able to deliver medication more effectively.

For the sake of completeness, epidural preparations should be briefly discussed as they are widely utilized in the perioperative and postoperative setting and have been shown to be more effective at controlling pain than intravenous administration [8, 27]. Epidural delivery of medication allows for targeted placement of opiates adjacent to the spinal afferent pain receptors which may diminish the systemic effects seen with oral and intravenous administration. This would initially appear promising for ED physicians as they are continually searching for ways to reduce the quantities of opiates being prescribed to their patients. Unfortunately this requires placement of an epidural catheter by a trained physician (often an anesthesiologist) which would not be feasible within the scope of the emergency department. Thus, the feasibility of its implementation in this setting is limited.

5. Special populations

5.1 Children

PCAD usage is considered safe for autonomous use in children over 6 who are experiencing acute pain [5]. Studies have demonstrated that PCAD use in this population results in decreased total opiate use, improved analgesia and decreased adverse effects, making it an ideal alternative to standard therapy [28]. One of the main determinants which govern its effective use in this population is the ability of the child to understand how and why the device is being used. The child must be able to understand basic principles regarding their pain as they will be required to follow instructions on how to self-administer medication. Studies have demonstrated that PCAD use in children under 4 is ineffective due to the aforementioned issues; however, children between 4 and 6 may use the device with the caveat that they maintain close nursing oversight. The need for additional monitoring is important for patient safety but this may not be feasible in a busy ED. Parental controlled patient analgesia has been offered as an alternative to this but in order to be effective it requires one-on-one education from nursing staff which also takes time and cooperation from a third party which may be cumbersome to facilitate. Parental controlled analgesia also has the added detractor that it removes the inherent benefits of patient autonomy which PCADs provide. Thus, it is unlikely to demonstrate a significant benefit over IV morphine for the purposes of acute pain management.

Morphine remains the most commonly used medication for patient-controlled analgesia in the pediatric population [28]. Typical dosing consists of a bolus of 10–20 μg/kg and a lockout period of 7–15 minutes [5]. As with all pain medications there are issues that may arise with prolonged administration of Morphine, which is especially concerning in the pediatric population. Cycling narcotics, especially in children who will be admitted, can help combat some of the sensitivities that are seen in relation to morphine utilization. Switching to medications such as hydromorphone can help decrease side effects like pruritus which may be both uncomfortable and alarming to many children. Hydromorphone, morphine and fentanyl are all considered safe for use in the pediatric population and they may be used interchangeably depending on response to treatment. A recent study found that hydromorphone to morphine switches for patient using PCADS was far more common (88.5% versus 11.5%) than vice versa. The most common reason for switching morphine to hydromorphone in this cohort was due to pruritus and inadequate pain control. Hydromorphone to morphine switches were more commonly due to nausea. Thus, physicians should monitor this population closely and change medications as necessary should any adverse events arise.

5.2 Geriatrics

Acute pain relief in the elderly can be challenging. Elderly patients presenting to the ED frequently have multiple comorbidities and physiologic issues which can affect the way in which analgesics are metabolized. Acute pain control in the geriatric population is an important topic to address because it is integral to their recovery. Studies have shown that unrelieved episodes of acute pain can result in decreased pulmonary function, sympathetic hyperactivity (including tachycardia and hypertension) and central neural sensitization which can lead to the development of chronic pain [29]. PCAD use is well suited for this population as it allows for individualized dosing, decreased fluctuations in opiate plasma concentration and improved pain control [30]. A recent study by Egbert which included 83 high-risk elderly men, demonstrated that PCAD use had improved analgesia without a concomitant increase in adverse events such as sedation. Additionally, the patient-controlled analgesia group reported that the PCAD was easier to use than traditional therapy [30].

Drug choice is important in the elderly as the pharmacokinetics and pharmacodynamic profile of opiate medications changes throughout the aging process. As we age there is an increase in body fat and decrease in total body water which alters drug metabolism. Therefore, fat soluble drugs such as fentanyl and meperidine have a higher volume of distribution and a longer duration of action which make them less attractive for use in this population [29]. Morphine is the most widely used medication for PCADs in the elderly and studies have demonstrated that the optimal loading dose is 1.0–1.5 mg/dose which should be followed by similar bolus dosing after a 5–7 minutes lockout period. It is important to note that water soluble drugs such as morphine have a higher plasma concentration in elderly patients due to their redsuced volume of distribution as well as increased levels of free active drug due to reduced albumin synthesis. As such, continuous infusions are contraindicated in this population as there is an increased frequency of adverse events, namely respiratory depression and hypotension [29].

5.3 Chronic opiate users

Pain control is notoriously difficult in patients who chronically use opiates and they often remain undertreated [31]. Although PCAD use in this population remains controversial, it may prove effective when used selectively [32]. Unlike patients who are opiate naive, bolus dosing in chronic opioid users may necessitate periodic re-adjustments, as larger doses are usually required with shorter lockout periods [31]. By providing these patients with a more uniform dose of medication ED physicians can avoid sedation while also decreasing the propensity for anxiety and cravings that occur frequently with IV therapy. Some physicians may also be worried about the potential for increased medication administration, should patients attempt to tamper with the device. This is usually not possible with standard pumps though, as they contain safety precautions and redundancies within the structure of the device which limit the potential for abuse. It should be noted however, that the "wrist-watch" type of PCAD contains a reservoir which is less secure than standard devices and it has a fixed lockout schedule which makes it less attractive for use in this population [31].

In regards to medication selection, morphine is a commonly used medication which remains effective, albeit at higher concentrations, even in patients that have developed a tolerance. Studies which directly evaluated morphine use in ED patients receiving patient-controlled analgesia are limited but, as noted previously, there is a clear benefit to using morphine over other alternatives for numerous reasons [19]. Hydromorphone is another alternative that might initially seem appealing, however there is a push to limit its use in the ED, especially for chronic opioid users, so it is unlikely that it would gain widespread acceptance. Alternatively, one medication which has shown good efficacy for the treatment of acute pain is oral transmucosal fentanyl. Studies show that this medication is effective in chronic opioid users with breakthrough pain and may be a viable alternative for patients where morphine is initially ineffective or patient sensitivities preclude its use [10].

6. Benefits of patient-controlled analgesia use in the ED

6.1 Opiate utilization

One of the more divisive topics relating to PCAD implementation in the emergency room relates to risk of abuse and reliance on opiates by patients provided with opiate analgesia. Initial systematic reviews regarding this subject demonstrated that patients using PCADs in the postoperative setting required less opiates than those undergoing standard therapy [8]. Unfortunately this does not appear to be the case for patients presenting to the ED. Evaluation of the most current randomized controlled trials for PCAD use in this population have demonstrated that patients receiving this therapy utilize a greater quantity of opiates than those receiving intravenous morphine [11, 33]. A recent study done by Bijur which included 636 patients presenting to the ED in acute pain, demonstrated that patients utilizing a PCAD required significantly more morphine (12.0 mg ± 4.3 versus 6.1 mg ± 2.9; 95% CI: 5.9 [5.2–6.4]) than those in the standard therapy group [11]. This data may seem worrisome at first but, as previously discussed, patients presenting to the ED with acute pain are notoriously undertreated. As such, the increased utilization of opiates in this population may reflect that patients need higher levels of analgesia than provided by standard measures of nurse administered analgesia.

In an effort to mollify this effect, recent studies have evaluated the efficacy of adding non-opiate medications to traditional PCAD formulations, with the expectation there would be a level of opiate sparing and analgesic synergy. One of the most commonly studied of these additives is the NMDA inhibitor, Ketamine. This medication is of particular interest to emergency physicians as it is widely available and used frequently in both the pediatric and adult populations in procedures such as rapid-sequence intubation and procedural sedation. It has a favorable pharmacokinetic profile in terms of pain management as it has both intrinsic analgesic properties and opiate sparing effects via antagonism of NMDA receptors [5, 34]. Unfortunately, research on this subject has been mixed as some studies have shown that it may not provide a significant reduction in pain scores and has an increased incidence of deleterious side effects [5, 35, 36]. Clonidine has also been used as an additive in PCADs and initially showed some benefits in regard to nausea reduction in certain post-operative patients but this has not been reliably reproduced in subsequent studies [5, 34, 37].

One medication which has shown promise for use with PCADs is dexmedetomidine. This medication is a "highly selective α2-adrenoreceptor agonist, with analgesic, anxiolytic, and sedative properties, but without effects on respiratory function." [5, 38] In a recent study it was shown that adding dexmedetomidine to PCADs with morphine resulted in improved analgesia, decreased nausea and significant morphine sparing, without significantly impacting patients hemodynamic status [5, 39]. Thus, it would appear that this medication would be particularly well-suited for use in the ED. Optimal dosing of this medication has not been definitively established, however the concentration used in this study consisted of 5 μg/mL with the PCAD being programmed to deliver 1 mL per demand bolus followed by a 5-minute lockout period. Formulations such as this are determined by the pharmacokinetic properties of the medication being studied and mixtures of these medications generally require additional assistance by pharmacy staff. This would likely add additional hard costs with regard to medication preparation but this may be a viable option for patients with a labile hemodynamic status (such as the elderly, septic or traumatically injured) where the analgesic benefits of increased dosing may be tempered by the fear of respiratory depression or hypotension. Additionally, these additives would offer a clear benefit for chronic opiate users where opiate sparing may be of increased importance.

6.2 Pain reduction

The perception of pain is highly subjective and varies greatly among individuals and makes it difficult to measure in precise terms. That being said, multiple formal measures have been created to objectively measure reductions in pain, namely the Visual Analogue Scale score (VAS score) and Numeric Rating Scales (NRS). These tools are of primary importance to both patients and physicians in objectifying levels of pain. Studies show that improvement in pain scores are directly correlated with patient satisfaction which can significantly influence the clinical course of patients experiencing an episode of acute pain [40]. Although it is well established that PCADs reduce pain scores in the post-operative setting there has been some controversy as to whether this would hold true for ED patients, as they often do not have as much time to convalesce from injuries. In reviewing the literature it appears that eight randomized controlled trials have been done which specifically examined the effect that patient-controlled analgesia had on pain scores in patients presenting to the ED. Five out of the eight studies in question have shown statistically significant results which favor PCAD use over conventional intravenous therapy. Two of the remaining studies demonstrated a downward trend which favored PCADs (although this did not reach the threshold for statistical significance) and only one study showed no difference [9, 11, 33, 41–46]. Unfortunately there is significant heterogeneity among these studies and due to the wide range of presenting complaints there are many confounding factors which must be accounted for. That being said, the initial data appears to support the use of PCADs over standard therapy for patients presenting to the ED with acute pain.

6.3 Patient autonomy and patient satisfaction

Patient satisfaction is becoming ever more important in clinical medicine. It is imperative that physicians maximize their ability to take care of patients in an empathetic manner which utilizes principles of patient autonomy and shared decision making. Studies have demonstrated that PCADs are preferred by many patients in comparison with both IV and IM preparations and patient satisfaction with this type of treatment is generally high [5, 9, 11, 33, 41–46]. In a recent systematic review of 21 trials which included 1260 postoperative patients, it was shown that patients had increased satisfaction with PCAD use in all of the studies that were included in the cohort [8]. Additionally, a meta-analysis done on the same group showed that patients preferred PCADs significantly more than standard therapy [8]. Studies which have been conducted that have evaluated patient satisfaction for patients presenting to the emergency room have also shown similar results, with the overwhelming majority of studies showing a clear preference for PCADs [9, 11, 33, 41–46]. This is likely due to several factors including faster time to analgesia, decreased need of nursing assistance and an increased sense of autonomy and control over one's pain [44].

In addition to patient satisfaction it is important to remember that proper implementation of this technology requires cooperation across multiple disciplines. As such, the support of physician extenders, nurses, and hospital pharmacists is integral to patient care and should not be overlooked. Relatively few studies have addressed this issue directly but current evidence shows that PCADs are generally well received by nursing staff. One study in particular demonstrated that patient-controlled analgesia regiments were rated as "good to excellent" more frequently than those utilizing traditional intravenous therapy (69% versus 54%) and the majority of nursing staff would use them again in the future (77%) [41].

7. Drawbacks of patient-controlled analgesia use

The majority of studies which have examined PCAD use in the emergency setting have found that there were similar rates of side effects such as nausea, vomiting, pruritus and drowsiness when compared to those receiving standard therapy [9, 11, 33, 41–46]. However, two studies showed PCADs to have a slightly increased risk of adverse events, including hypotension and hypoventilation, although neither group experienced any long-term sequelae in connection with these events. Additionally, these effects were transient and did not require the use of reversal with naloxone [9, 11]. When evaluating the literature it appears that the preponderance of adverse events associated with PCAD use have been due to factors which are inherent to all sustained opioid use and would likely be minimized with appropriate monitoring by staff. It is important to note that certain subgroups of patients may be prone to respiratory depression with patient-controlled analgesia. Studies have shown that elderly patients, patients with obstructive sleep apnea, and those using concurrent analgesics are at particular risk, and are vulnerable to the sedative effects which occur with repeated dosing [22].

Although it appears that PCADs are safe in this patient population, there are unique characteristics associated with this technology which require special attention and education for both patients and staff. Programming errors can occur, especially when staff are unfamiliar with the equipment which can lead to over-sedation and respiratory depression. In a large randomized study conducted in the ED by Bijur et al. there were a similar number of adverse events among patients assigned to the PCAD group versus those receiving standard IV therapy. However, the PCAD group had 11 pump programming errors, 10 of which were due to nursing staff unintentionally giving patients background infusions. None of the patients in question were subject to any long-term side effects. Additionally, following staff remediation and education, no additional errors were seen [11]. One way to address this in the ED would be to have special teams which are trained specifically in PCAD usage and implementation. Studies which have examined the effect of using specially trained support staff have demonstrated that there are less adverse events and a greater likelihood of being able to transition to oral opiates (rather than IM) when staff are trained appropriately [5, 47]. Thus, it appears that many of these events may be mitigated by improving education and regular training among providers and support staff.

There are some additional factors relating to patient perceptions which are unique to this modality and may influence its effectiveness in regard to pain control. Chumbley and colleagues found that many patients had reservations about using PCADs with 22% of patients fearing addiction and 30% fearing overdose [44, 48]. The study goes on to explain that lack of education likely played a large role in this and a patient's psychological background and coping abilities were also involved in influencing their response to treatment [44]. Intrinsic issues such as these are more difficult to control for in an acute setting and are largely related to preconceived notions that patients have prior to presenting to the ED. It is likely that these variables could be minimized if providers were to make an effort to first educate the patients regarding PCAD use and set reasonable expectations regarding pain control prior to the initiation of care.

8. Economics

Although patient safety maintains primacy in the hierarchy of prioritization with regard to the implementation of new technology, economic considerations play an important role when determining the feasibility of its widespread clinical utility. With regard to PCADs there are both hard costs, in terms of the device itself, length of stay and medication, as well as soft costs, such as time saved by staff and patient satisfaction, which must be considered when analyzing the cost-effectiveness of this modality. Although current research clearly demonstrates that there are improvements in patient satisfaction and an objective reduction in pain scores in patients receiving patient-controlled analgesia, it is difficult to quantify how these benefits translate in terms of savings. As such, clear cost-benefit ratios remain difficult to establish. Due to this complexity, a multivariate approach must be used when evaluating the benefits that PCADs offer in an acute care setting.

Although device costs vary among distributors it is safe to assume that the cost of obtaining the device and subsequent maintenance would be greater than that of traditional therapy. A study by Pritchard et al., which evaluated specific costs associated with the device including depreciation, electrical testing, calibration/rebuild costs, and servicing demonstrated that the annual costs of a PCAD was approximately $1573 which equates to $4.34 per day [49]. In addition to these initial capital expenditures relating to acquiring the device, there is mounting evidence that patients receiving patient-controlled analgesia in the ED also require a greater quantity of opiates than those receiving IV therapy [9, 33, 42, 44, 46]. These increased costs are also compounded by additional administrative challenges which require nursing staff, physicians and pharmacy to coordinate care in a novel manner which may be difficult to implement in many EDs.

One factor which clearly favors the use of PCADs in patients experiencing acute pain is the ability of this modality to save valuable staff time. This translates to increased productivity for both nursing staff and physicians which has the propensity to further increase RVUs and improve overall savings. For example, a recent study by Chan et al., demonstrated that PCAD utilization could save an average of 10–13 minutes of treatment time within specific post-operative groups [50]. Literature on costs related to length of stay, on the other hand, appears equivocal. A review of the literature shows that four randomized controlled trials have been done which specifically evaluated length of stay in the ED relative to PCAD use. Two studies reported an increase in length of stay and two reported a reduction [9, 33, 41, 43]. None of the studies reached statistical significance, therefore the question of whether patient-controlled analgesia reduces length of stay remains unanswered.

The PASTIES study was a large scale randomized trial which evaluated the effectiveness of patient-controlled analgesia in the ED for patients suffering from traumatic injuries and non-traumatic abdominal pain [9, 33]. This study evaluated patients presenting to the ED who were subsequently admitted to the hospital, thus, providing important follow-up information on patient outcomes after their initial ED care. Subsequent PASTIES studies have since been published which have evaluated the costs associated with PCAD use in this cohort. These studies are important to this discussion as they are the only studies to date which have specifically evaluated the economic feasibility of patient-controlled analgesia in the ED. According to the study there were significant reductions in pain, particularly in patients with acute abdominal pain, however, this came at increased cost. Patients with traumatic injuries incurred an additional $21.79–$23.10 per 12 hours; and non-traumatic abdominal pain incurred an additional $23.67–$25.09 per 12 hours [49]. Although these costs were significant within the scope of this study, they may be negligible as improvements in patient satisfaction may eventually translate into improved reimbursement. As such, further studies must be done in the future to determine the true financial feasibility of PCAs in this type of setting.

9. Conclusion

Use of patient-controlled analgesia has been demonstrated to be both safe and effective for acute pain management in the ED. It offers a means of pain control which is more patient-centered and allows for a greater degree of shared decision making while simultaneously improving baseline analgesia. Recently, a few small scale studies have shown that the use of patient-controlled analgesia in the acute care setting may improve objective pain scores and increase both patient and nurse satisfaction. However, the economic feasibility for utilization of this modality within the scope of the emergency room remains unclear. As always, medication selection should be guided by clinical presentation and patient response. In conclusion, this technology appears to provide a promising alternative to standard therapy, however, additional studies must be done before more broad recommendations can be made regarding widespread implementation.

Conflict of interest

The authors have no affiliations with or involvement in any organization or entity with any financial interest or non-financial interest in the subject matter or materials discussed in this manuscript.

Author details

Mark Bender and Linda Papa*
Orlando Health, Orlando, FL, United States

*Address all correspondence to: lpstat@aol.com

References

[1] Motov SM, Nelson LS. Advanced concepts and controversies in emergency department pain management. Anesthesiology Clinics. 2016;**34**(2):271-285

[2] McCaig LF, Stussman BJ. National Hospital Ambulatory Medical Care Survey: 1996 Emergency department summary. Advance Data;**1997**(293):1-20

[3] Motov S, Strayer R, Hayes B, et al., editors. AAEM White Paper on Acute Pain Management in the Emergency Department. Vol. 2018. Milwaukee: American Academy of Emergency Medicine; 2017. Position Statement

[4] Specifications Manual for National Hospital Inpatient Quality Measures. Emergency Department. Version 5.4 ed., Vol. 2018: Centers for Medicare & Medicaid Services and the Joint Commission, 2018; The Specifications Manual for National Hospital Inpatient Quality Measures includes the measure sets: ED, IMM, STK, SUB, TOB, and VTE. https://www.jointcommission.org/specifications_manual_for_national_hospital_inpatient_quality_measures.aspx

[5] Ellen M, Soffin MD, Spencer S, Liu MD. Patient-controlled analgesia. In: Benzon H, Raja SN, editors. Essentials of Pain Medicine. Philadelphia: Elsevier; 2018. pp. 117-122, e2

[6] Chapman CR, Fosnocht D, Donaldson GW. Resolution of acute pain following discharge from the emergency department: The acute pain trajectory. The Journal of Pain. 2012;**13**(3):235-241

[7] Rockett M, Creanor S, Squire R, et al. The impact of emergency department patient-controlled analgesia (PCA) on the incidence of chronic pain following trauma and non-traumatic abdominal pain. Anaesthesia. 2018;**74**:69-73. https://www.ncbi.nlm.nih.gov/pubmed/30367688

[8] McNicol ED, Ferguson MC, Hudcova J. Patient controlled opioid analgesia versus non-patient controlled opioid analgesia for postoperative pain. Cochrane Database of Systematic Reviews. 2015;**6**:CD003348

[9] Smith JE, Rockett M, Creanor S, Squire R, et al. PAin SoluTions In the Emergency Setting (PASTIES)—Patient controlled analgesia versus routine care in emergency department patients with pain from traumatic injuries: Randomised trial. British Medical Journal. 2015;**350**:h2988

[10] Fine PG, Marcus M, De Boer AJ, Van der Oord B. An open label study of oral transmucosal fentanyl citrate (OTFC) for the treatment of breakthrough cancer pain. Pain. 1991;**45**(2):149-153

[11] Bijur PE, Mills AM, Chang AK, et al. Comparative effectiveness of patient-controlled analgesia for treating acute pain in the emergency department. Annals of Emergency Medicine. 2017;**70**(6):809-818, c2

[12] FDA. Prescribing information for Morphine Sulfate Injection. Vol. 2018. Lake Forest: FDA; 2011

[13] Hong D, Flood P, Diaz G. The side effects of morphine and hydromorphone patient-controlled analgesia. Anesthesia and Analgesia. 2008;**107**(4):1384-1389

[14] Fookes C, Puckey M, Stewart J, Anderson LA. Fentanyl, Fentanyl Citrate, Fentanyl Hydrochloride. AHFS DI Essentials™. Vol. 2018. Bethesda: American Society of Health-System Pharmacists; 2018. Selected Revisions October 22, 2018. https://www.drugs.com/monograph/fentanyl-fentanyl-citrate-fentanyl-hydrochloride.html#moreResources

[15] Lehmann KA, Heinrich C, van Heiss R. Balanced anesthesia and

patient-controlled postoperative analgesia with fentanyl: Minimum effective concentrations, accumulation and acute tolerance. Acta Anaesthesiologica Belgica. 1988;**39**(1):11-23

[16] Lindley P, Ding L, Danesi H, Jones JB. Meta-analysis of the ease of care from a patients' perspective comparing fentanyl iontophoretic transdermal system versus morphine intravenous patient-controlled analgesia in postoperative pain management. Journal of Perianesthesia Nursing. 2017;**32**(4):320-328

[17] Viscusi ER, Grond S, Ding L, Danesi H, Jones JB, Sinatra RS. A comparison of opioid-related adverse events with fentanyl iontophoretic transdermal system versus morphine intravenous patient-controlled analgesia in acute postoperative pain. Pain Management. 2016;**6**(1):19-24

[18] Alvarado-Rivera O. Meperidine: Friend or foe? Pharmacy Times. 2016;**2018**. https://www.pharmacytimes.com/contributor/orlando-alvarado-rivera-pharmd-ms/2016/09/meperidine-friend-or-foe

[19] Solhi H, Sanaei-Zadeh H, Solhi S, Azizi Nadian MA, Gharibi M, Sadeghi Sedeh B. Meperidine (pethidine) versus morphine in acute pain management of opioid-dependent patients. Open Access Emergency Medicine. 2016;**8**:57-59

[20] Fogarty T, Murray GB. Psychiatric presentation of meperidine toxicity. Journal of Clinical Psychopharmacology. 1987;**7**(2):116-117

[21] Simopoulos TT, Smith HS, Peeters-Asdourian C, Stevens DS. Use of meperidine in patient-controlled analgesia and the development of a normeperidine toxic reaction. Archives of Surgery. 2002;**137**(1):84-88

[22] Macintyre PE. Safety and efficacy of patient-controlled analgesia. British Journal of Anaesthesia. 2001;**87**(1):36-46

[23] Katz P, Takyar S, Palmer P, Liedgens H. Sublingual, transdermal and intravenous patient-controlled analgesia for acute post-operative pain: Systematic literature review and mixed treatment comparison. Current Medical Research and Opinion. 2017;**33**(5):899-910

[24] Minkowitz HS. A review of sufentanil and the sufentanil sublingual tablet system for acute moderate to severe pain. Pain Management. 2015;**5**(4):237-250

[25] Jove M, Griffin DW, Minkowitz HS, Ben-David B, Evashenk MA, Palmer PP. Sufentanil sublingual tablet system for the management of postoperative pain after knee or hip arthroplasty: A randomized, placebo-controlled study. Anesthesiology. 2015;**123**(2):434-443

[26] Thipphawong JB, Babul N, Morishige RJ, et al. Analgesic efficacy of inhaled morphine in patients after bunionectomy surgery. Anesthesiology. 2003;**99**(3):693-700; discussion 6A

[27] Block BM, Liu SS, Rowlingson AJ, Cowan AR, Cowan JA Jr, Wu CL. Efficacy of postoperative epidural analgesia: A meta-analysis. Journal of the American Medical Association. 2003;**290**(18):2455-2463

[28] DiGiusto M, Bhalla T, Martin D, Foerschler D, Jones MJ, Tobias JD. Patient-controlled analgesia in the pediatric population: Morphine versus hydromorphone. Journal of Pain Research. 2014;**7**:471-475

[29] Lavand'Homme P, De Kock M. Practical guidelines on the postoperative use of patient-controlled analgesia in the elderly. Drugs & Aging. 1998;**13**(1):9-16

[30] Egbert AM, Parks LH, Short LM, Burnett ML. Randomized trial of postoperative patient-controlled analgesia vs intramuscular narcotics in frail elderly men. Archives of Internal Medicine. 1990;**150**(9):1897-1903

[31] Mehta V, Langford R. Acute pain management in opioid dependent patients. Reviews in Pain. 2009;**3**(2):10-14

[32] Iocolano CF. Perioperative pain management in the chemically dependent patient. Journal of Perianesthesia Nursing. 2000;**15**(5): 329-344; quiz 344-7

[33] Smith JE, Rockett M, Creanor S, et al. PAin SoluTions In the Emergency Setting (PASTIES)—Patient controlled analgesia versus routine care in emergency department patients with non-traumatic abdominal pain: Randomised trial. British Medical Journal. 2015;**350**:h3147

[34] Petrenko AB, Yamakura T, Baba H, Shimoji K. The role of N-methyl-D-aspartate (NMDA) receptors in pain: A review. Anesthesia and Analgesia. 2003;**97**(4):1108-1116

[35] Burstal R, Danjoux G, Hayes C, Lantry G. PCA ketamine and morphine after abdominal hysterectomy. Anaesthesia and Intensive Care. 2001;**29**(3):246-251

[36] Reeves M, Lindholm DE, Myles PS, Fletcher H, Hunt JO. Adding ketamine to morphine for patient-controlled analgesia after major abdominal surgery: A double-blinded, randomized controlled trial. Anesthesia and Analgesia. 2001;**93**(1):116-120

[37] Striebel WH, Koenigs DI, Kramer JA. Intravenous clonidine fails to reduce postoperative meperidine requirements. Journal of Clinical Anesthesia. 1993;**5**(3):221-225

[38] Khan ZP, Ferguson CN, Jones RM. Alpha-2 and imidazoline receptor agonists. Their pharmacology and therapeutic role. Anaesthesia. 1999;**54**(2):146-165

[39] Lin TF, Yeh YC, Lin FS, et al. Effect of combining dexmedetomidine and morphine for intravenous patient-controlled analgesia. British Journal of Anaesthesia. 2009;**102**(1):117-122

[40] Brown T, Shetty A, Zhao DF, Harvey N, Yu T, Murphy M. Association between pain control and patient satisfaction outcomes in the emergency department setting. Emergency Medicine Australasia. 2018;**30**(4):523-529

[41] Gonzalez ER, Bahal N, Hansen LA, et al. Intermittent injection vs patient-controlled analgesia for sickle cell crisis pain. Comparison in patients in the emergency department. Archives of Internal Medicine. 1991;**151**(7):1373-1378

[42] Evans E, Turley N, Robinson N, Clancy M. Randomised controlled trial of patient controlled analgesia compared with nurse delivered analgesia in an emergency department. Emergency Medicine Journal. 2005;**22**(1):25-29

[43] Melzer-Lange MD, Walsh-Kelly CM, Lea G, Hillery CA, Scott JP. Patient-controlled analgesia for sickle cell pain crisis in a pediatric emergency department. Pediatric Emergency Care. 2004;**20**(1):2-4

[44] Rahman NH, DeSilva T. A randomized controlled trial of patient-controlled analgesia compared with boluses of analgesia for the control of acute traumatic pain in the emergency department. The Journal of Emergency Medicine. 2012;**43**(6):951-957

[45] Birnbaum A, Schechter C, Tufaro V, Touger R, Gallagher EJ, Bijur P. Efficacy

of patient-controlled analgesia for patients with acute abdominal pain in the emergency department: A randomized trial. Academic Emergency Medicine. 2012;**19**(4):370-377

[46] Rahman NH, DeSilva T. The effectiveness of patient control analgesia in the treatment of acute traumatic pain in the emergency department: A randomized controlled trial. European Journal of Emergency Medicine. 2012;**19**(4):241-245

[47] Stacey BR, Rudy TE, Nelhaus D. Management of patient-controlled analgesia: A comparison of primary surgeons and a dedicated pain service. Anesthesia and Analgesia. 1997;**85**(1):130-134

[48] Chumbley GM, Hall GM, Salmon P. Patient-controlled analgesia: An assessment by 200 patients. Anaesthesia. 1998;**53**(3):216-221

[49] Pritchard C, Smith JE, Creanor S, et al. The cost-effectiveness of patient-controlled analgesia vs. standard care in patients presenting to the Emergency Department in pain, who are subsequently admitted to hospital. Anaesthesia. 2017;**72**(8):953-960

[50] Chan VW, Chung F, McQuestion M, Gomez M. Impact of patient-controlled analgesia on required nursing time and duration of postoperative recovery. Regional Anesthesia. 1995;**20**(6):506-514

Section 2

Chronic Pain: Advanced Treatments

Chapter 5

The Use of Neurotoxins for Palliative Treatment of Chronic Joint Pain

Hollis Krug

Abstract

Osteoarthritis is a significant public health problem and is rapidly increasing in prevalence with the aging population. Pain is the most disabling consequence of osteoarthritis. Treatment for pain is inadequate and needs to be addressed with new therapeutic modalities. Chronic pain is often the result of peripheral and central pain sensitization which reduces the pain threshold and increases the perceived pain response to noxious and even non-noxious stimuli. Neurotoxins can reduce this sensitization by various mechanisms and are a fertile area of research for the treatment of chronic pain. Botulinum toxins, vanilloids, and conotoxin have all been studied for the treatment of chronic pain. Botulinum toxins and vanilloids have the greatest potential as analgesics for chronic joint pain thus far. Monoclonal antibodies directed against nerve growth factor have also been developed for the treatment of chronic joint pain due to osteoarthritis. These antibodies are not technically neurotoxins but have significant analgesic potential. However, they may have undesirable side effects and are still being evaluated as possible therapies for chronic osteoarthritis pain.

Keywords: osteoarthritis, chronic pain, arthritis, neurotoxins, anti-nerve growth factor

1. Introduction

Chronic joint pain is a world-wide problem. Osteoarthritis (OA) is the most common cause of chronic joint pain and is increasing in prevalence. In the United States alone, osteoarthritis affects approximately 27 million adults and is expected to exceed 67 million by the year 2030 [1, 2]. Although disability due to osteoarthritis varies, pain is the most disabling symptom affecting OA patients [3, 4]. To date, there are no disease modifying treatments for osteoarthritis. Treatment goals are focused on relief of symptoms and minimizing disability. The direct costs of treatment of OA combined with the indirect costs due to lost wages are substantial. According to one estimate, this cost accounts for 2% of the annual gross domestic product [5, 6]. Management of chronic pain from OA is challenging. Non-pharmacologic options include education, exercise, weight reduction, acupuncture, and joint protection, but these practices are generally insufficient to provide joint pain relief. Pharmacologic options include systemic and intraarticular therapies [7]. Insufficient pain relief, intolerable drug side effects and drug interactions increase the risk-benefit ratio for

IntechOpen

available pharmaceutical therapies [8]. Even surgical therapies for degenerative joint disease may not be effective. Knee joint lavage has been shown to be no more effective for alleviation of pain than placebo [9, 10].

In particular, end stage disease provides challenges for effective therapy. Opioids can sometimes be effective when other therapies have lost efficacy, but the use of narcotics for chronic pain is undesirable due to eventual dependence and loss of efficacy, the need for dose escalation to maintain effectiveness, and the rising problem of opioid abuse and overdose that has occurred since the use of long-acting narcotics have been available [11]. In addition, unacceptable side effects, particularly in the elderly who are more likely to have end stage osteoarthritis pain, makes the use of opioids a poor choice [12]. Finally, opioids may not have any increased efficacy for chronic OA pain compared with non-narcotic therapies [13]. The efficacy of intra-articular treatments such as corticosteroids and hyaluronic acid preparations have not been clearly demonstrated. For this reason the American Academy of Orthopedic Surgeons recommends against viscosupplementation and felt the evidence to be inclusive regarding corticosteroid injections for osteoarthritis [14].

Surgical treatment for end stage osteoarthritis is limited. Total joint replacement is generally considered to be effective for short and long-term pain relief and usually achieves positive clinical and functional outcomes [15, 16]. However, surgical treatments are not without risk of complications. These include systemic complications such as pulmonary embolism, but also local complications such as dislocation of hips, wound and joint infection, periprosthetic fracture, aseptic loosening, patellar maltracking, rupture of the extensor mechanism, stiffness with reduced range of motion, heterotopic ossification, metal hypersensitivity, vascular injury or bleeding, or nerve palsy. Success rates vary but as many as 1 in 5 patients undergoing total knee arthroplasty (TKA) are not satisfied with the outcome [16]. Obese patients are at increased risk for complications following TKA. Pre-operative management including weight loss, optimization of diabetes treatment, venous thromboembolism prevention, and physical therapy can help to minimize these complications [17]. Even so, some individuals will not be surgical candidates. Clearly other options are needed for effective pain relief to minimize disability and optimize function in patients who are not candidates for surgery and for whom standard analgesics have not been helpful.

Palliative therapy is specialized medical care focused on providing relief from the symptoms and stress of a serious illness. The goal is to improve quality of life and enhance physical function, but without treating or attempting to cure the underlying disease. Palliative therapy for end stage osteoarthritis is a concept that has been explored but due to a lack of effective therapies has not been very successful [18].

2. Neurobiology of chronic pain

Pain is the result of nerves transmitting a noxious signal, usually the result of some sort of injury, to the brain where it is perceived as pain. This is an important signal for the organism experiencing the injury to withdraw or avoid the stimulus that is producing the pain. Chronic pain results when nociceptive systems are altered so that there is no longer a direct relationship between a noxious stimulus and pain perception. These alterations are due to plasticity of the nervous system whereby peripheral nerves become sensitized, or spinal cord neurons become increasingly excitable. Projections from the spinal cord to higher centers can result in changes to descending inhibitory controls that are initiated in the midbrain and brainstem. All these changes together tend to alter the perceived response to any stimulus and thus lead to persistent pain states. This plasticity appears to be reversible and thus amenable to pharmacologic therapies [19].

Peripheral sensitization is thought to be the result of inflammation or nerve injury which alters nociceptive receptors causing increased intracellular calcium and activated intracellular protein kinase C and tyrosine kinases. These mediators phosphorylate sensory neuron-specific sodium channels and Transient Receptor Potential Vanilloid 1 (TRPV1) receptors causing a reduction in the depolarization threshold and reduced pain threshold. Nociceptive neurons themselves release chemical stimulants such as substance P (SP) and calcitonin gene-related peptide (CGRP) which amplify the local inflammatory response by interacting with local inflammatory cells and nearby blood vessels. This "neurogenic inflammation" causes vasodilation and edema, and increases local inflammation adding to peripheral sensitization [20]. Pharmacologic inhibition of this sensitization process is an attractive target for analgesia, as reducing sensitization would be expected to reduce the pain perception without eliminating the important pain defense mechanisms. Given the critical involvement of neuropeptides in the development of sensitization, the efficacy of neurotoxins was hypothesized for treatment of chronic pain.

3. Botulinum toxins as analgesics

3.1 Botulinum toxin background and human studies

There are eight serotypes of botulinum toxin. All are products of the bacterial genus *Clostridium*. Types A-G have been fully characterized and have varying durations of action, and enzymatic targets. They all cleave components of the soluble N-ethylmaleimide-sensitive fusion protein (NSF) attachment protein receptor (SNARE) proteins. The inability of the disrupted SNARE proteins to bring the synaptic vesicle membrane and the terminal plasma membrane of the peripheral nerve in close proximity results in an inability of the two membranes to fuse and failure of the nerve to release neurotransmitter such as acetylcholine (ACh). This produces the dramatic paralytic activity of botulinum toxin [21]. The eighth serotype, H, has been recently described, but its gene sequence has been withheld due to public safety concerns since it is considered the deadliest substance in the world [22].

Botulinum toxins A and B have been used for some time to treat painful muscle dystonias such as torticollis. It was thought that the paralytic effect of the toxin on motor units in the dystonic muscle was responsible for the pain relief that accompanied this treatment. But it was observed that pain relief preceded the muscle weakness that was expected with these treatments. This observation led to early studies of the use of intra-articular onabotulinum toxin (Type A) for end stage osteoarthritis [23]. Subsequent similar studies have been done and summarized in meta-analyses and systematic reviews. Their findings suggest that even for end stage arthritis pain, intra-articular botulinum toxin has modest beneficial effects in patients with refractory joint pain [24–27]. Studies of shoulders and knees predominated but one study treated refractory ankle osteoarthritis pain and one treated refractory pain after total knee arthroplasty. Doses used were between 100 and 200 IU onabotulinum toxin A (BOTOX), 200–500 IU abobotulinum toxin A (Dysport) and 2500 IU rimabotulinum toxin B (Myobloc). Controls in these studies were variable ranging from triamcinolone to saline to unspecified placebo. Some studies used botulinum toxin diluted with lidocaine and compared to saline with lidocaine. One small study of 75 patients compared intra-articular (IA) botulinum toxin A to injection with 2 ml sodium hyaluronate in patients with symptomatic ankle OA and found no difference in effectiveness between the two interventions [28]. Since the American

Academy of Orthopedic Surgeons has stated in their evidence based guidelines for the treatment of OA of the knee that viscosupplementation cannot be recommended, this comparison may be less than appropriate [29].

Studies of IA botulinum toxin use in humans have not reported significant safety issues. Although weakness was initially a concern, it was not found in extensive safety evaluations [23, 26]. Since a single injection provides pain relief for up to 6 months, fewer injections may be required as compared to corticosteroid or viscosupplementation injections and therefore, the risk of infection is minimized.

3.2 Botulinum toxin studies in preclinical models of joint pain

In an effort to better understand the mechanism of action of pain relief seen with botulinum toxin and to precisely define functional outcomes, a variety of animal studies have been done (**Table 1**). Botulinum toxins have been given intraarticularly for joint pain in mice, rats and dogs. IA botulinum toxin appears to be effective for chronic arthritis pain but not acute joint pain in mice, supporting the idea that botulinum toxin reduces peripheral sensitization by inhibiting neuropeptide release in the periphery [30, 31]. Only one study evaluated efficacy of rimabotulinum toxin for osteoarthritis pain in mice and found that it reduced both spontaneous and evoked pain behaviors [32]. In dogs with chronic lameness due to stifle, hip or elbow osteoarthritis IA onabotulinum toxin produced improvement in several force platform variables including vertical impulse, peak vertical force and in the Helsinki chronic pain index compared to the placebo group after 12 weeks. The secondary outcomes of subjective pain score and the need for rescue analgesics were not significantly improved in the botulinum toxin treated group compared to placebo. No major adverse events were detected [33]. A second study in dogs designed to detect adverse effects of IA botulinum toxin compared toxin injection to placebo in healthy beagle dogs. This study evaluated dynamic and static weight bearing, range of motion, joint tenderness, synovial fluid, neurologic function and electrophysiologic recordings, and histopathology of joint structures and adjacent muscles and nerves. Intra-articular botulinum toxin A did not produce significant clinical, cytological, or histopathological adverse effects in healthy dogs, but based on the electrophysiological recordings that found low compound muscle action potentials in 2 dogs in the botulinum toxin injected limb, the authors concluded that toxin may spread from the joint, but that its clinical impact is probably low [34]. In rats with inflammatory arthritis of the temporal mandibular joint (TMJ) produced by immunization with bovine serum albumin (BSA) and subsequent intra-articular challenge with BSA, injecting the joint with botulinum toxin A significantly reduced nociceptive behaviors that resulted from IA injection of low dose formalin into these inflamed joints. These authors demonstrated that the trigeminal ganglion of botulinum A treated arthritic animals released less substance P (SP) and calcitonin gene related peptide (CGRP) than saline treated arthritic animals but glutamate release was not affected. Glutamate receptors AMPA and NMDA were also unchanged in botulinum treated ganglia compared to saline treated controls. Periarticular tissues from the arthritic TMJs released increased amounts of interleukin 1-β (IL-1β) and tumor necrosis factor α (TNFα). Treatment with botulinum toxin reduced IL-1β release but had no effect on TNFα [35]. In another study of rats with adjuvant-induced arthritis induced in the tibial-tarsal joint, mechanical and thermal hyperalgesia and TRPV1 expression in the L4-5 dorsal root ganglia (DRG) were measured. DRGs were also stained for the presence of cleaved synaptosomal-associated protein of 25 kDa (SNAP-25)—the cleavage product of botulinum toxin A—and for transient receptor potential vanilloid 1 and put TRPV1 in parentheses TRPV1 and CGRP. TRPV1 expression increased significantly in

Arthritis model	Experiment	Results	Reference
Murine CFA, COL	IA BoNT/A vs. sham	Reduced spontaneous and evoked pain behaviors in CFA arthritis, reduced spontaneous pain behavior in COL arthritis	[30, 31]
Murine COL	IA BoNT/B vs. saline or sham injection	Improved visual gait analysis, improved joint tenderness	[32]
Dog, OA, multiple joints	IA BoNT/A vs. placebo Outcome measured after 12 weeks	Improved peak vertical force, improved Helsinki chronic pain index	[33]
Healthy beagles (safety study)	IA BoNT vs. placebo	No adverse clinical, cytological, or histopathological effects. Some EMG evidence for spread outside the joints to muscle	[34]
Rat BSA TMJ inflammatory arthritis	IA BoNT/A followed by pain induction with formalin injection	Significantly reduced pain behaviors, reduced SP and CGRP release, no change in glutamate release, reduced release of IL-1β but not TNFα	[35]
Rat CFA tibiotarsal joint	IA BoNT/A (dose ranging) compared to CFA alone and saline control	All pain outcomes improved in a dose dependent fashion. (Mechanical and thermal hyperalgesia) TRPV1 expression reduced but not transcription, thought due to the observed reduced movement of TRPV1 to the cell membrane	[36]
Rat CFA ankle arthritis Plantar injection of capsaicin and formalin and plantar incision as standardized pain models. Also included SNI model	BiTox—unique nonparalyzing botulinum toxin molecule	CFA induced swelling reduced, mechanical hyperalgesia but not thermal hyperalgesia reduced. No effect on acute pain from capsaicin or formalin but reduced secondary mechanical hyperalgesia after plantar capsaicin injection. Plantar incision pain response reduced after day 2. Reduced neuropathic pain in the SNI model	[37]
ACIA model in mice	Genetic modification of mice to express the conotoxin ω-conopeptide MVIIA vs. wild type	Pain was suppressed but joint inflammation was increased and more destructive in genetically modified mice	[55]

CFA—complete freund's adjuvant induced arthritis, COL—collagenase-induced osteoarthritis, BoNT/A—onabotulinum toxin type A, BoNT/B—rimabotulinum toxin type B, BSA—bovine serum albumin, TMJ—temporal mandibular joint, SNI—spared nerve injury, ACIA—antigen and collagen-induced arthritis.

Table 1.
Preclinical studies of botulinum and other toxins as analgesics for arthritis pain.

the arthritic animals' DRGs and arthritic animals demonstrated mechanical and thermal hyperalgesia. Botulinum toxin A increased the paw withdrawal threshold and latency to both mechanical and thermal stimuli and reduced TRPV1 expression in a dose-dependent manner. TRPV1 transcription was likewise increased with Complete Freund's Adjuvant (CFA) induced arthritis but botulinum toxin A did not alter this increased transcription. Using immunofluorescent staining, these authors found that the increase in TRPV1 and CGRP co-expressing neurons which was the result of CFA arthritis was reduced by botulinum toxin in a dose dependent manner. Since botulinum toxin exerts its effects by cleaving SNAP-25 and thus preventing release of neuropeptide by preventing fusion of vesicles with the terminal membrane, the presence of cleaved SNAP 25 localized with TRPV1 in the DRG was analyzed. Co-localization of cleaved SNAP-25 with TRPV1 in the botulinum toxin A group was clearly seen 5 days after botulinum toxin injection. This was not seen in the sham and CFA saline control groups. These authors speculated that botulinum toxin A may prevent TRPV1 expression on DRG neurons by inhibition of TRPV1 trafficking to the cell membrane after retrograde transport of botulinum toxin from the periphery to the DRG since the expression of the TRPV1 receptor has been shown to be dependent on exocytosis that requires interactions with proteins of the soluble N-ethylmaleimide-sensitive factor attachment protein receptor (SNARE) complex consisting of SNAP-25 [36]. The presence of botulinum toxin in the DRG would prevent the SNARE complex from functioning normally to move TRPV1 to the cell membrane. A botulinum toxin A based molecule—BiTox—has been synthesized that is reported to retain neuronal silencing capacity without causing paralysis. This molecule reduces plasma extravasation and inflammatory edema but is not transported to the DRG ganglia or dorsal horn and does not inhibit pain behaviors in response to formalin or capsaicin and does not inhibit formalin-induced c-Fos expression in the dorsal horn. It was found to strongly reduce A-nociceptor mediated secondary mechanical hyperalgesia due to CFA joint inflammation or capsaicin injection and decreased hypersensitivity from nerve injury. The authors concluded that this botulinum toxin based molecule could reduce local release of neuromodulators from C fibers without impairing C nociceptive signaling function [37].

4. Vanilloids as analgesics

4.1 Vanilloids and their receptors background

Vanilloids such as capsaicin (the active ingredient in hot chili peppers) and resiniferatoxin (a product of the plant *Euphorbia resinifera*) were first notable for their ability to produce burning pain when administered topically. Later, both molecules were found to have analgesic potential and subsequent work identified the non-selective cation channel to which these compounds bind. This receptor was found to be located on the dorsal root and trigeminal ganglia of various species. Subsequent work identified the channel, allowed cloning and cDNA characterization, and revealed that the channel could be activated not only by vanilloids but also by heat suggesting a role in thermosensation. The receptor was named transient receptor potential vanilloid 1 (TRPV1) and other ligands were identified making it a transducer of many types of noxious stimuli [38].

Because of the variety of ligands, TRPV1 was considered a likely target for analgesia. Agonists such as vanilloids were noted to cause desensitization of these channels and in rodents as well as humans, pain behaviors could be alleviated with vanilloid treatment. TRPV1 knockout mice demonstrated reduced thermal hypersensitivity with inflammation. TRPV1 antagonists were shown to reverse pain behavior in rodents with a wide variety of painful conditions including inflammation, osteoarthritis and cancer. Both agonists and antagonists have been considered as analgesic therapies. Although systemic administration of vanilloids demonstrated analgesic efficacy in preclinical pain models, because of the undesirable systemic side effects of these compounds, most therapeutic trials have focused on local or topical administration of these compounds. Undesirable effects include hypotension, respiratory compromise and other negative effects on reflex pathways. Less pungent analogs were found to be less efficacious with respect to analgesia [38].

4.2 Vanilloids as analgesics—Human and pre-clinical studies

In humans, current treatment of joint pain with vanilloids is limited to topical therapies. Pain relieving creams such as Zostrix® and patches such as Salonpas Hot Capsicum Patch® are available over the counter and contain capsaicin as the active ingredient. Multiple clinical trials have found modest benefit for osteoarthritis from low dose topical capsaicin [39–41]. More recently, a high dose 8% capsaicin patch has been approved for the treatment of post-herpetic neuralgia. According to the package insert, application of the patch requires careful adherence to application instructions by the health care professional and local anesthesia for the patient prior to application and systemic analgesics as needed in the post-application period. Interestingly, results from clinical trials of this drug for treatment of painful HIV neuropathy did not show clinical benefit [42, 43].

Resiniferatoxin (RTX) is an ultra-potent capsaicin (CAP) analogue [44], that is several thousand-fold more potent than CAP [45]. RTX in low concentrations produces a slow and sustained depolarization of membrane potential, preventing the generation of action potentials but causing less toxicity. A single IA injection in rats has been found to reduce hyperalgesia due to carrageenan induced joint pain [46].

RTX has been studied in clinical trials for other painful conditions. When given intravesicularly for interstitial cystitis and painful bladder syndrome, it did not improved overall symptoms of pain, urgency, frequency or nocturia [47, 48]. Adlea™ (4975) is another CAP analogue under development for the treatment of post-operative musculoskeletal pain, osteoarthritis and tendinopathy. Phase II trials of intra-articular injection of this compound were encouraging but no further clinical trials appear to have been performed [38]. Zucapsaicin (Civamide) is the cis-isomer of capsaicin, and functions as a TRPV1 blocker. Phase III trials have been done with topical civamide for OA knee pain [49]. This topical therapy is not absorbed systemically, is well tolerated, and produced significant improvement in Western Ontario and McMaster Universities Arthritis Index (WOMAC) physical function score, pain score and subject global evaluation. Improvement was maintained for a year. This drug has not yet been approved by the US FDA.

4.3 TRPV1 antagonists as analgesics

Several TRPV1 antagonists have also been identified that act as analgesics [50]. Some are more selective than others, complete nonselectivity producing inhibition of all modes of TRPV1 activation (protons, heat and capsaicin). More selectivity

Arthritis model	Experiment	Results	Reference
Rat carrageenan-induced acute joint pain	IA RTX vs. vehicle given 24 hours after arthritis induction in a dose ranging study	Significant reduction in pain behavior with RTX treatment	[46]
Rat MIA model—early phase	A-425619 given IP in a dose range during acute inflammatory phase	47% reduction in weightbearing asymmetry. Prolonged benefit	[50, 51]
Rat MIA model—late phase	A-889425 and A-995662 given orally	Reduced loss of grip force within 1 hour and maintained up to 8 hours	[50, 52, 53]

IA—intra-articular, RTX—resiniferatoxin, MIA—monosodium iodoacetate.

Table 2.
Preclinical studies of vanilloid agonists and antagonists as analgesics for arthritis pain.

appears to improve the side effect profile. Centrally active TRPV1 antagonists appear to provide greater analgesia when given systemically or intrathecally in preclinical models of OA pain. Most preclinical studies of OA have been done in the monosodium iodoacetate (MIA) model in the rat (**Table 2**). Rats with MIA-induced arthritis pain demonstrate reduced weightbearing of the affected limb, pain with movement of the joint and hypersensitivity of uninjured tissues (secondary allodynia of the hind paw). These pain behaviors are thought to be due to both central and peripheral sensitization. TRPV1 antagonists appeared to be analgesic during both the acute inflammatory phase of MIA pain and later during the chronic phase [50–53]. Analgesia appears to improve with repeated dosing and side effects such as hyperthermia abate with some of the investigational TRPV1 antagonists. The potency of hyperthermia induction seems to relate most closely to the blockade of proton-induced TRPV1 activation [50].

Only a few TRPV1 antagonists have been used in clinical trials. ADZ1386 given orally in two different doses did not reduce OA pain more than placebo. A study in dogs with hip OA using oral ABT116 did not improve the total pain score, pain severity or pain interference score, but did reduce rescue medication use, increased night time activity levels and briefly produced an acute hyperthermic effect. NEO 6860, which is specific for blocking capsaicin activation of the target, with little or no effect against pH or heat activation, underwent a first-in-human phase I trial of the safety and efficacy of the drug in healthy human subjects [54]. The dose ranging study included 64 subjects and measured pharmacodynamics with a intradermal capsaicin test as well as pharmacokinetics. The drug was rapidly absorbed with a half-life of between 4 and 8 hours. Side effects included headache, paresthesia, nausea, and dizziness. Study participants were monitored specifically for increase in temperature and heat pain threshold/tolerance, but these were not noted. At all doses, most subjects reported a rapid onset, transient sensation of "feeling hot". The authors concluded that this compound had potential for development for treating OA-associated pain and future clinical studies were planned but have not yet been initiated.

5. Other potentially analgesic neurotoxins

5.1 Conotoxin

Ziconotide (ω-conopeptide MVIIA) is a synthetic compound of the neurotoxin ω-conopeptide derived from the Conus Magus fish hunting marine snail found in the Pacific Ocean. It selectively binds to the N-type voltage-gated calcium channels found in the laminae of the spinal cord's dorsal horn and blocks these channels. This blockade prevents calcium influx and halts neurotransmission thereby preventing nociceptive signaling. Pain transmission messages are prevented from arriving at the brain. It is FDA approved for intrathecal use for severe chronic pain in individuals who are intolerant of or refractory to other treatments including intrathecal (IT) morphine, but has demonstrated some serious side effects such as suicidal ideation and psychosis [55].

In a study of transgenic mice bred to express a membrane-tethered form of the conotoxin ω-conopeptide MVIIA under control of a nociceptor-specific gene, who were subjected to unilateral induction of joint inflammation with the antigen- and collagen- induced arthritis (ACIA) model, pain was effectively suppressed, but joint inflammation became persistent and more destructive. The authors concluded that blockade of $Ca_V2.2$-mediated calcium influx and nociceptive signaling by this toxin impaired recovery from induced inflammatory arthritis. They concluded that this blockade could lead to potentially deleterious and devastating effects if used during inflammation [55].

5.2 Tetrodotoxin

Another neurotoxin studied as a potential analgesic is tetrodotoxin (TTX). Voltage-gated sodium channels (VGSCs) are critical for neuronal function and dysfunctional VGSCs have been implicated in several pain states. There are nine isoforms of the sodium channel alpha-subunit (Nav1.1–1.9 in mammals). Only Nav1.1–1.4 and Nav1.6–1.7 subtypes (TTX-sensitive channels) can be blocked by nanomolar concentrations of tetrodotoxin. Micromolar concentrations are required to block Nav1.5 and Nav1.8–1.9 subtypes (TTX-resistant channels) [56]. Although it appears to have little effect on acute pain further studies are needed. Analgesic efficacy in preclinical inflammatory pain models demonstrated promising effects of systemic administration for mechanical hyperalgesia and the neurogenic inflammatory response to injury. There are contradictory results for TTX efficacy for neuropathic pain. Effectiveness in preclinical models of neuropathic pain varied depending on dose, route of application, and appeared more effective in acute neural injury than in chronic neuropathic pain. In one clinical trial of tetrodotoxin for chemotherapy-induced neuropathic pain, injected TTX did not have a significant effect on pain [57]. There have been no specific studies evaluating tetrodotoxin for the treatment of chronic joint pain.

6. Anti-nerve growth factor

Thought not technically neurotoxins, several monoclonal antibodies have been developed against nerve growth factor (NGF) specifically for the treatment of chronic pain, and specifically for pain from OA. Tanezumab was the first of these to be developed. Three other companies have now created similar antibodies. Tanezumab was in phase III studies when the US FDA placed a hold on further clinical trials after an increase in joint destruction was observed in patients who had been given this drug. After that, preclinical studies suggested that this class of drugs could damage the autonomic nervous system, which delayed further research [58]. Since the hold was released in 2015, phase III clinical trials are being repeated. Results from those that have been published show that these biologic therapies appear to be effective with acceptable side effect profiles [59–61]. These therapies are administered parenterally, and therefore are systemically active. These antibodies have significant potential to improve analgesia for chronic arthritis pain. Alternative routes of administration such as IA will be of interest.

7. Conclusions

Chronic joint pain is a significant public health problem that will only increase along with the aging population. In the absence of disease modifying treatments for OA, the need for better pain therapies will continue to increase. Neurotoxins can be helpful as adjunct treatments for pain, particularly in cases where peripheral sensitization has lowered pain thresholds and increased pain perception. Advances in understanding of the pathophysiologic mechanisms of nociception and sensitization and elucidation of the specific functions of the various neurotoxins will allow more advanced development of toxins that may avoid potential side effects and more specifically reduce pain perception.

Acknowledgements

Thanks to Maren Mahowald who first introduced me to the concept of neurotoxins as therapy for joint pain.

Conflict of interest

The author has no conflict of interest to declare.

Author details

Hollis Krug
Minneapolis VA Health Care System, University of Minnesota, Minneapolis, Minnesota, USA

*Address all correspondence to: hollis.krug@va.gov

References

[1] Hootman JM, Helmick CG, Barbour KE, Theis KA, Boring MA. Updated projected prevalence of self-reported doctor-diagnosed arthritis and arthritis-attributable activity limitation among US adults, 2015-2040. Arthritis & Rhematology. 2016;**68**(7):1582-1587

[2] Hootman JM, Helmick CG. Projections of US prevalence of arthritis and associated activity limitations. Arthritis and Rheumatism. 2006;**54**(1):226-229

[3] Malfait AM, Schnitzer TJ. Towards a mechanism-based approach to pain management in osteoarthritis. Nature Reviews Rheumatology. 2013;**9**(11):654-664

[4] Neogi T. The epidemiology and impact of pain in osteoarthritis. Osteoarthritis and Cartilage. 2013;**21**(9):1145-1153

[5] Kotlarz H, Gunnarsson CL, Fang H, Rizzo JA. Osteoarthritis and absenteeism costs: Evidence from US National survey data. Journal of Occupational and Environmental Medicine. 2010;**52**(3):263-268

[6] Yelin E, Murphy L, Cisternas M, Foreman A, Pasta D, Helmick C. Medical care expenditures and earnings losses among persons with arthritis and other rheumatic conditions in 2003, and comparisons to 1997. Arthritis and Rheumatism. 1997;**56**(5):1397-1407

[7] Wenham CY, Conaghan PG. New horizons in osteoarthritis. Age and Ageing. 2013;**42**(3):272-278

[8] Zhang W, Nuki G, Moskowitz RW, Abramson S, Altman RD, Arden NK, et al. OARSI recommendations for the management of hip and knee osteoarthritis, part III: Changes in evidence following systematic cumulative update of research published through January 2009. Osteoarthritis and Cartilage. 2010;**18**(4):476-499

[9] Kirkley A, Birmingham TB, Litchfield RB, Giffin JR, Willits KR, Wong CJ, et al. A randomized trial of arthroscopic surgery for osteoarthritis of the knee. The New England Journal of Medicine. 2008;**359**(11):1097-1107

[10] Mosely JB, O'Malley K, Petersen NJ, Menke TJ, Brody BA, David H, et al. A controlled trial of arthroscopic surgery for osteoarthritis of the knee. The New England Journal of Medicine. 2002;**347**:81-88

[11] Manchikanti L, Helm S 2nd, Fellows B, Janata JW, Pampati V, Grider JS, et al. Opioid epidemic in the United States. Pain Physician. 2012;**15**(3 Suppl):ES9-E38

[12] Rolita L, Spegman A, Tang X, Cronstein BN. Greater number of narcotic analgesic prescriptions for osteoarthritis is associated with falls and fractures in elderly adults. Journal of the American Geriatrics Society. 2013;**61**(3):335-340

[13] Krebs EE, Gravely A, Nugent S, Jensen AC, DeRonne B, Goldsmith ES, et al. Effect of opioid vs nonopioid medications on pain-related function in patients with chronic back pain or hip or knee osteoarthritis pain: The SPACE randomized clinical trial. Journal of the American Medical Association. 2018;**319**(9):872-882

[14] Jevsevar D, Brown GA, Jones DL, Matzin EG, Manner P, Mooar P, et al. Treatment of Osteoarthritis of the Knee: Non-Arthroplasty Treatment. 2nd ed. Rosemont, IL: American Academy of Orthopaedic Surgeons; 2013

[15] Varacallo M, Johanson NA. Hip, replacement. In: Treasure Island. FL: StatPearls Publishing LLC; 2018

[16] Varacallo M, Johanson NA. Total knee arthoplasty. In: Treasure Island. FL: StatPearls Publishing LLC; 2018

[17] Feng JE, Novikov D, Anoushiravani AA, Schwarzkopf R. Total knee arthroplasty: Improving outcomes with a multidisciplinary approach. Journal of Multidisciplinary Healthcare. 2018;**11**:63-73

[18] Pavelka K. Treatment of pain in osteoarthritis. European Journal of Pain. 2000;**4**(Suppl A):23-30

[19] Dickenson A. The neurobiology of chronic pain states. Anaesthesia and Intensive Care Medicine. 2016;**17**(9):436-439

[20] Mahowald ML, Krug HE. Chronic musculoskeletal pain. In: Firestein GS, Budd RC, Harris ED Jr, McInnes IB, Ruddy S, Sergent JS, editors. Kelly's Textbook of Rheumatology. I. 8th ed. Philadelphia, PA: Saunders Elsevier; 2009. pp. 963-992

[21] Montecucco C, Molgo J. Botulinal neurotoxins: Revival of an old killer. Current Opinion in Pharmacology. 2005;**5**(3):274-279

[22] Barash JR, Arnon SS. A novel strain of clostridium botulinum that produces type B and type H botulinum toxins. The Journal of Infectious Diseases. 2014;**209**(2):183-191

[23] Mahowald ML, Singh JA, Dykstra D. Long term effects of intra-articular botulinum toxin A for refractory joint pain. Neurotoxicity Research. 2006;**9**(2-3):179-188

[24] Wu T, Fu Y, Song HX, Ye Y, Dong Y, Li JH. Effectiveness of botulinum toxin for shoulder pain treatment: A systematic review and meta-analysis. Archives of Physical Medicine and Rehabilitation. 2015;**96**(12):2214-2220

[25] Wu T, Song HX, Dong Y, Ye Y, Li JH. Intra-articular injections of botulinum toxin a for refractory joint pain: A systematic review and meta-analysis. Clinical Rehabilitation. 2017;**31**(4):435-443

[26] Singh JA, Fitzgerald PM. Botulinum toxin for shoulder pain: A cochrane systematic review. The Journal of Rheumatology. 2011;**38**(3):409-418

[27] Khenioui H, Houvenagel E, Catanzaritia JF, Guyota MA, Agnania O, Donzea C. Usefulness of intra-articular botulinum toxin injections. A systematic review. Joint, Bone, Spine. 2016;**83**:149-154

[28] Sun SF, Hsu CW, Lin HS, Chou YJ, Chen JY, Wang JL. Efficacy of intraarticular botulinum toxin A and intraarticular hyaluronate plus rehabilitation exercise in patients with unilateral ankle osteoarthritis: A randomized controlled trial. Journal of Foot and Ankle Research. 2014;**7**(1):9

[29] Sanders JO, Murray J, Gross L. Non-arthroplasty treatment of osteoarthritis of the knee. The Journal of the American Academy of Orthopaedic Surgeons. 2014;**22**(4):256-260

[30] Krug HE, Frizelle S, McGarraugh P, Mahowald ML. Pain behavior measures to quantitate joint pain and response to neurotoxin treatment in murine models of arthritis. Pain Medicine. 2009;**10**(7):1218-1228

[31] Blanshan N, Mahowald ML, Dorman C, Frizelle S, Krug HE. The analgesic effect of intraarticular OnabotulinumtoxinA in a female murine model of collagenase induced chronic degenerative monoarthritis. Toxicon. 2018;**158**:8-15

[32] Anderson S, Krug H, Dorman C, McGarraugh P, Frizelle S, Mahowald M. Analgesic effects of intra-articular

botulinum toxin type B in a murine model of chronic degenerative knee arthritis pain. Journal of Pain Research. 2010;**3**:161-168

[33] Heikkila HM, Hielm-Bjorkman AK, Morelius M, Larsen S, Honkavaara J, Innes JF, et al. Intra-articular botulinum toxin A for the treatment of osteoarthritic joint pain in dogs: A randomized, double-blinded, placebo-controlled clinical trial. Veterinary Journal. 2014;**200**(1):162-169

[34] Heikkila HM, Jokinen TS, Syrja P, Junnila J, Hielm-Bjorkman A, Laitinen-Vapaavuori O. Assessing adverse effects of intra-articular botulinum toxin A in healthy beagle dogs: A placebo-controlled, blinded, randomized trial. PLoS One. 2018;**13**(1):e0191043

[35] Lora VR, Clemente-Napimoga JT, Abdalla HB, Macedo CG, Canales GT, Barbosa CM. Botulinum toxin type A reduces inflammatory hypernociception induced by arthritis in the temporomadibular joint of rats. Toxicon. 2017;**129**:52-57

[36] Fan C, Chu X, Wang L, Shi H, Li T. Botulinum toxin type A reduces TRPV1 expression in the dorsal root ganglion in rats with adjuvant-arthritis pain. Toxicon. 2017;**133**:116-122

[37] Mangione AS, Obara I, Maiaru M, Geranton SM, Tassorelli C, Ferrari E, et al. Nonparalytic botulinum molecules for the control of pain. Pain. 2016;**157**(5):1045-1055

[38] Wong GY, Gavva NR. Therapeutic potential of vanilloid receptor TRPV1 agonists and antagonists as analgesics: Recent advances and setbacks. Brain Research Reviews. 2009;**60**(1):267-277

[39] Deal CL, Schnitzer TJ, Lipstein E, Seibold JR, Stevens RM, Levy MD, et al. Treatment of arthritis with topical capsaicin: A double-blind trial. Clinical Therapeutics. 1991;**13**(3):383-395

[40] Kosuwon W, Sirichatiwapee W, Wisanuyotin T, Jeeravipoolvarn P, Laupattarakasem W. Efficacy of symptomatic control of knee osteoarthritis with 0.0125% of capsaicin versus placebo. Journal of the Medical Association of Thailand. 2010;**93**(10):1188-1195

[41] McCarthy GM, McCarty DJ. Effect of topical capsaicin in the therapy of painful osteoarthritis of the hands. The Journal of Rheumatology. 1992;**19**(4):604-607

[42] Brown S, Simpson DM, Moyle G, Brew BJ, Schifitto G, Larbalestier N, et al. NGX-4010, a capsaicin 8% patch, for the treatment of painful HIV-associated distal sensory polyneuropathy: Integrated analysis of two phase III, randomized, controlled trials. AIDS Research and Therapy. 2013;**10**(1):5

[43] Clifford DB, Simpson DM, Brown S, Moyle G, Brew BJ, Conway B, et al. A randomized, double-blind, controlled study of NGX-4010, a capsaicin 8% dermal patch, for the treatment of painful HIV-associated distal sensory polyneuropathy. Journal of Acquired Immune Deficiency Syndromes. 2012;**59**(2):126-133

[44] Rosenbaum T, Simon SA. TRPV1 receptors and signal transduction. In: Liedtke WB, Heller S, editors. TRP Ion Channel Function in Sensory Transduction and Cellular Signaling Cascades. Frontiers in Neuroscience. Boca Raton, FL: CRC Press/Taylor & Francis; 2007

[45] Szolcsanyi J, Szallasi A, Szallasi Z, Joo F, Blumberg PM. Resiniferatoxin: An ultrapotent selective modulator of capsaicin-sensitive primary afferent neurons. The Journal of Pharmacology

and Experimental Therapeutics. 1990;**255**(2):923-928

[46] Kissin EY, Freitas CF, Kissin I. The effects of intraarticular resiniferatoxin in experimental knee-joint arthritis. Anesthesia and Analgesia. 2005;**101**(5):1433-1439

[47] Chen TY, Corcos J, Camel M, Ponsot Y, Tu le M. Prospective, randomized, double-blind study of safety and tolerability of intravesical resiniferatoxin (RTX) in interstitial cystitis (IC). International Urogynecology Journal and Pelvic Floor Dysfunction. 2005;**16**(4):293-297

[48] Payne CK, Mosbaugh PG, Forrest JB, Evans RJ, Whitmore KE, Antoci JP, et al. Intravesical resiniferatoxin for the treatment of interstitial cystitis: A randomized, double-blind, placebo controlled trial. The Journal of Urology. 2005;**173**(5):1590-1594

[49] Schnitzer TJ, Pelletier JP, Haselwood DM, Ellison WT, Ervin JE, Gordon RD, et al. Civamide cream 0.075% in patients with osteoarthritis of the knee: A 12-week randomized controlled clinical trial with a longterm extension. The Journal of Rheumatology. 2012;**39**(3):610-620

[50] Kelly S. TRPV1 antagonists in the treatment of osteoarthritis pain. International Journal of Clinical Rheumatology. 2015;**10**(3):161-175

[51] Honore P, Chandran P, Hernandez G, Gauvin DM, Mikusa JP, Zhong C, et al. Repeated dosing of ABT-102, a potent and selective TRPV1 antagonist, enhances TRPV1-mediated analgesic activity in rodents, but attenuates antagonist-induced hyperthermia. Pain. 2009;**142**(1-2):27-35

[52] Chu KL, Chandran P, Joshi SK, Jarvis MF, Kym PR, McGaraughty S. TRPV1-related modulation of spinal neuronal activity and behavior in a rat model of osteoarthritic pain. Brain Research. 2011;**1369**:158-166

[53] Puttfarcken PS, Han P, Joshi SK, Neelands TR, Gauvin DM, Baker SJ, et al. A-995662 [(R)-8-(4-methyl-5-(4-(trifluoromethyl)phenyl) oxazol-2-ylamino)-1,2,3,4-tetrahydr onaphthalen-2-ol], a novel, selective TRPV1 receptor antagonist, reduces spinal release of glutamate and CGRP in a rat knee joint pain model. Pain. 2010;**150**(2):319-326

[54] Brown W, Leff RL, Griffin A, Hossack S, Aubray R, Walker P, et al. Safety, pharmacokinetics, and pharmacodynamics study in healthy subjects of oral NEO6860, a modality selective transient receptor potential vanilloid subtype 1 antagonist. The Journal of Pain. 2017;**18**(6):726-738

[55] Brookes ME, Eldabe S, Batterham A. Ziconotide monotherapy: A systematic review of randomised controlled trials. Current Neuropharmacology. 2017;**15**(2):217-231

[56] Nieto FR, Cobos EJ, Tejada MA, Sanchez-Fernandez C, Gonzalez-Cano R, Cendan CM. Tetrodotoxin (TTX) as a therapeutic agent for pain. Marine Drugs. 2012;**10**(2):281-305

[57] Kavoosi M. The Purpose of this Study Is to Determine if Tetrodotoxin (TTX) Is Effective in the Treatment of Pain Resulting from Chemotherapy Treatment (TTX-CINP-201). Bethesda, MD: U.S. National Library of Medicine; 2012. Available from: https://clinicaltrials.gov/ct2/show/results/NCT01655823?term=tetrodotoxin&rank=2 [Accessed: June 1, 2019]

[58] Mullard A. Drug developers reboot anti-NGF pain programmes. Nature Reviews. Drug Discovery. 2015;**14**(5):297-298

[59] Mayorga AJ, Wang S, Kelly KM, Thipphawong J. Efficacy and safety of

fulranumab as monotherapy in patients with moderate to severe, chronic knee pain of primary osteoarthritis: A randomised, placebo- and active-controlled trial. International Journal of Clinical Practice. 2016;**70**(6):493-505

[60] Tiseo PJ, Kivitz AJ, Ervin JE, Ren H, Mellis SJ. Fasinumab (REGN475), an antibody against nerve growth factor for the treatment of pain: Results from a double-blind, placebo-controlled exploratory study in osteoarthritis of the knee. Pain. 2014;**155**(7):1245-1252

[61] Ekman EF, Gimbel JS, Bello AE, Smith MD, Keller DS, Annis KM, et al. Efficacy and safety of intravenous tanezumab for the symptomatic treatment of osteoarthritis: 2 randomized controlled trials versus naproxen. The Journal of Rheumatology. 2014;**41**(11):2249-2259

Chapter 6

Features and Clinical Effectiveness of the Regenerative Injection Treatments: Prolotherapy and Platelet-Rich Plasma for Musculoskeletal Pain Management

Ilker Solmaz and Aydan Orscelik

Abstract

Pain is a symptom caused by a disease process and/or tissue injury. With the prolongation of life expectancy in humans, the incidence of degenerative joint diseases and as a result pain has increased. Unfortunately, a method of treatment that stops or reverses progression by affecting the pathogenesis in these diseases has not been developed. Physical therapeutics such as medicine and physical rehabilitation often are prescribed for patients suffering with pain. Recently, in addition to these routine therapies used in pain treatment, many regenerative injection-based therapies, including prolotherapy (PrT) or platelet-rich plasma (PRP) have been widely used. PrT is using for damaged or degenerated connective tissue healing, such as ligaments, tendons, and cartilage. The combination of local inflammatory effect, stimulation of local growth factor release, and down regulation of neuropathic inflammation can be defined as the mechanism. As a result of these, joint instability and ligament laxity reduce and pain decrease. PRP is the cellular component of the plasma. Although PRP is used for the same reasons as PrT, it can be used in acute cases unlike PrT. This chapter is intended to understand the use of regenerative injection therapies (PrT and PRP) better in the treatment of pain.

Keywords: regenerative injection treatments, prolotherapy, platelet-rich plasma, musculoskeletal pain

1. Introduction

New developments are taking place every day in every field of medicine. Disease prevention, early diagnosis, and the definite treatment method call has become the target of scientists. With the prolongation of life expectancy in humans, the incidence of degenerative joint diseases and as a result pain has increased. Unfortunately, a method of treatment that stops or reverses progression by affecting the pathogenesis in these diseases has not been developed.

Pain is a symptom caused by a disease process and/or tissue injury. Physical therapeutics, such as medicine and physical rehabilitation, often are prescribed for patients suffering with pain [1]. Recently, in addition to these routine therapies used in pain treatment, many regenerative injection based-therapies, including prolotherapy (PrT) or platelet-rich plasma (PRP) have been widely used. The evidence for these treatments has arisen from the basic sciences and has been transformed into clinical research through controlled researches [2].

2. Regenerative injection treatments

2.1 Prolotherapy

PrT is derived from the words "proliferation" and "therapy" in Latin [3]. In the 1930s, it was introduced in the USA first, but the word "Prolotherapy" was first used by George Hackett in 1950. Dr. Hemwall's studies reported that 82% of the patients provided pain remission [4]. George Hackett formed the injection protocols for PrT in the 1950s depending on his clinical experience [4, 5]. Death of a case has been reported due to an allergic reaction due to phenol injection during PrT in 1959. After this negativity, this method has been removed to history [6].

PrT is an increasingly popular regenerative injection-based therapy and using for damaged or degenerated connective tissue healing, such as ligaments, tendons, and cartilage [7–10]. Following injury, chronic musculoskeletal pain develops if connective tissue repair is insufficient [4, 5]. Chronic musculoskeletal pain and disability often result from degeneration associated with these structures. PrT treatment can help us to correct this degeneration at the tissue level [4, 9]. We can correct this degeneration at the tissue level with the help of PrT. Pain reduction and regeneration mechanism are not clearly understood yet [7, 8]. However, the combination of local inflammatory effect, stimulation of local growth factor release, and down regulation of neuropathic inflammation can be defined as the mechanism [8, 11]. As a result of these, both joint instabilities with ligament laxity may reduce and also pain may reduce [12].

The proliferant solutions are used for injection into tender ligamentous and tendinous attachments and adjacent joint spaces. Irritants, osmotics, and chemotactics are proliferants commonly used in PrT. Irritants are phenol, guaiacol, and tannic acid. These damage cells. Particulates, that is, pumice flour, are also irritants but make cellular trauma and attract macrophages directly. Sodium morrhuate is a chemotactic and attract inflammatory cells. Glucose, glycerin, and zinc sulphate are the osmotic proliferants and cause osmotic shock to cells [12]. The most common injectant used in the randomized controlled trials (RCTs) is hypertonic dextrose [7, 11, 13]. Proliferant solutions may cause osmotic rupture of cells in the area in which they are applied and may direct to growth factor increase in various cells of human. Also, a hypertonic environment may lead to the release of DNA-encoding growth factors [11, 14]. Furthermore, various proliferant solutions cause fibroblast stimulation. Growth factors activate and also release the fibroblasts. The active fibroblasts secrete new collagen fibrils. Collagen fibrils are essential for the repair of damaged ligament and tendons and support healing [4, 10]. PrT tighten and strengthen the ligaments, tendons, and joint stabilizing structures. So, PrT could improve the stability of the joints [4, 10, 12, 15]. Increased joint stabilization could be associated with tissue healing process by increasing local blood flow and the excitability of mechanoreceptors and also by decreasing the excitability of pain receptors [4].

Instead of phenol, hypertonic dextrose solution can be done safely for PrT nowadays. The risk of side effects and complications is very low. As a result of this, hypertonic dextrose solutions with different concentrations (10–30%) have been commonly used in studies and books to date for PrT treatments. In these studies, greater than 10% of dextrose solutions proposed to use inflammatory response and proliferation. An animal study is designed for determining the optimal concentrations of dextrose solutions. This claimed that under the concentration of 10% only induce cell proliferation; however, do not have any effectivity on inflammation histology [16]. However, 5% dextrose solution increased gene expression in angiogenetic factors (platelet-derived growth factor (PDGF)-A and B, insulin-like growth factor-I, and vascular endothelial growth factor-A) and in apoptotic factors (caspase-3 and -8) in adult fibroblast culture [17]. High concentrations of glucose stimulate the PDGF activation. PDGF has two effects; first, it induces TGF-beta gene expression in mesangial cells, and second, it stimulates DNA synthesis [18]. Above the glucose concentrations of 10% make stimulus for the connective tissue growth factor and other genes expression in mesangial cells [19]. Cartilage volume stability improved by PrT injections, and this can be evaluated by magnetic resonance imaging [16].

Excessive pain and fatigue due to inflammatory reaction can occur after the PrT injections. According to this rarely, treatment can be abandoned. To reduce the pain, hypertonic dextrose commonly combined with lidocaine, sensorcaine, and xylocaine as local anesthetics [20]. The local anesthetics delay and disrupt wound healing by inhibiting collagen synthesis in fibroblast tissue [21]. However, this condition disrupts the outcome of the treatment.

2.1.1 Classification

PrT can be classified as enthesofascial, myofascial, and neurofascial according to injection location.

2.1.1.1 Enthesofascial/intra-articular PrT

Enthesofascial/intra-articular PrT is the classic and traditional method of PrT. The injection location is on to the bony cortex/enthesis where the ligaments attach to or into joints.

2.1.1.2 Myofascial PrT

Myofascial PrT is the other type of PrT. In this type, injection location is soft tissue of the bony cortex and below the subcutaneous fascia. This is used for degeneration of muscle and tendon, tears of muscle, defects of fascia. It prevents function of muscle, or fascia surrounded by neovessels or neonerves.

2.1.1.3 The neurofascial PrT

The neurofascial PrT is another type for PrT. Injection location is near to the peripheral sensory nerves and particularly their fascial penetrations. So this is performed to subcutaneous tissue. The goal of PrT is repairment or functional restoration of soft tissue, and neurofascial PrT produces the restoration of full function in small nerves. The reparative proteins and their correlation with nerve repairment are less well known. Nerves and ligament and tendon are covering with mainly collagen-based structure (i.e., perineurium). Nerves must take place in repair of soft tissue faults and that rather probably are planned to behave a similar order of growth factors. According to these reasons, dextrose is potentially therapeutic to small nerves [3]. However, this classification of neurofacial PrT is not widely accepted.

2.1.2 Indications and contraindications of PrT

Indications of PrT are chronic musculoskeletal disorders such as chronic low back pain, osteoarthritis, epicondylitis, and rotator cuff lesions.

Contraindications of PrT are hereditary or acquired bleeding tendency, osteomyelitis, systemic infection, chronic infection history or active infection in the treatment region, rheumatic or other systemic inflammatory disease, oncological diseases, having been injected local corticosteroid within 12 weeks and allergy to the solution that is using for PrT.

2.1.3 Disorders for PrT

2.1.3.1 Chronic low back pain

Chronic low back pain is a common disease in the population. It causes temporary or permanent disability [12]. The results of the studies on this subject contain contradictions. Intra-articular PrT injection is significantly superior to corticosteroid injection in sacroiliac joint pain [22]. A RCT of sclerosing injections reported that PrT has similar result as saline plus lignocaine in chronic low back pain [23]. Injections performed once a week for 3 weeks unlike to normal use. Another RCT for nonspecific chronic low back pain compared PrT injections, saline injections, and exercises. All ligament injections caused meaningful decreases in pain and disability along the follow-up. Results are similar for PrT and saline or for exercises and daily life [24]. When integrated to spinal manipulation, exercise, and other interventions, PrT may have better impact on chronic low back pain and disability [12]. Also vitamin B12 usage increases the effectiveness of the treatment [25].

2.1.3.2 Osteoarthritis

Knee osteoarthritis is an important disease with increasing rate of pain, functional disability, and stiffness. A systematic review and meta-analysis compare the effect of dextrose PrT against control injections and exercise in the treatment of osteoarthritis. Dextrose PrT is superior to exercise, local anesthetics, and corticosteroids in 6 month follow-up [26]. Similar to this, a 3-arm, blinded, RCT compared dextrose PrT, saline, and at-home exercise, and PrT is better clinical enhance of pain, function, and stiffness than saline injections and at-home exercises [27]. There are more studies showing the success of PrT in knee osteoarthritis. Injection locations are different according to researchers; a combination of extra and intra-articular injection [28, 29], and only intra-articular [30, 31]. Combination of injections is thought to be an important treatment in young people with connective tissue disorders and also in elderly patients with severe knee osteoarthritis alternative to knee prosthesis. In these studies, it is reported that it not only reduced the pain but also corrected knee mechanical instability and cartilage damage.

Corticosteroid injections are an important treatment modality in symptomatic hand osteoarthritis [32]. The short-term effectiveness is well but the long-term effect is temporary. In carpometacarpal joint osteoarthritis, corticosteroid injection is superior to PrT at 1 month follow-up. Symptoms repeated with corticosteroid injection at the end of the sixth month, but improvement continued with PrT in the long-term and recurrence was less. PrT had better results in long term than corticosteroid injections [33].

2.1.3.3 Epicondylitis

Although PrT is a promising method for the treatment of epicondylitis, there are contradictions in a limited number of studies. In a randomized double-blind study PrT and placebo injections in patients with lateral epicondylitis compared PrT and placebo injections in patients with lateral epicondylitis. PrT was found to be significantly successful in pain and function [13]. A three-arm RCT reported PrT with dextrose and PrT with dextrose and sodium morrhuate were similar successful results for pain and function than wait and see group [7]. Subsequently, a double blinded RCT compared PrT and the corticosteroid injections, and no difference was found between groups in the same indication.

2.1.3.4 Rotator cuff injuries

PrT injection to the shoulder region was first reported by Lee et al., and successful results have shown in patients with resistant to conservative treatment [34]. Similar results were obtained in RCT's [14, 35].

2.1.4 Adverse events

Adverse events change according to the localization of injections. Pain and stiffness may increase temporary, and these are the most common events. Also post-injection headache, postmenopausal spotting, pain with neurological features, nausea, and diarrhea may occur, but transiently [12].

2.2 Platelet-rich plasma

PRP is the cellular component of the plasma. It has a higher platelet concentration than whole blood [36]. Platelets are obtained by fragmentation of precursor megakaryocytes [37]. Activated platelets release clotting and growth factors in the α-granules. The main growth factors secreted by α-granules of platelets and effective in wound healing are known as PDGF, IGF-1, VEGF, TGF-β, and b-FGF [38]. Other factors such as serotonin, adenosine, dopamine, calcium, histamine, ADP, ATP, and catecholamine in the dens granules of platelets also play a role in tissue regeneration [39].

Growth factors assure the release of other growth factors, enhancing healing process in chronic injuries and quickening repair in acute lesions [38–40]. It was first used to accelerate the wound healing of cutaneous ulcers in the 1980s [41]. The potential of regeneration and curative effect of PRP in oral implantology has been demonstrated [42]. The usage of PRP has spread to other clinics [43].

Cellular components of plasma consist of 93% erythrocytes, 6% platelet, and 1% leukocytes. PRP contains platelets 3–5 times higher than whole blood. Depending on this, it contains growth factors in hyperphysiological rate [36].

There is no accepted clear platelet concentration value for PRP. However, there are studies that report the healing effect when the number of platelets up to 150,000/μl, and 350,000/μl in whole blood is above 1,000,000/μl in 5 ml plasma [42].

PRP is provided by centrifugation of autologous anticoagulant whole blood. Prior to centrifugation, citrate is added to whole blood for bounding ionized calcium and coagulation is prevented. After centrifugation, whole blood is divided into three layers according to gravity. The top layer consists of plasma, the middle layer called as "buffy coat" consists of platelets and leukocytes, and the lowest layer consists of erythrocytes [43]. A second centrifuge is applied to the buffy coat and plasma section, indicating that PRP and platelet poor plasma may lead to further separation [44, 45].

According to preparation technique and the resulting product ingredients, PRP is classified as: pure-PRP (P-PRP), leukocyte and leucocyte and PRP (L-PRP), and pure platelet-rich fibrin (P-PRF), leucocyte and platelet-rich fibrin (L-PRF). Nowadays, leukocytes can increase local inflammation, and leucocyte-poor content is shown to be superior to rich content. Centrifugation and activation methods are two important determinants of PRP quality and growth factor release. To date, there is no worldwide accepted PRP preparation protocol [45].

2.2.1 Indications and contraindications of PRP

Indications of PRP can be summarized as the acute/chronic musculoskeletal, cartilage and bone diseases such as chronic tendinopathies and enthesitis, acute/chronic ligament injuries, acute/chronic muscle tears and strains, osteoarthritis, osteochondritis dissecans, arthroplasty operations, meniscus injuries, delayed fracture healing, nonunions, intervertebral disc injuries.

PRP's being an autologous graft minimizes the risk of allergic reaction and infectious disease. The side effects are pain formation due to local inflammatory response at the injection site, scar formation, and calcifications as infection and further possibilities at the rate of risk at all injections. Patient selection should be performed carefully as there is a risk of serious allergic reaction to bowel thrombin. The contraindications of PRP are the presence of tumors and metastatic disease, active infection, thrombocytopenia, anemia, pregnancy and lactation, and bowel thrombin allergy [46].

Acetaminophen and narcotic analgesics can be administered against pain, while nonsteroidal anti-inflammatory drugs are often banned for 2–4 weeks. It is thought that nonsteroidal anti-inflammatory drugs can inhibit the prostaglandin pathway and the beneficial effects of growth factors. Furthermore, in patients who received systemic steroids or immunosuppressive drugs, steroid injections were used instead of lesions in the last 6 weeks, and PRP injections were not preferred for NSAIDs in the last 7–10 days [36].

2.2.2 Disorders for PRP

2.2.2.1 Rotator cuff injuries

The recovery process in massive chronic rotator cuff tears often results with failure. PRP injection is not more effective than saline [47]. During the arthroscopic repair of full-thickness rotator cuff tears, PRP induces reduction in the pain level at the early postoperative period, a significant increase in shoulder function tests, and shoulder external rotation muscle strength in the short term; but there is no significant difference in pain, function, and MRI results in the long-term [48]. While PRP usage did not create a difference in arthroscopic repair of full-thickness rotator cuff tears, PRP was better for improvement in the arthroscopic repair of small and medium rotator cuff tears [49].

2.2.2.2 Lateral epicondylitis

The common feature of the lateral epicondylitis studies is the standardization of patient selection. PRP treatment is performed by the patients with chronic lateral epicondylitis who did not benefit from conservative treatment. Therefore, unlike to other disorders, standardization of the patient selection seems to be provided in the lateral epicondylitis.

PRP is superior to steroid injections for reducing pain and improving function [50–52]. Steroid injections have better results in the first weeks, deterioration occurs especially after 26 weeks [50], and at the end of the second year, patients return to the baseline level [51]. PRP has a progressive improvement effect [50, 51], and this effect continues in the long term [51].

In two studies conducted by the same author applying the same diagnosis and treatment, the total number of patients can be considered as 350. PRP by using the peppering technique is applied to extensor carpi radialis brevis tendon and vicinity. Success of PRP was found more than 80% after 6 months of treatment [53].

Repeated injections are not superior to single dose administration in the treatment of chronic lateral epicondylitis [54].

2.2.2.3 Patellar and Achilles tendinopathy

PRP provides healing in pain and function even in patients with resistant patellar tendinopathy. Unlike the other injuries, 5 ml of PRP is injected into the tendon three times with an interval of 15 days [55, 56]. Even, ultrasound-guided PRP (by using peppering technique and ~2 ml/2 times/2 weeks intervals) was found to be superior from ESWT in the treatment of patellar tendinopathy [57].

While PRP treatment was shown to be significant in patellar and Achilles tendinopathy case series, it was similar as saline injection in RCTs. However, it is indicated that saline injection cannot be considered as placebo because of the mechanical effect caused by the needle and bleeding [58].

PRP injections were considered successful in the treatment of chronic refractory Achilles tendinitis [59–61].

2.2.2.4 Osteoarthritis

Intra-articular PRP and hyaluronic acid provide similar clinical improvement. The success rate was higher in the joints with low degeneration at 6 and 12 month

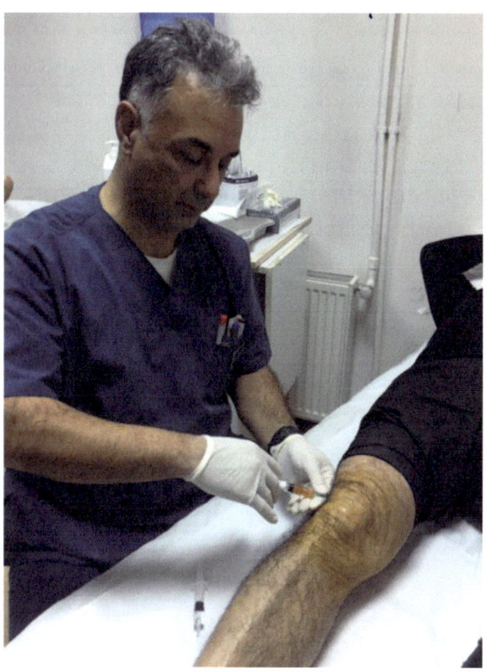

Figure 1.
Intra-articular PRP applications to the knee joint.

Application	Indications	Contraindications
PrT	Chronic musculoskeletal disorders; Chronic low back pain, Osteoarthritis, Epicondylitis, Rotator cuff lesions.	Hereditary or acquired bleeding tendency, Osteomyelitis, Systemic infection, Chronic infection history or active infection in the treatment region, Rheumatic or other systemic inflammatory disease, Oncological diseases, Having been injected local corticosteroid within 12 weeks, Allergy to the solution that is using for PrT.
PRP	Acute/chronic musculoskeletal, cartilage and bone diseases; Chronic tendinopathies and enthesitis, Acute/chronic ligament injuries, Acute/chronic muscle tears and strains, Osteoarthritis, Osteochondritis dissecans, Arthroplasty operations, Meniscus injuries, Delayed fracture healing, Nonunions, Intervertebral disc injuries	Presence of tumors and metastatic disease, Active infection, Thrombocytopenia, Anemia, Pregnancy and lactation, Bowel thrombin allergy (if it is used as an activator)

Table 1.
Indications and contraindications of PrT and PRP applications.

follow-up of PRP [62]. PRP is superior to placebo in the treatment of early stage knee osteoarthritis. Interestingly, a similar improvement is observed between single and two doses of PRP [63] (**Figure 1**).

Indications and contraindications of PrT and PRP applications are shown in **Table 1**.

3. Conclusion

It is obvious that increasing of the regenerative injection treatment types will continue progressively in the future. At the present time, PrT can be used as a simple, reliable, fast-acting treatment method in patients resistant to conservative treatment. Although PRP is used for the same diseases as PrT, it can also be used in acute cases unlike PrT. Both methods can be used with confidence in pain management. Proper patient selection is the most important issue to obtain effective results from methods.

Declaration of conflicting interests

The authors declared no conflicts of interest with respect to the authorship and/or publication of this article.

Funding

The authors received no financial support for the research and/or authorship of this article.

Author details

Ilker Solmaz[1]* and Aydan Orscelik[2]

1 Health Sciences University Gulhane Education and Research Hospital Complementary Medicine Center, Ankara, Turkey

2 Health Sciences University Gulhane Medical Faculty, Department of Sports Medicine, Ankara, Turkey

*Address all correspondence to: ilkersolmaz72@hotmail.com

References

[1] Adams ML, Arminio GJ. Non-pharmacologic pain management intervention. Clinics in Podiatric Medicine and Surgery. 2008;**25**(3):409-429. DOI: 10.1016/j.cpm.2008.02.003

[2] Sanapati J, Manchikanti L, Atluri S, Jordan S, Albers SL, Pappolla MA, et al. Do regenerative medicine therapies provide long-term relief in chronic low back pain: A systematic review and metaanalysis. Pain Physician. 2018;**21**(6):515-540

[3] Waldman SD. Pain Management. 2nd ed. Philadelphia: Saunders (Elsevier); 2011. 1027p

[4] Hackett GS, Hemwall GA, Montgomery GA. Ligaments and Tendon Relaxation Treated by Prolotherapy. 5th ed. USA: Hackett Hemwall Foundation; 2008

[5] Rabago D, Best TM, Beamsley M, Patterson J. A systematic review of prolotherapy for chronic musculoskeletal pain. Clinical Journal of Sport Medicine. 2005;**15**:376

[6] Schneider RC, Williams JJ, Liss L. Fatality after injection of sclerosing agent to precipitate fibro-osseous proliferation. Journal of the American Medical Association. 1959;**170**(15):1768-1772

[7] Rabago D, Lee KS, Ryan M, Chourasia AO, Sesto ME, Zgierska A, et al. Hypertonic dextrose and morrhuate sodium injections (prolotherapy) for lateral epicondylosis (tennis elbow): Results of a single-blind, pilot-level, randomized controlled trial. American Journal of Physical Medicine & Rehabilitation. 2013;**92**(7):587-596

[8] Louw F. The occasional prolotherapy for lateral epicondylosis (tennis elbow). Canadian Journal of Rural Medicine. 2014;**19**(1):31-33

[9] Childress MA, Beutler A. Management of chronic tendon injuries. American Family Physician. 2013;**87**(7):486-490

[10] Carayannopoulos A, Borg-Stein J, Sokolof J, Meleger A, Rosenberg D. Prolotherapy versus corticosteroid injections for the treatment of lateral epicondylosis a randomized controlled trial. PM & R : The Journal of Injury, Function, and Rehabilitation. 2011;**3**(8):706-715

[11] Yildiz Y, Apaydin AH, Seven MM, Orscelik A. The effects of prolotherapy (hypertonic dextrose) in recreational athletes with patellofemoral pain syndrome. Journal of Experimental and Integrative Medicine. 2016;**6**(2):53-56

[12] Dagenais S, Yelland MJ, Del Mar C, Schoene ML. Prolotherapy injections for chronic low-back pain. Cochrane Database of Systematic Reviews. 2007;**18**(2):CD004059

[13] Scarpone M, Rabago D, Zgierska A, Arbogest J, Snell E. The efficacy of prolotherapy for lateral epicondylosis: A pilot study. Clinical Journal of Sport Medicine. 2008;**18**(3):248-254

[14] Seven MM, Ersen O, Akpancar S, Ozkan H, Turkkan S, Yıldız Y, et al. Effectiveness of prolotherapy in the treatment of chronic rotator cuff lesions. Orthopaedics & Traumatology, Surgery & Research. 2017;**103**(3):427-433. DOI: 10.1016/j.otsr.2017.01.003

[15] Linetsky FS, Rafael M, Saberski L. Pain management with regenerative injection therapy (RIT). In: Weiner RS, editor. Pain Management: A Practical Guide for Clinicians. Washington, DC: CRC Press; 2002. pp. 381-402

[16] Jensen KT, Rabago DP, Best TM, Patterson JJ, Vanderby R. Early

inflammatory response of knee ligaments to prolotherapy in a rat model. Journal of Orthopaedic Research. 2008;**26**(6):816-823. DOI: 10.1002/jor.20600. [PubMed: 18240327]

[17] Guran S, Coban ZD, Karasimav O, et al. Dextrose solution used for prolotherapy decreases cell viability and increases gene expressions of angiogenic and apopitotic factors. Gulhane Medical Journal. 2018;**60**(2):42-46

[18] Di Paolo S, Gesualdo L, Ranieri E, Grandaliano G, Schena FP. High glucose concentration induces the overexpression of transforming growth factor-beta through the activation of a platelet-derived growth factor loop in human mesangial cells. The American Journal of Pathology. 1996;**149**(6):2095-2106

[19] Murphy M, Godson C, Cannon S, Kato S, Mackenzie HS, Martin F, et al. Suppression subtractive hybridization identifies high glucose levels as a stimulus for expression of connective tissue growth factor and other genes in human mesangial cells. The Journal of Biological Chemistry. 1999;**274**(9):5830-5834

[20] Akpancar S, Seven MM, Tuzun HY, Gurer L, Ekinci S. Current concepts of prolotherapy in orthopedic surgery. Archives of Trauma Research. 2017;**6**(2):e40447. DOI: 10.5812/atr.40447. DOI: 10.5812/atr.40447 Inpress

[21] Drucker M, Cardenas E, Arizti P, Valenzuela A, Gamboa A. Experimental studies on the effect of lidocaine on wound healing. World Journal of Surgery. 1998;**22**(4):394-397. Discussion 397-398. PubMed PMID: 9523522

[22] Kim WM, Lee HG, Jeong CW, Kim CM, Yoon MH. A randomized controlled trial of intra-articular prolotherapy versus steroid injection for sacroiliac joint pain. Journal of Alternative and Complementary Medicine. 2010;**16**(12):1285-1290

[23] Dechow E, Davies RK, Carr AJ, Thompson PW. A randomized, double-blind, placebo-controlled trial of sclerosing injections in patients with chronic low back pain. Rheumatology. 1999;**38**:1255-1259

[24] Yelland M, Glasziou P, Bogduk N, Schluter P, McKernon M. Prolotherapy injections, saline injections, and exercises for chronic low back pain: A randomized trial. Spine. 2004;**29**(1):9-16

[25] Staal JB, de Bie R, de Vet HC, Hildebrandt J, Nelemans P. Injection therapy for subacute and chronic low-back pain. Cochrane Database of Systematic Reviews. 2008;**16**(3):CD001824

[26] Hung CY, Hsiao MY, Chang KV, Han DS, Wang TG. Comparative effectiveness of dextrose prolotherapy versus control injections and exercise in the management of osteoarthritis pain: A systematic review and meta-analysis. Journal of Pain Research. 2016;**9**:847-857. eCollection 2016

[27] Rabago D, Patterson J, Mundt M, Kijowski R, Grettie J, Segal N. Dextrose prolotherapy for knee osteoarthritis: A randomized controlled trial. Annals of Family Medicine. 2013;**11**:229-237

[28] Rabago D, Zgierska A, Fortney L, Kijowski R, Mundt M, Ryan M. Hypertonic dextrose injections (prolotherapy) for knee osteoarthritis: Results of a single-arm uncontrolled study with 1-year follow-up. Journal of Alternative and Complementary Medicine. 2012;**18**:408-414

[29] Rezasoltani Z, Taheri M, Mofrad MK, Mohajerani SA. Periarticular dextrose prolotherapy instead of intra-articular injection for pain and functional improvement in knee

osteoarthritis. Journal of Pain Research. 2017;**10**:1179-1187. DOI: 10.2147/JPR. S127633. eCollection 2017

[30] Topol GA, Podesta LA, Reeves KD, Giraldo MM, Johnson LL, Grasso R, et al. Chondrogenic effect of intra-articular hypertonic-dextrose (prolotherapy) in severe knee osteoarthritis. PM & R : The Journal of Injury, Function, and Rehabilitation. 2016;**8**(11):1072-1082. DOI: 10.1016/j. pmrj.2016.03.008. Epub: April 4, 2016

[31] Reeves K, Hassanein K. Long-term effects of dextrose prolotherapy for anterior cruciate ligament laxity. Alternative Therapies in Health and Medicine. 2003;**9**:58-62

[32] Zhang Y, Niu J, Kelly-Hayes M, Chaisson CE, Aliabadi P, Felson DT. Prevalence of symptomatic hand osteoarthritis and its impact on functional status among the elderly the Framingham study. American Journal of Epidemiology. 2002;**156**(11):1021-1027

[33] Jahangiri A, Moghaddam FR, Najafi S. Hypertonic dextrose versus corticosteroid local injection for the treatment of osteoarthritis in the first carpometacarpal joint: A double-blind randomized clinical trial. Journal of Orthopaedic Science. 2014;**19**(5):737-743

[34] Lee DH, Kwack KS, Rah UW, Yoon SH. Prolotherapy for refractory rotator cuff disease: Retrospective case-control study of 1-year follow-up. Archives of Physical Medicine and Rehabilitation. 2015;**96**(11):2027-2032

[35] Bertrand H, Reeves KD, Bennett CJ, Bicknell S, Cheng AL. Dextrose prolotherapy versus control injections in painful rotator cuff tendinopathy. Archives of Physical Medicine and Rehabilitation. 2016;**97**(1):17-25

[36] Nguyen RT, Borg-Stein J, McInnis K. Applications of platelet-rich plasma in musculoskeletal and sports medicine: An evidence-based approach. PM & R : The Journal of Injury, Function, and Rehabilitation. 2011;**3**(3):226-250

[37] Ahmad Z, Howard D, Brooks RA, Wardale J, Henson FMD, Getgood A, et al. The role of platelet rich plasma in musculoskeletal science. JRSM Short Reports. 2012;**3**(6):40

[38] Sanchez M, Anitua E, Orive G, Mujika I, Andia I. Platelet-rich therapies in the treatment of orthopaedic sport injuries. Sports Medicine. 2009;**39**:345-354

[39] Foster TE, Puskas BL, Mandelbaum BR, Gerhardt MB, Rodeo SA. Platelet-rich plasma: From basic science to clinical applications. The American Journal of Sports Medicine. 2009;**37**(11):2259-2272

[40] Marx RE. Platelet-rich plasma: Evidence to support its use. Journal of Oral and Maxillofacial Surgery. 2004;**62**:489-496

[41] Margolis DJ, Kantor J, Santanna J, Strom BL, Berlin JA. Effectiveness of platelet releasate for the treatment of diabetic neuropathic foot ulcers. Diabetes Care. 2001;**24**:483-488

[42] Marx RE. Platelet-rich plasma (PRP): What is PRP and what is not PRP? Implant Dentistry. 2001;**10**(4):225-228

[43] Anitua E, Sanchez M, Orive G, Andia I. The potential impact of the preparation rich in growth factors (PRGF) in different medical fields. Biomaterials. 2007;**28**:4551-4560

[44] Mishra A, Woodall J, Vieira A. Treatment of tendon and muscle using platelet-rich plasma. Clinics in Sports Medicine. 2009;**28**(1):113-125

[45] Jain A, Bedi RK, Mittal K. Platelet-rich plasma therapy: A novel application in regenerative medicine.

Asian Journal of Transfusion Science. 2015;**9**(2):113-114

[46] Sampson S, Gerhardt M, Mandelbaum B. Platelet rich plasma injection grafts for musculoskeletal injuries: A review. Current Reviews in Musculoskeletal Medicine. 2008;**1**(3-4):165-174

[47] Kesikburun S, Tan AK, Yılmaz B, Yaşar E, Yazıcıoğlu K. Platelet-rich plasma injections in the treatment of chronic rotator cuff tendinopathy. The American Journal of Sports Medicine. 2013;**41**(11):2609-2616

[48] Randelli P, Arrigoni P, Ragone V, Aliprandi A, Cabitza P. Platelet rich plasma in arthroscopic rotator cuff repair: a prospective RCT study, 2-year follow-up. Journal of Shoulder and Elbow Surgery. 2011;**20**(4):518

[49] Cai YZ, Zhang C, Lin XJ. Efficacy of platelet-rich plasma in arthroscopic repair of full-thickness rotator cuff tears: A meta-analysis. Journal of Shoulder and Elbow Surgery. 2015;**24**(12):1852-1859

[50] Peerbooms JC, Sluimer J, Bruijn DJ, Gosens T. Positive effect of an autologous platelet concentrate in lateral epicondylitis in a double-blind randomized controlled trial: Platelet-rich plasma versus corticosteroid injection with a 1-year follow-up. The American Journal of Sports Medicine. 2010;**38**:255-262

[51] Gosens T, Peerbooms JC, van Laar W, den Oudsten BL. Ongoing positive effect of platelet-rich plasma versus corticosteroid injection in lateral epicondylitis: A double-blind randomized controlled trial with 2-year follow-up. The American Journal of Sports Medicine. 2011;**39**(6):1200-1208

[52] Yadav R, Kothari SY, Borah D. Comparison of local injection of platelet rich plasma and corticosteroids in the treatment of lateral epicondylitis of humerus. Journal of Clinical and Diagnostic Research. 2015;**9**(7):RC05-RC07

[53] Mishra AK, Skrepnik NV, Edwards SG, Jones GL, Sampson S, Vermillion DA, et al. Platelet-rich plasma significantly improves clinical outcomes in patients with chronic tenis elbow. The American Journal of Sports Medicine. 2014;**42**(2):463-471

[54] Glanzmann MC, Audige L. Platelet-rich plasma for chronic lateral epicondylitis: Is one injection sufficient? Archives of Orthopaedic and Trauma Surgery. 2015;**135**(12):1637-1645

[55] Kon E, Filardo G, Delcogliano M, Presti ML, Russo A, Bondi A, et al. Platelet-rich plasma: New clinical application: A pilot study for treatment of jumper's knee. Injury. 2009;**40**(6):598-603

[56] Filardo G, Kon E, Della Villa S, Vincentelli F, Fornasari PM, Marcacci M. Use of platelet-rich plasma for the treatment of refractory jumper's knee. International Orthopaedics. 2010;**34**(6):909-915

[57] Vetrano M, Castorina A, Vulpiani MC, Baldini R, Pavan A, Ferreti A. Platelet-rich plasma versus focused shock waves in the treatment of jumper's knee in athletes. The American Journal of Sports Medicine. 2013;**41**(4):795-803

[58] Di Matteo B, Filardo G, Kon E. Platelet-rich plasma: Evidence for the treatment of patellar and Achilles tendinopathy—A systematic review. Musculoskeletal Surgery. 2015;**99**:1-9

[59] Creaney L. Platelet-rich plasma for treatment of Achilles tendinopathy. JAMA. 2010;**303**(17):1696. Author reply: 1697-1698

[60] Paoloni J, de Vos RJ, Hamilton B, Murrell GA, Orchard J. Platelet-rich plasma treatment for ligament and tendon injuries. Clinical Journal of Sport Medicine. 2011;**21**(1):37-45

[61] Filardo G, Kon E, Di Matteo B, Di Martino A, Tesei G, Pelotti P, et al. Platelet-rich plasma injections for the treatment of refractory Achilles tendinopathy: Results at 4 years. Blood Transfusion. 2014;**12**(4):533-540

[62] Filardo G, Kon E, Di Matteo B, Merli ML, Cenacchi A, Fornasari PM, et al. Platelet-rich plasma vs hyaluronic acid to treat knee degenerative pathology: Study design and preliminary results of a randomized controlled trial. BMC Musculoskeletal Disorders. 2012;**13**:229

[63] Patel S, Dhillon MS, Aggarwal S, Marwaha N, Jain A. Treatment with platelet-rich plasma is more effective than placebo for knee osteoarthritis: A prospective, double-blind, randomized trial. The American Journal of Sports Medicine. 2013;**41**(2):354-364

Section 3

Cancer Pain

Chapter 7

Cancer Pain

Arūnas Ščiupokas, Liuda Brogienė and Dalia Skorupskienė

Abstract

In 1986, the World Health Organization (WHO) has published a document entitled "A Declaration of the Rights of Patients with Chronic Cancer," which says that according to the WHO, three-step analgesic ladder pain relief should be adequate for 70–90% of patients. However, despite increased attention on assessment and management, pain continues to be a prevalent symptom for patients with cancer. That is why refreshment of knowledge in cancer pain is necessary for every active practitioner. Broad overview of current understanding in cancer pain is presented in the chapter. Cancer pain syndromes are analyzed in between acute or chronic, and in among various causes occurred. Cancer pain assessment was presented with challenges meeting clinical practitioners. For cancer pain treatment, principles of multimodal approach are used. The pharmaceutical treatment presented in detail included rational use of opioids. Big attention is paid on palliative care of cancer pain patients and hospice-based palliative care model is presented too. New technologies of breakthrough cancer pain management are disclosed in detail including special questionnaire for patients. Cancer survivors' pain treatment and general practitioner's role among cancer pain problems are new topics presented in the chapter.

Keywords: cancer pain syndromes, assessment and treatment principles, multimodal approach, basic and breakthrough cancer pains, palliative care

1. Introduction

Cancer is diagnosed for more than 10 million people worldwide each year, and the illness of a malignant tumor is often associated with pain. The consequences of unrelieved cancer pain are devastating [1]. During the established diagnosis of cancer, the pain is present for 40% of tumor patients. The number increases up to 75–80% with the disease spread. About 4 million people in the world each day suffer from pain that comes due to oncological diseases, meaning that almost half of them do not receive proper treatment, and one-third live in severe or unbearable pain [2].

Despite increased attention on assessment and management, pain continues to be a prevalent symptom in patients with cancer. With reference to types of cancer, lower pain prevalence rates were demonstrated in prostate cancer compared to head and neck, lung, and breast cancer. Higher prevalence rates were seen in studies from Asia compared to Europe, in studies that used point or week prevalence rates compared to recall periods of a month or year [3].

Over the past few decades, we succeeded a better understanding of mechanisms underlying cancer pain, new developments achieved in pharmacologic cancer pain management, and increase in global opioid consumption becoming evident. Nevertheless, one-third of the patients worldwide still did not receive pain medication proportional to their pain intensity levels [4]. Data from Asia and North America revealed comparable prevalence rates, which imply that opioid availability alone is not an explanation for the high prevalence rates [3]. Even after implementation into clinical practice of rapid release opioids (ROOs), which provide faster relief than immediate-release preparations of other opioids, the prevalence of breakthrough pain is still 59% [5]. All these mean the importance of skilled use of opioid analgesics in the relief of cancer pain but also acknowledge the lack of evidence to support clinical practice and guidelines, which in turn causes recommendations in practice guidelines to be based on expert consensus.

In 1986, the World Health Organization (WHO) has published a document entitled "A Declaration of the Rights of Patients with Chronic Cancer." According to the WHO three-step analgesic ladder, in combination with appropriate dosage guidelines, pain relief should be adequate for 70–90% of patients. A systematic review on pain relief based on the WHO ladder, 20 years after its introduction, demonstrated adequate pain relief in 45–100% of patients [6, 7]. Among subjects of debates to improve the analgesic ladder the benefit of paracetamol (acetaminophen) with Step III opioids for which the evidence is "weak if any," as well as the use of adjuvant analgesics for which outcomes are generally modest [8]. On the other hand, not only drugs are a guarantee of success in the cancer pain. It is widely accepted that a biopsychosocial approach in assessment and management is needed for treatment of pain in patients with cancer. Cicely Saunders elaborated on the concept of "total pain," stating that pain is not purely a physical experience but involves various other components of human functioning including personality, mood, behavior, and social relations. A systematic review has identified an association between psychological distress, lack of social support, and cancer pain [9].

Different barriers have been acknowledged in relation to adequate pain management in patients with cancer. One of the most important reasons is lack of knowledge regarding the assessment and management of cancer pain. Health professionals are cautious when prescribing opioids because of fear of adverse effects, tolerance, and addiction. Otherwise, patients struggle with misconceptions about analgesic use, concerns about pain communication, and a belief that pain is inevitable and uncontrollable [10]. All reasons for the lack of adequate pain control are varied: (a) personal—fear of drug addiction, (b) legal issues by issuing a higher dose of these medicines, (c) material—with regard to the price and quantity of medicinal products, (d) organizational—regular supply and storage of medicines, (e) psychological—the conviction of the patient or his family members that narcotic analgesics can be used only in the last stages of the illness, (f) causes of medical staff in the absence of sufficient knowledge of analgesia and the principles for its administration, and (g) poor adherence to pain medication and poor pain relief, which appear to be more country-specific problems [11].

2. Cancer pain syndromes

Pain is an unpleasant sensory and emotional experience associated with actual or potential tissue damage, or described in terms of such damage. Pain is always subjective [the International Association for the Study of Pain (IASP)]. Cancer-induced pain may be acute or chronic. Cancer-induced pain may be nociceptive or neuropathic or psychogenic, but often it is mixed because there are several causes causing it to occur. The main (basic) is constant pain of controlled intensity. A breakthrough pain occurs when a basic pain is controlled. Breakthrough pain is a temporary exacerbation with high intensity pain, which is felt in patients whose basic pain was adequately treated with opioids [12].

Cancer pain is not a single entity. It incorporates a range of etiological, pathophysiological, and anatomical subtypes, all requiring unique descriptive terminology, assessment techniques, and treatment modalities [13]. Among patients with cancer, there is substantial heterogeneity in how pain is experienced and in how it appears. In many cases, the constellation of symptoms and signs can suggest a specific cancer pain syndrome [14]. The identification of such a syndrome may help to elucidate the etiology of the pain, direct the diagnostic evaluation, clarify the prognosis for the pain or the disease itself, and guide therapeutic intervention.

2.1 Acute pain syndromes

Most acute cancer pain syndromes are primary as related to a diagnostic test or treatment. However, some are secondary as they are disease related, such as pain due to acute hemorrhage into a tumor, bone pain from a pathologic fracture, etc. Although some tumor-related pains have an acute onset (as after pathological fracture), most of these will persist unless effective treatment for the underlying lesion is provided. Generally, acute cancer pain syndromes are divided: (1) directly related to cancer, (2) cancer diagnostics related, and (3) associated with antineoplastic treatments.

A clinical picture of directly related to various cancer syndromes depends on cancer's etiology, location, surrounding tissues involved, growing speed, and other factors. Cancer-diagnostic-related syndromes also have miscellaneous presentation and can be presented as: (a) headache after lumbar puncture, (b) prostate pain after biopsy, (c) breast pain after mammography; (d) pain after any other intervention, and some others. Acute pain associated with antineoplastic treatments can be presented as: (a) pain related to chemotherapy and (b) pain after radiotherapy [15].

Related to chemotherapy pain has various causes depending on an agent used, a method of inclusion into organism, etc. Most typical are intravenous infusion pain (due to venous spasm, chemical phlebitis, vesicant extravasation, and anthracycline-associated flare), intraperitoneal chemotherapy pain (chemical serositis or infection), mucositis (due to cytotoxicity of cytarabine, doxorubicin, methotrexate, and others), painful peripheral neuropathy (toxicity associated with vinca alkaloids, cisplatinum, oxaliplatin, and paclitaxel), headache (after intrathecal methotrexate), myalgias/arthralgias interferon induced, and others. Pain after radiotherapy can be incident pain precipitated by transport and positioning of the patient for radiotherapy, or it can be caused by acute radiation toxicity. Most typical are: oropharyngeal mucositis, early-onset brachial plexopathy, subacute radiation myelopathy, radiation enteritis and proctitis, and others. Some more acute cancer pain syndromes can be related to infection (herpes zoster) or venous thrombotic events.

2.2 Chronic pain syndromes

Chronic cancer pain syndromes usually are directly related to the neoplasm itself or to an antineoplastic therapy. The classification is presented in **Table 1** [16].

Bone metastases are the most common cause of chronic pain in cancer patients. Bone pain should be differentiated from non-neoplastic causes including osteoporotic fractures (such as associated with multiple myeloma), focal osteonecrosis (due to chemotherapy or corticosteroids, or radiotherapy), and osteomalacia. Vertebrae are the most common sites of bony metastases pain. Typical locations are atlantoaxial destruction and odontoid fracture, C7–T1 syndrome, and T12–L1 (thoracolumbar junction) syndrome. Epidural compression of the spinal cord or cauda equina is a common neurologic complication

Chronic cancer pain syndromes	Clinical presentation
Tumor-related somatic pain syndromes	Multifocal bone pain
	Soft tissue pain
Tumor-related visceral pain syndromes	
Tumor-related neuropathic pain	Leptomeningeal metastases
	Cranial neuralgias
	Radiculopathies
	Plexopathies
	Peripheral mononeuropathies
	Paraneoplastic syndromes
Headache	
Pain related to antineoplastic treatments	Chemotherapy-related neuropathy
	Bone complications and glucocorticoids
	Antiandrogens and gynecomastia
Postsurgical pain syndromes	Pain and phantom sensation after amputation
Postradiation pain syndromes	Plexopathies
	Myelopathy
	GI tract disorders
	Lymphedema
	Osteonecrosis

Table 1.
The classification of cancer chronic pain syndromes.

of cancer. Breast, lung, and prostate cancers each account for 20–25% of events [17]. And back pain is the initial symptom in almost all patients with epidural compression. The pelvis and hip are also common sites of metastatic involvement. Lesions may involve any of the three anatomic regions of the pelvis (ischiopubic, iliosacral, or periacetabular), the hip joint itself, or the proximal femur [18]. Leptomeningeal metastases, which are characterized by diffuse or multifocal involvement of the subarachnoid space by metastatic tumor, occur in 1–8% in patients with systemic cancer [19]. The most common presenting symptoms are headache, cranial nerve palsies, and radicular pain in the low back and buttocks. Gadolinium-enhanced MRI imaging of the neuroaxis is the investigation of choice when leptomeningeal metastases are suspected. Base of skull metastases can be presented with various syndromes: orbital syndrome, parasellar syndrome, middle cranial fossa syndrome, jugular foramen syndrome, trigeminal neuralgia, and others. Neuropathic pains can be presented as painful radiculopathy, postherpetic neuralgia, malignant brachial plexopathy (lymphoma, beast, lung cancers). Brachial plexopathy also is typical for radiation-induced syndromes. Radiation changes in the skin and lymphoedema are commonly associated. Malignant lumbosacral plexopathy is most frequently associated with colorectal, cervical, breast cancers, sarcoma, and lymphoma [20]. Paraneoplastic painful peripheral neuropathy can be related to injury to the dorsal root ganglion (also known as subacute sensory neuronopathy or ganglionopathy) or injury to peripheral nerves [21]. Subacute sensory neuronopathy is usually associated with small cell carcinoma of the lung. Even in the absence of involvement of the chest wall or parietal pleura, lung tumors can produce a visceral pain syndrome, being unilateral or bilateral (less common).

Most treatment-related pains are caused by tissue-damaging procedures. Chronic-treatment-related pain syndromes are associated with either a persistent nociceptive complication of an invasive treatment (such as a postsurgical abscess), or more commonly, neural injury. Toxic peripheral neuropathy, avascular (aseptic) necrosis of femoral, or humeral head are among most common treatment-related chronic cancer pain syndromes. Breast surgery pain syndromes are very prevalent, too. Chronic neuropathic pain of variable severity is common for those patients, and severity of pain is correlated positively with the number of lymph nodes removed [22] both with tumor location (upper outer quadrant of the breast).

3. Cancer pain assessment

Despite significant medical, pharmacological, and technological advances in the area of cancer pain assessment and management, up to 90% of patients with advanced cancer experience pain [23], which means careful pain assessment is essential for successful pain management. Cancer pain assessment is a complex undertaking. The evaluation begins with a thorough history of both the pain and the underlying malignancy as well as its treatment. A localization and intensity of pain have to be analyzed in detail, constantly indicating it in the diary. After initial treatment, the effect of treatment pain intensity is to be re-evaluated. Because of the potential impact of pain on quality of life, it is also essential to determine the adverse effects of pain on physical and psychosocial well-being, as well as the spiritual impact of the pain. Also, it is important to remember that cancer pain may linger after the cancer is removed (as examples, postmastectomy, postamputation, or postthoracotomy syndrome), and this may have important psychological and spiritual impact. Other factors that may influence the pain experience should be overestimated and discussed with the patient and his family.

Current recommendations advise that pain severity should be assessed on an 11-point numerical rating scale (NRS) (0–10), with more comprehensive tools including the Brief Pain Inventory (BPI) and McGill Short Form Questionnaire reserved for occasions when more detailed assessment is required [24, 25]. Newer tools including the Alberta Breakthrough Pain Assessment Tool, specifically designed for breakthrough pain, also could be used in the clinical trial setting [26].

3.1 Pain measurement scales

Numerical rating scale (NRS)—the intensity of pain is measured by asking the patient to select a number from 0 to 10 that describes the intensity of his pain: "0" means "no pain" and "10" means "unbearable pain." The numbers are arranged in one line. This method is easily understood by many patients, eliminates linguistic and cultural barriers between the investigator and patient, and is most often recommended for pain assessment. The lingual version of NRS can be easily adapted to ill patients who cannot write. In Verbal Rating Scale (VRS), patients are asked to choose the word best suited to describe their pain: no pain, mild pain, moderate pain, severe pain, and unbearable pain.

In Faces pain scale (FPS), five smileys are given, starting from a smiley face to the left (no pain) to a sad, and crying right ("unbearable pain") (**Figure 1**). The patient points out the smile that most reflects the pain. The researcher compares the chosen smile with the expression of the patient's face.

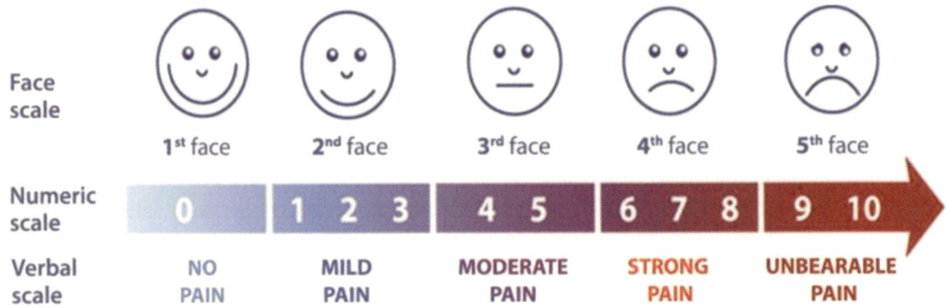

Figure 1.
Lithuanian pain scales (Decree of the Lithuanian MOH V-608, 26-08-2004 [27], English version).

These three pain scales (NRS, VRS, and FPS) are useful clinical tools to assess pain intensity if they are integrated in **Table 1**, which allows a comparative assessment of the patient's pain intensity [27].

In Visual analogue scale (VAS), patients are asked to pinpoint their pain in the 10 cm section (in the straight line) as accurately as possible. The end of the left line indicates "no pain" and the right is "unbearable pain." The method is widely used in scientific research, but not all patient groups are easy to understand.

Inferred pathophysiology or types of cancer pain (nociceptive/neuropathic) are also core in diagnostics, that is why neurological somatosensory examination using specific sensory stimuli tools (von Frey filament, brush, pin prick, hot/cold water tubes, tuning fork) is essential.

In diagnosing a breakthrough in cancer pain, first is necessary to ask the patient to describe his/her baseline pain over 24 hours, including description of location, intensity, quality, and other features. If continuous pain has fluctuations and breakthrough pain suspected, it is necessary to ask the patient how many different types of breakthrough pains the patient experiences in a 24 hour period following pain variables: location, provocation, quality, etiology, etc. Finally, asking the patient about three most bothersome breakthrough pains allows us to determine what is a breakthrough pain really wearying the patient. Breakthrough pain intensity should be rated by NPS and filled in the pain diary. It also have to be investigated in detail including such characteristics as localization, number of episodes, possible irritant, beginning of pain outbreak, strength, quality, distribution, effectiveness of the medication used. It is also important to evaluate other symptoms of the patient's pain breakthrough: psychological stress, spiritual suffering, craving for chemicals and medications, and cognitive function.

To conclude the evaluation of cancer pain, it is necessary to agree with the patient what the aim of the intended treatment is, what is the analgesia (score from...to), and what pain intensity is tolerated.

3.2 Challenges in cancer pain assessment

There are a number of significant challenges associated with the precise assessment of a cancer patients' pain [28]. They include: (1) multiple cancer pain mechanisms, patients often have multiple coexiting pain disorders even in the one cancer as the example of breast cancer, pain can be caused by surgical outcome, tumor spread, chemotherapy and bony metastases to the spine, (2) lack of a universal cancer pain classification system, (3) lack of objective testing modalities, (4) time constraints of staff that failing in continuous reassessment of pain as this is a vital sign to be fully controlled, and (5) individual differences in cancer pain sensitivity.

The National Cancer Institute (NIH, USA) has funded a Patient Reported Outcome Measurement System (PROMIS). This aims to develop a widely available set of standardized instruments to measure subjective outcomes in illnesses, including cancer [29].

4. Cancer pain treatment principles

Adequate pain relief can be achieved in 70–90% of patients when well-accepted treatment guidelines for cancer pain are followed (World Health Organization [30]). Therefore, pain management techniques should be implemented as early as possible to prevent the development of persistent pain, which can lead to a significant reduction in quality of life. Unfortunately, the availability of effective therapy and updated guidelines from reliable leading societies has not eliminated the problem of undertreatment of cancer pain [3]. The causes of undertreatment are multifactorial and reflect the combined effects of clinician-, patient-, and system-related barriers as been provided in this chapter previously (p.2, Introduction).

Methods of pain control in cancer pain can be divided into: (a) pharmacological, (b) oncological, (c) surgical, (d) interventional, (e) psychological, (f) physiotherapy, and (g) complementary.

Medications are mainstream in the treatment of cancer pain and taken on a regular basis to provide pain relief. They are mostly given by oral administration as this increases ease of use and is usually the most cost-effective solution. Other forms of pain relief medication may be required in some cases, including rectal suppositories, transdermal patches, or injections.

The WHO analgesic ladder provides a structured starting point for the pharmacological treatment of the patient with cancer pain. It is not without controversy, however, some authors questioning the need to start all patients with severe pain on the bottom rung (i.e., managing with paracetamol alone rather than proceeding directly to stronger drugs). Some also have suggested that the second step (weak opioids) should be omitted in favor of low-dose strong opioids for the sake of both clinical effectiveness and simplicity [31]. For mild to moderate cancer pain, simple analgesic medications such as paracetamol or nonsteroidal anti-inflammatory medications (e.g., ibuprofen or aspirin) can usually provide effective pain relief. Nevertheless, opioid analgesics are mainstream in treating the cancer pain as in most cases it is severe or even unbearable [32]. Some important rules must be followed before starting with the prescription with opioids. Careful assessment of the pain and its effect on function, and of the possible risks associated with use of an opioid, are the first step. When opioids are considered, providers should assess every patient for risk factors for addiction. Providers should also employ strategies to reduce the risk of misuse for all patients who are taking opioids. These strategies may include urine testing, checking state prescription drug monitoring programs to evaluate a person's history of filling prescriptions for controlled substances, doing pill counts, and using patient-provider agreements or contracts.

Long-acting opioids may be administered orally or can be given in the form of a transdermal patch. Long-acting opioids are usually started at an initial low dose and titrated upward every 2–3 days for oral formulations and 5–6 days for patches. Short-acting opioid preparations may be used to treat breakthrough pain. One-sixth of the daily opioid requirement is commonly prescribed, and is often a useful starting point. Well-documented side-effects of opioid therapy include sedation, constipation, confusion, nausea and vomiting, pruritus, urinary retention, and occasionally, respiratory depression is necessary. Chronic administration may lead to problems such as tolerance, physical dependence, and addiction. It must be noticed that by case, opioids may worsen pain—a phenomenon known as opioid-induced hyperalgesia. Management principles of side effects include: (a) opioid reduction or cessation, (b) opioid rotation, where one therapeutic opioid is substituted for an equivalent dose of another, (c) symptomatic treatment, and (d) administration of a specific antagonist.

Another group of pharmaceuticals used for the treatment of cancer pain is adjuvants (**Table 1**). Common adjuvants are antidepressants, anticonvulsant, biphosphonates, and others [33]. An adjustment of adjuvants to the treatment plan of cancer pain is typical if the pain has a neuropathic element or is wholly neuropathic. In such cases, antidepressants and anticonvulsants may be more effective in providing balanced analgesia and better tolerance than the high doses of opioids. Bisphosphonates are helpful in reducing the severity of bone pain secondary to both osteoporotic vertebral collapse and metastatic deposit. They are incorporated into the structure of mineralized bone as pyrophosphate analogues, to be then taken up by active osteoclasts, which are then inhibited. High-dose steroids can be given to reduce inflammation and edema associated with tumor growth, and to partially mitigate local mass effect. Capsular distension of intra-abdominal visceral can be very painful, and steroids may be helpful in this situation. They are also used for the immediate management of metastatic spinal cord compression and in the palliation of intracerebral lesions.

Chemotherapy, radiotherapy, endocrinotherapy, and immunotherapy are oncological methods used for cancer pain relief. Chemosensitive tumors include small-cell lung carcinoma, myeloma, colorectal, and breast cancers. These drugs are designed to target rapidly dividing cells, but can lead to the well-known side-effects of hair loss, mucositis, and diarrhea. Also, many chemotherapeutic agents are neurotoxic and cause varying degrees of temporary and permanent nerve damage, resulting in peripheral neuropathy.

Radiotherapy is particularly useful in the treatment of bony metastases and nonoperable pathological fractures, but may be used in various other contexts where the tumor type is known to be radiosensitive. Several types of radiotherapy exist: (a) localized external beam radiotherapy, (b) wide-field external beam radiotherapy, (c) brachytherapy, and (d) radioisotope treatment. Certain types of tumor may be dependent on circulating hormones to affect growth, and therefore susceptible to manipulation of the endocrine system, for example, prostate cancer. The use of immunotherapy in cancer treatment has shown to improve survival even in some advanced cancers, such as breast tumor.

Surgery can be undertaken with curative or palliative intent. If a cancerous tumor is responsible for causing the pain, techniques to reduce the size or obstruction of the tumor offer the greatest benefit. This may involve surgical removal of the tumor or shrinking of the tumor with radiation therapy. Neurosurgery to cut or block the nerves involved in the pain pathways can also help to reduce severe neuropathic pain. Bone fixation may be necessary to palliate a pathological fracture or decompress the spinal cord.

The aim of interventional cancer pain management is to interrupt nociceptive transmission at one or more points between periphery and cortex to achieve adequate analgesia. This can be achieved via reversible, nondestructive techniques for diagnostic purposes and short-term analgesia, or offer a longer-lasting solution via the physical or chemical destruction of the nervous tissue.

The diagnosis of a life-threatening illness has a huge psychological impact on patients and their families. Grief reactions, anxiety, and depression are particularly problematic at nodal points in the cancer pathway: at diagnosis, starting treatment, recurrence, failure of treatment, and facing the prospect of dying. Such psychological states exacerbate, and also are exacerbated by, uncontrolled pain, and addressing them is often of paramount importance in beginning to manage pain and improve the quality of life. Multidisciplinary input, with the use of evidence-based interventions such as cognitive behavioral therapy, distraction and relaxation techniques, graded exercise, and goal setting can be delivered with the involvement of psychologists, physiotherapists, and occupational therapists.

There are some complimentary medicinal techniques that can be used as additional complex in the treatment of cancer pain. These include: (a) acupuncture, which can help to relieve pain through the manipulation of pressure points in the body, (b) biofeedback is a technique that promotes awareness of bodily processes such as heart rate and blood pressure to influence the severity of the pain, (c) distraction techniques such as music therapy can be useful to shift attention away from the pain to a more pleasant stimulus, (d) hot or cold packs can be helpful to regulate pain and provide relief, (e) hypnosis can be used to manage pain by focusing the patient's consciousness to process pain information more effectively, and (f) relaxation exercises can be used to refocus the attention of the patient on a specific task, such as breathing, to lessen the pain.

In general, an effective strategy for cancer pain management is predicated on several broad principles [34]:

- A detailed assessment of the pain should be performed initially; careful reassessment is indicated whenever a change occurs. The initial assessment of the patient with cancer pain always includes a history and examination, and often requires imaging or laboratory tests. The approach may be conceptualized as collecting data are sufficient to characterize key elements of the pain (a specific pain syndrome, the inferred pathophysiology, the etiology of pain, etc.).

- The second principle recognizes that pain may be addressed by disease-modifying antineoplastic therapy and other interventions directed against the etiology of the pain. Treatments that address the underlying etiology of pain, such as radiation therapy, surgery, or in some cases, chemotherapy can be integrated into a broader plan of care for symptom control. Treatment of cancer-related pain usually requires close consultation with an oncology specialist, who can provide the necessary information about the availability of antineoplastic therapy.

- Whether or not primary disease-modifying therapy is possible, a large proportion of patients with pain due to active cancer require symptomatic treatment. Beginning in the early 1980s, a worldwide consensus has evolved that considers opioid-based pharmacotherapy as the mainstay approach for the symptomatic treatment of cancer patients with active disease and pain that is moderate to severe. This conclusion was originally codified in the World Health Organization's (WHO) "analgesic ladder" approach, which was originally published in the mid-1980s and has had a global influence on clinical practice and policies pertaining to medication availability.

5. WHO analgesic ladder in twenty-first century

In 1986, the World Health Organization (WHO) declared cancer pain management algorithm, so called three-step analgesic ladder (**Figure 2**) [35].

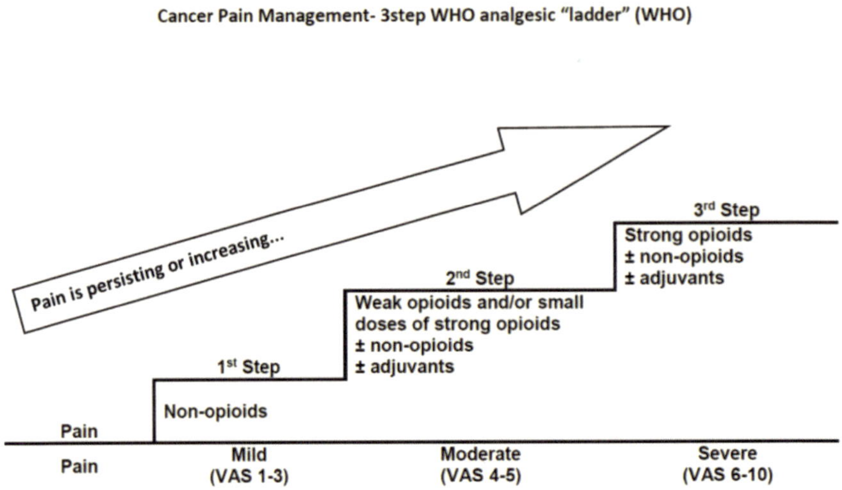

Figure 2.
Cancer pain management—three step WHO analgesic "ladder" [35].

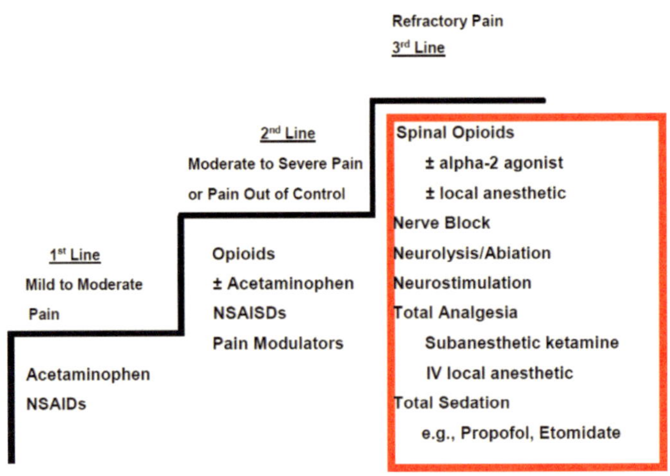

Figure 3.
Modified WHO ladder approach for cancer pain (Fine P G, 2005).

I step: main medication—aspirin, acetaminophen, and nonsteroidal anti-inflammatory drugs (NSAIDs) are used for the treatment of mild pain (score 1–3 in NAS). Nonopioids can be used as adjuvants in II and III steps analgesia.

II step: medication—weak opioids: codeine, dihydrocodeine, and tramadol are used for moderate intensity pain relief (4–6 by NAS). The upper tramadol daily (ceiling) dose is 400 mg. If oral or parental route of administration is not possible, for moderate pain treatment, one can use strong opioids in low doses, e.g., transdermal fentanyl patches.

III step: medication—strong opioids: morphine, fentanyl, methadone, and others are used for severe and intolerable cancer pain (NAS-7-10) relief [36].

Adjuvants may be administered in all steps together with main analgesics. They enhance pain relief and decrease or prevent opioids side effects. In 2000, algorithm was revised in decreasing limitations of opioid use, enabling to start treatment with strong opioids if patient is suffering from severe cancer pain. Other modifications of WHO three-step analgesic ladder were later applied (2005), introducing spinal opioids for refractory pain (see **Figure 3**).

6. Pharmaceuticals

There are two groups of medication for cancer pain management: (1) analgesics: opioids and nonopioids and (2) adjuvants.

6.1 Analgesics

Opioid analgesics are: (a) weak: tramadol, codeine (and dihydrocodeine) and (b) strong: morphine, fentanyl, methadone, buprenorphine, pethidine [37]. The route of administration are as follows: (a) noninvasive (oral, rectal, transdermal, nasal, sublingual), (b) invasive-parenteral (intramuscular, intravenous, subcutaneous, etc.), including long acting devices such as "morphine pumps "with subcutaneous or epidural catheters and PCA-patient-controlled analgesia option, allowing patient to determine and regulate the needed day and night doses of opioids. The day dose is determined by giving short-acting (immediate release) opioids, such as morphine hydrochloride 1% or morphine sulfate, 1–2% solution injections or tablets (e.g., 10 mg every 4 hours), day dose correction is made after 24–48 hours. After the needed day dosage is achieved (after 3–4 days), we switch to long-acting (slow release) (12–24 hours) morphine medication—tablets, suspension, suppositories, or fentanyl patches (72 hours) [38]. If morphine was administered parenterally, the needed daily oral or rectal dose of morphine should be three times bigger than the injected one earlier. Short-acting (immediate release) opioids should be used for breakthrough pain relief.

The use of opioid analgesics may induce [39]:

(a) tolerance—a state of adaptation in which exposure to a drug induces changes that result in diminution of one or more of the drugs' effects over time, which is while using opioid, one has to increase its dose after some time due to the decrease in analgesic effect;

(b) physiologic dependence—a state of adaptation that is manifested by a drug-class-specific withdrawal syndrome that can be produced by abrupt cessation, rapid dose reduction, decreasing blood level of the drug, and/or administration of an antagonist. It can be avoided by gradual opioid dose reduction;

(c) psychologic dependence (addiction)—a primary chronic, neurobiologic disease with genetic, psychosocial, and environmental factors influencing its development and manifestations. It is characterized by behavior that includes one or more of the following: impaired control over drug use, compulsive use, and continued use despite harm and craving (AAPM, APS, ASAM, 2001).

Adverse effects of opioids: constipation, nausea/vomiting, respiratory depression, urinary retention, pruritus, sedation, and more rarely, neurotoxic disorders-hallucinations, seizures, delirium, hyperalgesia. To evade or decrease these effects, one uses adjuvants (laxatives, antiemetics) or opioid rotation (changing one strong opioid to another and adapting the dosage).

Medication	Route of administration	Equivalent of 10 mg morphine dose
Codeine	Oral	100 mg
Tramadol	Oral/parenteral	50–100 mg/25–50 mg
Oxycodone	Oral/parenteral	5–7.5 mg/3.33–5 mg
Pethidine	Parenteral	25 mg
Methadone	Oral	5 mg*
Fentanyl	Patch	0.067 mg**
Morphine	Parenteral	3.33–5 mg

**Methadone/morphine, if morphine day dose: (a) >30 mg 1:4, (b) >100 mg 1:8, and (c) >300 mg 12:1.*
***Fentanyl/morphine, if morphine day dose: (a) 30 mg—12 mcg/hours, (b) 60 mg—25 mcg/hours, (c) 90 mg—37 mcg/hours, (d) 120 mg—50 mcg/hours, etc.*

Table 2.
Opioid equianalgesic day doses.

6.2 Opioid rotation

Opioid rotation is a change of one opioid drug to another due to acquired tolerance or unmanageable side effects. These are the rules of opioid rotation:

- additional clinical assessment of pain and its diagnostics;
- adaptation of the day dosage for the newly prescribed opioid (in 24 hours period);
- determine the equianalgesic dose of the new opioid (**Table 2**);
- decrease the determined dose of newly applied opioid by 25–50% to avoid cross-tolerance of both drugs and possible inadequacy of the dosage;
- if after applying new opioid, the pain relief is not enough and its dose is increased by 100–125%;
- titrate new drugs' dose for 24 hours until good pain control is achieved;
- evaluate side effects and drugs' effectivity; and
- pain re-assessment for every 2–3 days.

Opioid rotation is applied according to opioids equianalgesic doses table, thus changing the daily dose of the new drug [40].

In the event of opioid overdose antagonist, naloxone is applied.

The adequate pain control is achieved gradually, by dose titration and administration of various treatment options. Preliminary period of time to achieve:

- no awakening at night due to pain—2–3 days;
- no pain while not in movement (seated or lying in bed)—3–5 days;
- no pain while moving—3–7 days (not for patients with multiple vertebral and pelvic bone metastases—for them total pain control may not be achieved); and
- for patients experiencing anxiety and depression—3–4 weeks.

Nonopioids: aspirin, paracetamol, and nonsteroidal anti-inflammatory drugs (NSAIDs). They are effective in treating mild pain (score 1–3 by number analogue pain intensity scale (NAS)), due to bone metastases, soft tissue or muscular irritation, and damage. They are treating inflammation and decreasing fever and pain. NSAIDs are COX-1 and COX-2 also COX-3 inhibitors. They can be quite toxic to the GI tract (dyspepsia, erosions, ulcers, bleeding, constipation), slowing thrombocytes aggregation, impairing renal and liver function, enhancing hypervolemia, provoking rashes, headaches, dizziness, and allergic reactions. These drugs have their upper dose limit so-called "ceiling effect" when the analgesic effect cannot be increased but the adverse effects are progressing.

6.3 Adjuvant drugs

Glucocorticoids (dexamethasone, prednisolone, hydrocortisone)—indications: increased intracranial pressure, spinal cord compression, nerve compression or infiltration, bone metastases, extended liver capsule, soft tissue cancer infiltration (head and neck, abdominal, and pelvic tumors). Contraindications: no absolute contraindications, dose is limited by adverse effects, and being cautious with peptic ulcers, diabetes, cardiovascular dysfunction, and endemic situations. Adverse effects: Cushing syndrome, gastric ulcers, erosions, bleeding, increased appetite, weight, hyperglycemia, diabetes complications, muscle wasting, euphoria, dysphoria, emotional lability, depression, steroidal psychosis, edemas, hypertension, thrombosis, myopathies, decreased immunity to infections, potassium blood levels, liquid detention in the body, insomnia, skin purpura, etc.

Drugs for neuropathic pain: antidepressants, anticonvulsants, local anesthetics, and myorelaxants (baclofen).

Antidepressants—not always effective for neuropathic pain treatment and is better to prescribe tricyclic antidepressants (TCAs). Start with amitriptyline — 10–25 mg dose in the evening and then increase to 50–100 mg/day. If no effective pain relief is achieved, it is discontinued after 1 week of use. Adverse effects: somnolence and hypotension.

Anticonvulsants—for neuropathic pain—gabapentin, carbamazepine, and clonazepam. The starting dose is the same as treating epilepsy. Increase until pain relief is achieved, or unmanageable adverse effects (nausea, vomiting, somnolence, ataxia, dizziness, disorientation) occur.

Local anesthetics (lidocaine, mexiletine)—for neuropathic pain systemic treatment when other options are not working. Adverse effects: somnolence, nausea, tremor, dyspepsia (better use while eating).

NMDA receptors antagonists (ketamine)—for persistent neuropathic pain and other chronic pain when opioids are not tolerated. Routes of administration of ketamine: oral, intravenous, starting with 100 mg/day, and titration till 500 mg/day. Adverse effects: psychomimetic can be reversed by benzodiazepines and haloperidol.

According to medical literature, about 20% of women have neuropathic pain after mastectomy and about 1/3 of cancer patients suffer from neuropathic pain (or both—nociceptive and neuropathic—together).

Bisphosphonates (pamidronate, zoledronic acid)—decrease bone resorption, effective in treating cancer hypercalcemia, decrease bone pain and occurrence of pathologic bone fractures for the patients with bone metastases, inhibit activity of osteoclasts, and are useful with ineffective radiotherapy and analgesics.

Radionuclides—Stroncium 89 systemic administration effectively relieves pain due to bone metastases, better works for osteoblastic metastases, and helps about

80% of patients. The response lasts from 3 to 6 months and is evident already after 2–3 weeks. Adverse effects: myelosuppression, monitored by blood tests. Trials with radioisotopes of samarium and rhenium were also performed.

Psychotropic drugs—neuroleptics. Common neuroleptics (e.g., haloperidol) have no analgesic effect but decrease anxiety, insomnia, treat nausea, and delirium. Levopromazine has analgesic effect: 20 mg dose is equivalent to 10 mg of morphine. Adverse effects: somnolence and hypotension. Benzodiazepines (diazepam, lorazepam, oxazepam) are useful for muscle spasms or acute bone-muscular pain. Adverse effects: hypotension, somnolence, and fatigue. Psychostimulants: metilphenidate has no analgesic effect and may be used to decrease severe opioid-induced somnolence. Adverse effects: dysphoria, tolerance, and dependence.

Myorelaxants—baklofen (act on spinal cord level, start with 5 mg/day dose, and increase till 100 mg/day, for severe hiccup (hiccough)). Adverse effects: fatigue and somnolence. It should be discontinued slowly due to possible withdrawal syndrome and convulsions. Dantrolene—primary effect on muscles. Start with 25 mg/day, and continue with maximal titration till 400 mg/day. Adverse effects: fatigue, somnolence, and hepatotoxicity.

7. Invasive cancer pain management

In most patients, cancer pain can be adequately controlled with pain medication; however, in 5–14% of oncological patients', invasive pain management is needed [41]. Invasive procedures are the part of the option available for cancer pain management. Anesthetic, neurosurgical, or other invasive procedures can be given. Interventional pain management can improve pain control and reduce the amount of systemically administered drugs and their side effects. Also, invasive procedures can be an option when it is not possible to administer oral or parenteral medications. Final decision maker is a physician (anesthetist, pain specialist, and neurosurgeon) who will perform the procedure. He is main person that will decide about indications and contraindications for intervention treatment and will explain and talk with the patient or his relatives about the possibility of intervention and of course risk factors and possible complications. Invasive cancer pain procedures can be divided in to nondestructive and destructive.

Nondestructive procedures are such that the pain signal is modulated or interrupted (blocked) by the administration of a pharmacological agent to a source of pain. The pharmacological preparation may be administered by a single shot dose or via a catheter for long-term administration of the medication. Usually, the catheter is placed neuroaxially (into the spinal canal) or near the peripheral nerves or plexuses. Peripheral nerve blocks/injections can be used, but they are effective for short term and are usually performed in patients with limited survival when the pain source is one or more nerves or when the pain is caused by pathological fractures or vascular occlusion. As a first-line treatment, these blockades are rarely used and, if applicable, it is necessary to combine with systemic analgesics.

Neuraxial invasive procedures can be: intrathecal or epidural. For example, an epidural medication injection (transforaminal or translaminar) or catheter/devise placement is applied in most of the cases when the nerve structures are involved in pain cause.

In case of complicated cases and intolerable pain, opioid analgesics can also be delivered through neuraxial delivery systems. The use of neuraxial system for long term can range from simple percutaneous (tunneled) patient controlled to implantable complex programmable medication delivery systems. Implantable systems are expensive, but safe and their application is always justified, if patient need pain control longer than 3 months and other medical treatments are not effective [42, 43]. These techniques may be on an oncological pain management plan, but they do not generally apply to everyday cases.

Destructive procedures can be applied in cases where pharmacological preparations cannot modulate the pain signal. For example, in case of small cell lung cancer and mesothelioma, chest pain is poorly localized, severe, and intolerable. This is because intercostal nerves and their branches can be infiltrated in cancer cells, during metastatic spread and making it difficult to manage the source of pain. Then, the cordotomy can be applied—a neurosurgical procedure in which the spinal cord-spinothalamic tract ablation is performed in the area opposite to the pain. After the ablation pain disappears, but along with the disappearing of pain on the part of the body below, the ablation area develops temperature and paresthesia [44]. Another destructive procedure is rhizotomy, segmental or multisegmental destruction of spinal cord nerve roots. It can be done in several ways: (a) surgically, (b) chemical neurolysis (phenol), and (c) radio-frequency ablation [45, 46].

Chemical neurolysis is widely used in the treatment of intractable cancer-related pain, especially in abdominal and pelvic cancer-related pain. These procedures can provide prolonged pain relief (3–6 month) and decrease the need of opioids.

High evidence is for coeliac plexus neurolysis in pancreatic cancer-related pain [47].

Neurolytic agents that often used for chemical neurolysis are alcohol, phenol, and glycerol.

All procedures can be done under ultrasound, X-ray, or CT scan. After the procedure, patient may experience significant pain relief and opioid withdrawal symptoms [48].

8. Nonpharmacological cancer pain treatment

Palliative radiotherapy is effective for the treatment of cancer pain caused by bone and brain metastases, metastatic skin ulcerations, and infiltrative growth of tumor in soft tissues. The summary dose of palliative radiotherapy is smaller than the dose for radical radiotherapy; maximal effect is achieved giving minimal number of radiation fractions (1–5) [49].

Transcutaneous electroneurostimulation (TENS)-nerve stimulation via electrodes put on skin, thus, inhibits pain signal in spinal cord. Optimal dose varies for different patients. TENS is used for the treatment of mild and moderate cancer pain but is not effective for visceral pain. TENS is contraindicated for the patients with pacemaker (ECS). Pain relief effect is quick but usually not long-lasting (only for 15–20% of patients).

Psychotherapy-introducing patients psychological support groups, delivering enough information; relaxation therapies, meditation; cognitive therapy, autotraining, hypnosis, short psychotherapy seances with psychotherapist. Drug is administered if there is a need to correct renal, liver failure, and antidepressants for depression [50].

Acupuncture, physical therapy, mild massage can also be applied.

9. Cancer pain and palliative care

Palliative care includes palliative cancer treatment options, such as palliative radio therapy, palliative surgery, palliative chemotherapy, also pain relief and control of other symptoms caused by advanced cancer [51].

Palliative surgical procedures—palliative operations such as tumor mass reduction, stomas: colostomy, tracheostomy, gastrostomy, nephrostomy, etc., and drainage of pleural effusion and ascites.

Palliative chemotherapy is effective while treating pain, caused by chemotherapy-susceptible tumor and metastases. The main goal is to minimize its side-effects. Monotherapy of drug combination in reduced doses can be applied [52].

Most common symptoms control [53].

Anorexia is a loss of appetite, usually with decreased food intake. *Cachexia*-lack of nutrition and wasting. Causes maybe disease-related (bowel obstruction, etc.), psychological or treatment-related (intoxication due to chemotherapy, radiation esophagitis, etc.). Treatment-dietary consultation, parental/enteral nutrition, medications (e.g., megestrol acetate suspension), odor control, and counseling.

Constipation is a common symptom in palliative care. The key should be prevention. Causes can be diseases related to GI obstruction, neurologic (spinal cord compression), hypercalcemia, inactivity; or treatment related-opioids, other medication. Treatment-laxatives, other medication, increasing fluid intake, and dietary consultation.

Nausea and vomiting—common in advanced disease. Assessment of etiology is important, maybe acute, anticipatory (e.g. before chemotherapy) and delayed. Causes can be physiological (GI pathology, metabolic dysfunction, brain metastases, also-treatment related (opioids), psychological. Treatment—both pharmacological (anti-cholinergics, antihistamines, steroids, prokinetic agents, etc.) and non-drug treatment (small/slow feeding, dietary consultation, relaxation/distraction techniques).

Lymphedema—chronic, progressive swelling due to failure of lymph drainage. Patients limbs and whole body can be affected. Treatment—skin care, compression, limb elevation, education, etc. For those patients trophic ulcers and bedsores occur more often.

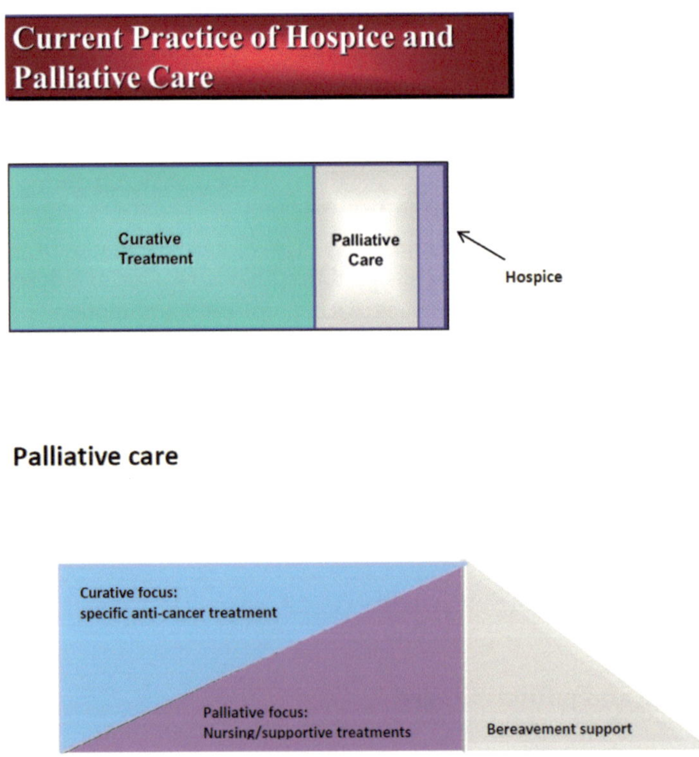

Figure 4.
Palliative care models (WHO directives, 2002) (adapted by Skorupskiene (2018)).

Advanced cancer patients at the end of life also often exhibit *delirium* (acute change in cognition/awareness) with *agitation and confusion* (disorientation, inappropriate behavior, hallucinations). The causes vary, most common-medications, infection, bladder distention, hypoxemia. As treatment option medication re-evaluation, hydration, oxygen therapy, reorientation, psychotropic drugs should be considered.

Aging population and increasing number of long time cancer survivors, some of them finally ending as advanced cancer patients, now especially increase the need of *hospice and palliative care* [54]. It should be patient-oriented, and not related to artificial prolongation of life and failure to acknowledge the limits of medicine with inappropriate use of aggressive curative treatment. Palliative care should help with all patients' problems (physical, psychological, social, spiritual), include interdisciplinary team approach (doctors, nurses, social workers, psychologists, other specialists and volunteers) and is oriented to achieve better quality of life for the patient and his/her family members. Palliative care should start for the cancer patients still receiving specific anti-cancer therapies, not waiting until all treatment options are exhausted (**Figure 4**).

General principles of palliative care:

1. patient and family as unit of care;
2. attention to physical, psychological, social, and spiritual needs;
3. interdisciplinary team approach;
4. education and support of patient and family;
5. extends across illnesses and settings; and
6. bereavement support [55].

The main idea of palliative care-no matter how much the disease is advanced, and what complex treatment has been applied, one always can do something more to improve the quality of life, still left for the patient.

10. Cancer basic pain relief

Planning pain relief for cancer pain patients one should take into the consideration possible mechanisms and types of pain (nociceptive, neuropathic, mixed), patients' wishes, former treatment. If psychological distress is present, talking about pain assessment is needed, if there is suffering, help from the clergymen may be useful. If the signs of drug addiction appear, drug release should be more controlled, physical aspects of pain relief introduced. With cognitive disorders depression and anxiety should be treated, also opioid rotation should be available.

Basic pain	Breakthrough pain
Start—slow, gradual increase in intensity	Start—acute, not predictable
Duration—no less 12 hours/day	Duration—from several seconds to 30 minutes
Type—dull, pressing, gnawing...	Type—acute, shooting, irradiating
Treatment—long acting, slow release opioids, fixed scheme	Treatment—short acting, immediate release opioids, on demand basis

Cancer pain treatment algorithm [2]:

1. assessment of pain reason, type, and intensity;
2. pharmacological pain treatment: basic pain relief, breakthrough pain relief, and adjuvants;
3. nonpharmacological treatment of pain;
4. evaluation of results and correction of treatment plan; and
5. providing constant pain relief and palliative care.

10.1 Basic cancer pain drug treatment principles

After the cause and type of cancer pain is determined, the constant analgesia is started by the easiest route, the patient-oral or transdermal, individualizing the dose, and also providing drugs for relief from other symptoms. The drug is selected taking into consideration the type and intensity of pain, WHO "analgesic ladder,", also drug combinations, but combined medications should not be used and no placebo drugs as well [56].

To prevent pain becoming chronic, cancer pain relief should be started as soon as pain appears, as it helps to reduce drugs doses, adverse effects, and achieve better drug tolerance. It also reduces the cost of pain treatment, enhances the trust between patient and doctor, and patient is socially active for a longer time. The pain relief effect should be quick, so we can start with stronger medications and later pass on the weaker ones. Different medication is used for different types of pain: (a) nociceptive pain, due to soft tissue, bone damage, and visceral pain are treated by combinations of nonopioids and opioids and (b) neuropathic pain, due to nerve compression—by opioids, glucocorticoids, when nerve is damaged—by antidepressants, anticonvulsants, and NMDA receptor antagonists [57].

11. Cancer breakthrough pain management

Breakthrough cancer pain (BTCP) is a transient exacerbation of pain that occurs either spontaneously or in relation to a specific predictable or unpredictable trigger, despite relatively stable and adequately controlled background pain [58]. The frequency is less than four times/day, if it takes more than four times/day, we need to think about lack in background cancer pain control.

Leading doctor in BTCP management should preform regular assessments and repeatedly investigate pain management after 1–4 weeks dependably on patient's complexity.

It is important to understand that the BTCP management is different compared with background cancer pain, which is managed according to the ladder and "by the clock," while for BTCP, "rescue medication" should be given as needed. Main feature is that the breakthrough cancer pain should be started when background cancer pain is well controlled (**Figure 5**) [59]. This type of pain can take about from 30 minutes but not more than 60 minutes. The highest intensity of the pain can be reached at tenth minute, and it can take 1–4 episodes/day [60]. For that reason, for BTCP should be given very strong, short-acting opioids.

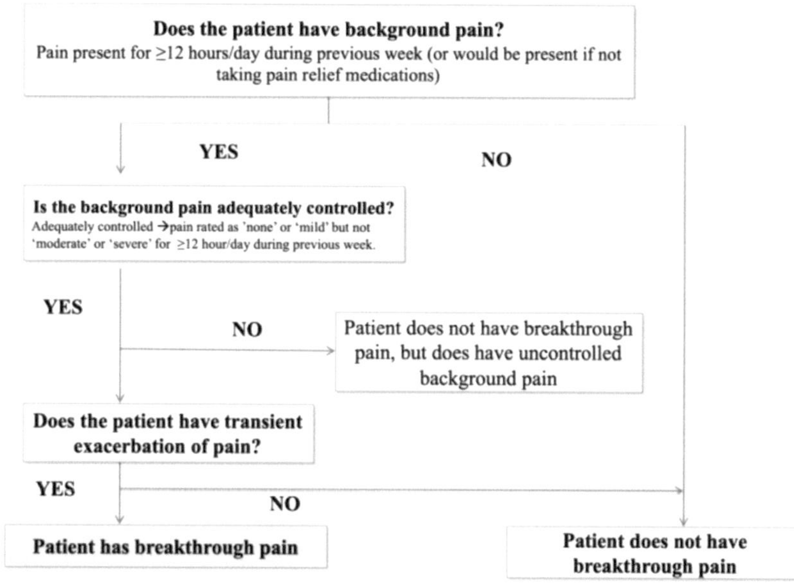

Figure 5.
Association of Palliative Medicine of Great Britain and Ireland (APM) algorithm for assessing breakthrough cancer pain.

It is better to use the same chemical opioid structure, which is chosen to manage background cancer pain.

When fentanyl plasters/patches is used, the short-acting medication (buccal or sublingual tablet) for BTCP control can be prescribed. The dose should be titrated up to effective one, because of the lipophilic structure and the absorption, which is through the mucous of the mouth and gastrointestinal tract. There is a variety of short-acting fentanyl forms (**Table 3**). For example, BTCP management can be started with 200 μg of oral transmucosal fentanyl citrate tablet or 100 μg buccal-soluble film [61].

If for BTP management, immediate-release morphine is chosen, usually one BTP episode is needed, part of 1/6 injecting medication of all morphine day dose. Their pharmacokinetic characteristics have limitations, with a relatively slow onset of action (30–45 minutes) and duration of action of up to 4–6 hours [62].

BTCP management consists of other approaches as setting of pain management goals, education of the patient, and depending on the cause of breakthrough pain, occupational therapist, physiotherapist can be involved. Other acute causes as

Formulation	Description
Nasal spray	Phosphate-buffered solution Fentanyl pectin intranasal spray
Sublingual	Sublingual fentanyl orally disintegrating tablet Sublingual fentanyl tablet
Oromucosal	Oral transmucosal fentanyl citrate
Buccal tablet	Effervescent formulation
Buccal soluble film	Fentanyl buccal soluble film

Table 3.
Fentanyl short acting formulations.

bone fractures, bowel perforation, etc. should be excluded, and if the BTCP can be predicted, pain medication should be given before the coming pain event.

The evaluation of the effectiveness of the pharmacological treatment of BTCP has a four-factor rule [63]:

1. pain relief;

2. day activity;

3. adverse effect of medications; and

4. possible inappropriate use of opioids.

Possible inappropriate use of opioids is very important factor in pain management, and it should be carefully investigated. It manifests as addiction or pseudoaddiction for strong opioids and can be associated with mental disease. Clinically, it can be seen as seeking for opioids and/or problematic opioid use. In order to correct the possible misconduct in the use of opioids, it is important that these requirements are met before they are given:

1. to distinguish between people with risk factors (drug users, alcohol dependent, gambling, having mental problems); and

2. modifying the use of drugs for the prevention of BTCP (by giving a slightly higher dose of slow-release opioid to relieve background pain, try to use nonopioids for BTCP reduction, and family support-controlled home care, etc.) [64].

12. Cancer pain treatment for children and elderly patients

While treating cancer pain in children and elder patients, one should take into consideration the differences in metabolism, concurrent diseases. Children receive different adapted opioid doses, and opioid rotation is also different (e.g., better pain relief with methadone and not morphine).

Elderly patients more easily overdose opioids; one cannot double their opioid dose quickly for them. Also, one should be aware of elder persons' liver and renal function; if there is some failure, the correction is essential before prescribing opioid medication. There are usually a lot of tablets and other oral drugs prescribed for the concurrent diseases, so there is necessary to determine daily opioid dosage very carefully.

13. Cancer survivors pain treatment

Chronic pain can be a serious, negative consequence of surviving cancer. As a result of remarkable advances in cancer diagnosis and therapy, today there are a record 14 million cancer survivors in the United States. However, an estimated 40% of survivors continue to experience persistent pain as a result of treatment, which can be detrimental to their quality of life [3]. Two-thirds of these individuals are surviving more than 5 years after diagnosis, supporting the need to study pain in this growing population [65]. National Cancer Institute's Office of Cancer Survivorship characterizes the survivor as a person with a history of cancer who is beyond the acute diagnosis and treatment phase. Risk factors for chronic pain in survivors include the type and invasiveness of the tumor, the treatment regimen used, the time since the cancer treatment has started, and the efficacy of initial pain therapy. Continuous pain is associated with impaired quality of life in this population [66]. As the population of cancer survivors expands, all clinicians, including oncologists, advanced practice providers, and primary care physicians who interact with these individuals, will require the knowledge and skills to implement best practices in the management of chronic pain. When analgesic drugs are used, the imperative to prescribe safely must expand beyond immediate adverse effects, such as the resulting respiratory depression or constipation associated with opioids, to incorporate awareness and mitigation of the long-term consequences of these and other analgesic agents.

Clinical practice guidelines are issued recently, and they deal comprehensively with the pain people experience after cancer treatment, and are unique in its focus on chronic pain among cancer survivors. Key guideline recommendations include: (1) clinicians should screen for pain at each encounter with a patient. Recurrent disease, second malignancy, or late onset treatment effects should be evaluated, treated, and monitored; (2) clinicians may prescribe nonpharmacologic interventions such as physical medicine and rehabilitation, integrative therapies (e.g., acupuncture and massage), interventional therapies, and psychological approaches (e.g., guided imagery, hypnosis, and meditation); (3) systemic nonopioid analgesics (NSAIDS, acetaminophen) and adjuvant analgesics (selected antidepressants and anticonvulsants), may be prescribed to relieve chronic pain and/or improve physical function; (4) clinicians may prescribe a trial of opioids in carefully selected cancer patients who do not respond to more conservative pain management and who continue to experience pain-related distress or impairment of physical function [67]. The management of cancer survivors suffering chronic pain requires greater consideration of a multimodality plan of care that balances pharmacologic and nonpharmacologic techniques and may necessitate the involvement of an interdisciplinary team; the goals of treatment in these populations may focus on improving function and limiting the long-term adverse effects of pain and of its treatment, as much or more as they do on improving comfort [68].

As therapeutic treatment options and outcomes improve, patients with cancer are living longer. Chronic pain can develop from a variety of sources: peripheral neuropathy, muscle or bone pain, surgery, radiation, and other conditions. Comorbidity with other conditions or syndromes can make assessing chronic pain more difficult. Different chronic pain syndromes may be present for cancer survivors. Chronic inflammatory polyneuropathy is one of many well-recognized pain disorders, together with other treatment-related pain syndromes, such as postsurgical and postradiation pain. Hormonal therapies, such as aromatase inhibitors, can produce arthralgias. As the use of hematopoietic stem-cell transplantation expands, graft-versus-host disease (GVHD) is seen with greater frequency, leading to pain syndromes that can affect almost any organ system. In addition, immunosuppressive agents used to treat GVHD can lead to painful complications (e.g., corticosteroids and avascular necrosis). The recent validation of a tool specific to musculoskeletal symptoms in hematopoietic stem cell transplantation will allow better characterization of this painful phenomenon [69–71]. The important consideration when designing an usage of analgesics is the potential for harm, and drug-drug interactions with cancer therapies, or other treatments should be considered. Cytochrome P450 CYP 3A and CYP2D6 inhibitors can increase concentrations of opioids, such as codeine, oxycodone, hydrocodone, fentanyl, tramadol, and methadone, metabolized by this system [72, 73]. Methadone and buprenorphine can prolong the QT interval, an effect that can be potentiated by many chemotherapeutic agents, notably doxorubicin [74]. If pain is severe and disabling, and long-term opioid therapy is being considered, the potential for opioid-related harm over time must also be evaluated. Persistent adverse effects such as constipation are well recognized, and risk of sleep-disordered breathing suggests that these conditions must be considered when opioid therapy is initiated and later during the course of treatment. The potential for neurotoxicities, such as persistent mental clouding, increased risk of falls in the elderly, and other phenomena may occur. Opioid-induced hyperalgesia is well described in preclinical models but has uncertain clinical importance; the potential is considered when a patient reports escalating pain in tandem with opioid dose escalation in the absence of identifiable worsening of a pain cause. Opioid-related harm may also result from misuse or abuse, the development of opioid addiction, or the occurrence of drug diversion within the community. The problem of prescription drug abuse is serious, leading to an increase in opioid-related deaths [75]. The treatment of patients with additional chronic conditions, a situation in which the patient may have two or more such conditions, referred to as multiple chronic conditions, is challenging. Insomnia and psychological distress are common conditions in patients with chronic pain, present in 17–90% of adult sufferers, respectively. The most common psychiatric disorders comorbid with chronic pain include depression, anxiety, personality disorders, and PTSD [76]. Evidence also suggests that patients with comorbid conditions are less likely to improve with standard chronic pain treatment [77].

Because cancer posttreatment pain is so complicated; good communication between patients and their medical providers is essential. Cancer survivors may have varying capacities to deal with a great source of information that can sometimes be overwhelming. Some patients may even be reluctant to discuss their pain, seeing it as a sign of weakness or fearing a recurrence; some may see it as an expected and untreatable complication of their cancer treatment. That is why a pain assessment is recommended at every visit. In teasing out how they are coping, clinicians need to ask patients how chronic pain is affecting them and suggest how they can work together to better manage their symptoms and improve their quality of life. The question arises regarding who should provide pain management for the cancer survivor: the oncologist and his or her team, the patient's primary care provider, a multidisciplinary pain service, or any other professional? Oncology teams providing ongoing care for cancer survivors may be the optimal group to address pain, because they routinely manage a complex regimen of cancer therapies and related symptoms.

Comprehensive assessment, including the impact of pain on function and quality of life, is warranted for all survivors. Long-term assessment is also needed after clinical trials to better recognize novel or previously unrecognized painful consequences of treatment, including those syndromes that may occur after treatment is completed. Carefully designed, extended studies of pharmacologic and nonpharmacologic interventions to relieve pain and improve function are indicated in this population. An especially relevant and urgent need is research identifying those cancer survivors who respond optimally to opioid therapy and those at greatest risk of adverse effects.

14. General practitioner's role

Cancer care generally requires the technical knowledge and skills of specialty physicians such as medical oncologists, surgeons, and radiation oncologists. General practitioners (GP) may play an essential role because they are often the initial point of contact for patients in obtaining screening or evaluating symptoms, and they may make referrals, coordinate care, and manage symptoms or comorbid conditions. One of the main role for GP also is counseling cancer patients about treatment options and monitoring treatment progress and side effects [78].

The roles of GP's for patients with cancer such as managing comorbid conditions, chronic pain, or depression, and referring patients to hospice were tested in the study and showed that 22% of GPs reported no direct involvement in cancer care roles, while 19% reported heavy involvement, and rural practice location was not associated with greater GP involvement in cancer care [79]. There is a gradual move toward shared care models with GPs playing a central role alongside other healthcare providers. In this context, it will be important to understand the factors influencing the involvement of GPs in cancer care and how to maximize their involvement throughout the spectrum of cancer care [80]. The studies also confirm that the great majority of GPs are familiar with the modern management of pain control problems commonly encountered in practice, but are less aware of the drug options available for less common situations, particularly the use of syringe drivers [81]. Fortunately, there is no evidence of a reluctance to start strong opioids for severe pain, as identified in previous works [82]. However, it is of concern that only minority of GPs still are suggesting immediate-release opioids for breakthrough pain, and laxatives or antiemetics when starting strong opioids, which is a recommended practice in community palliative care [83].

Most common mistakes in the treatment of cancer pain are as following:

- monotherapy (NSAIDs or opioid analgesics only);
- a prescription of slow release(SR)-form opioids for intake regime "as needed";
- improper treatment of side effects caused by medicines;
- medicine for breakthrough pain is added in the situation where basic pain is not controlled sufficiently;
- pain breakthrough is not treated at all;
- adjuvants (antidepressants, anticonvulsants) and related medicine are not used; and
- with the prescription of opioids, behavioral aspects of patients are not evaluated.

A general practitioner, who has diagnosed pain in a cancer patient, starts treatment with analgesics. A ladder analgesia scheme is used. Opioids may even be prescribed for moderate pain, and if the pain is severe and unbearable, the opioid analgesic is the main remedy for pain relief. A sufficient daily dose for baseline (basic) analgesia should be achieved by increasing the dose (titration) of the product [84]. When titrating the product, the following rules should be used: (a) pain is controlled and there are no side effects—treatment to continue the current dose, (b) pain is controlled, but there are side effects—reduce the dose of the product, (c) pain is uncontrolled and there are no side effects—increase the dose of the preparation, and (d) pain is uncontrolled, in case of side effects, change the medicine [85].

It goes without saying that controlling such a complex syndrome as cancer pain can lead to other problems that require the help and advice of the pain physician. Therefore, GP should refer the cancer patient to a pain clinic for a clear indication of the following cases (indications):

- when initiating opioid analgesics, basic pain control is not achieved and there is an unadjusted side effect of the drug;
- failure to achieve control over cancer breakthrough pain in cases where basic pain is well controlled;
- the control of basic pain by an opioid analgesic becomes ineffective, a tolerance to the preparation is suspected, and it needs to be changed to another opioid analgesic (opioid rotation);
- pain must be controlled by combining the pharmaceutical treatment and invasive procedures (patient controlled analgesia, pain relief block);
- inappropriate behavior with opioid analgesics is identified or developing of psychological dependence on them is suspected;
- repeated multidisciplinary pain assessment and specialized control (specialists' meeting) is necessary; and
- if a cancer patient is given a palliative care nursing home or nursing home and cannot physically access the pain clinic, according to the above indications, the pain clinic staff can consult on arrival at the place of destination.

15. Conclusion

Following the International Association for the Study of Pain cancer pain is "unpleasant sensory and emotional experience associate with actual or potential tissue damage resulting either from the treatment of cancer or the cancer itself." Due to the complexity of symptoms and multimodality of treatments, cancer pain is built in the most sophisticated field of medicine, where each patient's stage of disease and diagnosis will require an individualized pain treatment plan to optimize the quality of life. Such tasks can only be carried out using multidisciplinary approach. That is why basic knowledge about cancer pain is essential for every healthcare professional. We believe that the text you have just read will help you to be an active practitioner giving the patients the cancer pain relief.

Acknowledgements

The authors acknowledge Lithuanian Pain Society for text support.

Notes

Materials from "Cancer induced pain,"(Lithuanian Pain Society's guidelines) 2nd ed., 2018, are used in the text.

DOI: http://dx.doi.org/10.5772/intechopen.84452

Author details

Arūnas Ščiupokas[1,2]*, Liuda Brogienė[1,3] and Dalia Skorupskienė[4]

1 Pain Clinic, Lithuanian University of Health Sciences Hospital Kauno Klinikos, Kaunas, Lithuania

2 Department of Neurology, Lithuanian University of Health Sciences, Kaunas, Lithuania

3 Department of Anesthesiology, Lithuanian University of Health Sciences, Kaunas, Lithuania

4 Department of Oncology, Lithuanian University of Health Sciences, Kaunas, Lithuania

*Address all correspondence to: arunas.sciupokas@lsmuni.lt

References

[1] IASP. 2008-2009 Global Year Against Cancer Pain. 2008. Available from: https://www.iasp-pain.org/GlobalYear/CancerPain [Accessed: November 25, 2018]

[2] Portenoy RK, Conn M. Cancer pain syndromes. In: Bruerra E, Portenoy RK, editors. Cancer Pain: Assessment and Management. Cambridge University Press; 2003. pp. 89-108

[3] van den Beuken-van Everdingen MH, Hochstenbach LM, Joosten EA, et al. Update on prevalence of pain in patients with cancer: Systematic review and meta-analysis. Journal of Pain and Symptom Management. 2016;**51**:1070-1090

[4] Greco MT, Roberto A, Corli O, et al. Quality of cancer pain management: An update of a systematic review of under-treatment of patients with cancer. Journal of Clinical Oncology. 2014;**32**:4149-4154

[5] Deandrea S, Corli O, Consonni D, et al. Prevalence of breakthrough cancer pain: A systematic review and a pooled analysis of published literature. Journal of Pain and Symptom Management. 2014;**47**:57-76

[6] Felleiter P, Gustorff B, Lierz P, Hornykewycz S, Kress HG. Use of the World Health Organization guidelines on cancer pain relief before referral to a specialized pain service. Schmerz. 2005;**19**:265-271

[7] Azevedo Sao Leao Ferreira K, Kimura M, Jacobsen Teixeira M. The WHO analgesic ladder for cancer pain control, twenty years of use. How much pain relief does one get from using it? Support Care Cancer. 2006;**14**:1086-1093

[8] Nabal M, Librada S, Redondo MJ, et al. The role of paracetamol and nonsteroidal anti-inflammatory drugs in addition to WHO step III opioids in the control of pain in advanced cancer. A systematic review of the literature. Palliative Medicine. 2012;**26**:305-312

[9] Clark D. 'Total pain', disciplinary power and the body in the work of Cicely Saunders, 1958-1967. Social Science & Medicine. 1999;**49**:727-736

[10] Jacobsen R, Moldrup C, Christrup L, Sjogren P. Patient related barriers to cancer pain management: A systematic exploratory review. Scandinavian Journal of Caring Sciences. 2009;**23**:190-208

[11] Jacobsen et al. Barriers to Cancer pain Management in Danish and Lithuanian patients treated in pain and palliative care units. Pain Management Nursing. 2014;**15**(1):51-58

[12] Davies AN, Dickman A, Reid C, Stevens AM, Zeppetalla G, et al. The management of cancer–related breakthrough pain: Recommendations of task group of the science Committee of the Association for palliative medicine of Great Britain and Ireland. European Journal of Pain. 2009;**13**:331-338

[13] Hjermstad M, Fainsinger R, Kaasa S, European Palliative Care Research Collaborative (EPCRC). Assessment and classification of cancer pain. Current Opinion in Supportive and Palliative Care. 2009;**3**(1):24-30

[14] Foley KM. Acute and Chronic Cancer Pain Syndromes: Oxford Textbook of Palliative Medicine. 3rd ed. New York: Oxford University Press; 2004. p. 298

[15] Cherny N, Fallon M, Kaasa S, Portenoy RK, and Currow DC (Eds). Cancer Pain Syndromes: Overview: Oxford Textbook of Palliative

Medicine 5th ed. Printed From Oxford Medicine Online. Available from: www.oxfordmedicine.com [Accessed: December 5, 2018]

[16] Portenoy RK, Dhingra LK. Overview of Cancer Pain Syndromes. Available from: https://www.uptodate.com/contents/overview-of-cancer-pain-syndromes#H3 [Accessed: December 5, 2018]

[17] Loblaw DA, Laperriere NJ, Mackillop WJ. A population-based study of malignant spinal cord compression in Ontario. Clinical Oncology. 2003;**15**:211-217

[18] Panayiotis J et al. Evaluation and treatment of pelvic metastases. Injury. 2007;**38**(4):509-520

[19] Taillibert S et al. Palliative care in patients with brain metastases. Current Opinion in Oncology. 2005;**17**(6):588-592

[20] Jaeckle KA. Neurologic manifestations of neoplastic and radiation-induced plexopathies. Seminars in Neurology. 2010;**30**:254-262 [PubMed]

[21] Oki Y, Koike H, Iijima M, Mori K, Hattori N, Katsuno M, et al. Ataxic vs painful form of paraneoplastic neuropathy. Neurology. 2007;**69**: 564-572 [PubMed]

[22] Hack et al. Predictors of arm morbidity following breast cancer surgery. Psycho-Oncology. 2010;**19**(11):1205-1212

[23] Van den Beuken-van Everdingen MH, de Rijke JM, Kessels AG, Schouten HC, van Kleef M, Patijn J. Prevalence of pain in patients with cancer: A systematic review of the past 40 years. Annals of Oncology. 2007;**18**(9):1437-1449

[24] Daut RL, Cleeland CS, Flanery RC. Development of the Wisconsin brief pain questionnaire to assess pain in cancer and other diseases. Pain. 1983;**17**(2):197-210

[25] Melzack R. The short-form McGill Pain Questionnaire. Pain. 1987;**30**(2):191-197

[26] Hagen NA, Stiles C, Nekolaichuk C, Biondo P, Carlson LE, Fisher K, et al. The Alberta breakthrough pain assessment tool for cancer patients: A validation study using a Delphi process and patient think-aloud interviews. Journal of Pain and Symptom Management. 2008;**35**(2):136-152

[27] MOH LR Decree N. V–608. Valstybės žinios, 2004-09-02, Nr. 134-4882 (in Lithuanian)

[28] Stewart J. The challenges of Cancer pain assessment. The Ulster Medical Journal. 2014;**83**(1):44-46

[29] Garcia SF, Cella D, Clauser SB, Flynn KE, Lad T, Lai J, et al. Standardizing patient-reported outcomes assessment in cancer clinical trials: A patient-reported outcomes measurement information system initiative. Journal of Clinical Oncology. 2007;**25**(32):5106-5112

[30] Cancer Pain Relief. 2nd ed. Geneva: World Health Organization; 1996

[31] Oxberry SG, Simpson K Pharmacotherapy for cancer pain. Continuing Education in Anesthesia, Critical Care and Pain. 2005;**5**:203-206

[32] Mercadante S. Pharmacological management of cancer pain. In: Mogil J, editor. Pain 2010: An Updated Review. Seattle: IASP Press; 2010. pp. 37-41

[33] Fallon M, Hanks G, Cherny N. ABC of palliative care: Principles of control of cancer pain. British Medical Journal. 2006;**332**:1022-1024

[34] Portenoy RK, Mehta Z, Ahmed E. Cancer Pain Management: General Principles and Risk Management for

Patients Receiving Opioids. Available from: https://www.uptodate.com/contents/cancer-pain-management-general-principles-and-risk-management-for-patients-receiving-opioids [Accessed: December 1, 2018]

[35] World Health Organization. Traitement de la Douleur cancéreuse. Geneva, Switz: World Health Organization; 1987

[36] Davies AN et al. Dose titration to individualize treatment. European Journal of Pain. 2009;**13**:331-338

[37] Forbes K, editor. Opioids in Cancer Pain. In: Oxford Pain Management Library. Oxford University Press; 2007

[38] Quigley C, Ross J, and Riley J. Clinical pharmacology of opioids: Opioids switching and genetic basis for variability in opioid sensitivity. In: Sykes N, Bennett MI, Yuan C-S, editors. Clinical Pain Management: Cancer Pain, 2nd edition. Published by Hodder Arnold, 2008. p. 168-178

[39] Justins DM. Pain and Palliative Care in Cancer Patients. In: Justins DM, editor. Pain 2005—An updated review// Refresher Course Syllabus. Sydney, Australia: International Association for the Study of Pain/IASP Press; 2005

[40] Kishner S, Schraga ED. Opioid Equivalents and Conversions. Available from: https://emedicine.medscape.com/article/2138678–overview [Accessed: January 9, 2018]

[41] Zech DF, Grond S, Lynch J, Hertel D, Lehmann KA. Validation of World Health Organization guidelines for cancer pain relief: A 10-year prospective study. Pain. 1995;**63**(1):65-76

[42] Day R. The use of epidural and intrathecal analgesia in palliative care. International Journal of Palliative Nursing. 2001;**7**(8):369-374

[43] Smith TJ, Coyne PJ, Staats PS, Deer T, Stearns LJ, Rauck RL, et al. An implantable drug delivery system (IDDS) for refractory cancer pain provides sustained pain control, less drug-related toxicity, and possibly better survival compared with comprehensive medical management (CMM). Annals of Oncology. 2005;**16**:825-833

[44] Viswanathan A, Bruera E. Cordotomy for treatment of cancer-related pain: Patient selection and intervention timing. Neurosurgical Focus. 2013;**35**(3):E6

[45] Shah DR, Green S, Elliot A, et al. Current oncologic applications of radiofrequency ablation therapies. World Journal of Gastrointestinal Oncology. 2013;**5**:71-80

[46] Steel TR, Burchiel KJ. Ablative Neurosurgical Techniques in the Treatment of Chronic Pain: Overview. 1st ed. New York, NY: Thieme; 2002

[47] Puli SR, Reddy JB, Bechtold ML, et al. EUS-guided celiac plexus neurolysis for pain due to chronic pancreatitis or pancreatic cancer pain. A meta-analysis and systematic review. Digestive Diseases and Sciences. 2009;**54**:2330-2337

[48] Sharma M, Simpson KH, Bennet MI, Gupta S. Oxford specialist handbooks in oncology: Practical management of complex cancer pain. Oxford University Press. 2014

[49] Doyle D, Woodruff R. The IAHPC Manual of Palliative care. 3rd edition. IAHPC Press. ISBN 978-0-9834597-6-7. 2013

[50] Otis-Green S et al. Quick reference for oncology clinicians: The psychiatric and psychological dimensions of Cancer symptom management. In: Holland JC, Greenberg DB, et al., editors. American

Psychosocial Oncology Society (APOS). IPOS Press; 2006. pp. 77-85

[51] Fainsinger RL, Nekolaichuk CL. A "TNM" classification system for cancer pain: The Edmonton classification system for cancer pain (ECS-CP). Support Care Cancer. 2008;**16**:547-555

[52] ELNEC (end-of-life nursing education consortium) Core curriculum. On-line Education Course. USA: Relias Academy; 2016

[53] Symptom Relief in Terminal Illness. Geneva: World Health Organization; 1998

[54] Twycross R. Symptom Management in Advanced Cancer. 2nd ed. Oxford: Radcliffe Press; 1997

[55] Panke J, Ferrell B. Emotional problems in the family. In: Doyle D, Hanks GWC, MacDonald N, editors. The Oxford Textbook of Palliative Medicine. 2nd ed. Oxford, England: Oxford University Press; 1998. pp. 985-992

[56] Skorupskiene D. Conservative ways to treat cancer pain. Medicina (Kaunas, Lithuania). 2004;**40**(9):917-923 (in Lithuanian)

[57] Ščiupokas A. Cancer pain. In: Pain Diagnostics and Syndromology. University Textbook. UAB "Medicinos spaudos namai"; 2012. pp. 255-258 (in Lithuanian)

[58] Zeppetella G. Breakthrough pain in cancer patients. Clinical Oncology (Royal College of Radiologists). 2011;**23**(6):393-398. DOI: 10.1016/j.clon.2010.12.002 (Epub January 11, 2011)

[59] Davies AN. The management of breakthrough cancer pain. British Journal of Nursing;**20**(13). DOI: 10.12968/bjon.2011.20.13.803 (Epub Aug 16, 2013)

[60] Davies A, Sjolund KF, Stenberg M, et al. Breakthrough cancer pain: An observational study of 1000 European oncology patients. Journal of Pain and Symptom Management. 2013;**46**(5):619-628. DOI: 10.1016/j.jpainsymman.2012.12.009 (Epub March 22, 2013)

[61] Janknegt R, Van den Beuken M, Schiere S, Überall M, Knaggs R, Hanley J, et al. Rapid acting fentanyl formulations in breakthrough pain in cancer. Drug selection by means of the system of objectified judgement analysis. European Journal of Hospital Pharmacy: Science and Practice. 2018;**25**(3):e2. DOI: 10.1136/ejhpharm-2016-001127 (Epub January 11, 2017)

[62] Janknegt R, Steenhoek A. The system of objectified judgement analysis (SOJA). A tool in rational drug selection for formulary inclusion. Drugs. 1997;**53**(4):550-562

[63] Passik SD, Weinreb HJ. Managing chronic nonmalignant pain: Overcoming obstacles to the use of opioids. Advances in Therapy. 2000;**17**(2):70-83

[64] Núñez JM. Breakthrough cancer pain and rational drug use. Support Care Cancer. 2017;**25**(Suppl 1):11-17. DOI: 10.1007/s00520-017-3636-5 (Epub February 18, 2017)

[65] Henley SJ, Singh SD, King J, et al. Invasive cancer incidence and survival—United States, 2012. Morbidity and Mortality Weekly Report. 2015;**64**:1353-1358

[66] Green CR, Hart-Johnson T, Loeffler DR. Cancer related chronic pain: Examining quality of life in diverse cancer survivors. Cancer. 2011;**117**:1994-2003

[67] Paice JA et al. Management of chronic pain in survivors of adult cancers: American Society of Clinical Oncology clinical practice

guideline. Journal of Clinical Oncology;**34**:3325-3345

[68] Glare PA, Davies PS, Finlay E, et al. Pain in cancer survivors. Journal of Clinical Oncology. 2014;**32**:1739-1747

[69] Siegal T, Haim N. Cisplatin-induced peripheral neuropathy. Frequent off-therapy deterioration, demyelinating syndromes, and muscle cramps. Cancer. 1990;**66**:1117-1123

[70] Syrjala KL, Langer SL, Abrams JR, et al. Late effects of hematopoietic cell transplantation among 10-year adult survivors compared with case matched controls. Journal of Clinical Oncology. 2005;**23**:6596-6606

[71] Syrjala KL, Yi JC, Artherholt SB, et al. Measuring musculoskeletal symptoms in cancer survivors who receive hematopoietic cell transplantation. Journal of Cancer Survivorship. 2010;**4**:225-235

[72] Samer CF, Daali Y, Wagner M, et al. The effects of CYP2D6 and CYP3A activities on the pharmacokinetics of immediate release oxycodone. British Journal of Pharmacology. 2010;**160**:907-918

[73] Overholser BR, Foster DR. Opioid pharmacokinetic drug-drug interactions. The American Journal of Managed Care. 2011;**17**(Suppl 11):S276-S287

[74] Keller GA, Ponte ML, Di Girolamo G. Other drugs acting on nervous system associated with QT interval prolongation. Current Drug Safety. 2010;**5**:105-111

[75] Dart RC, Surratt HL, Cicero TJ, et al. Trends in opioid analgesic abuse and mortality in the United States. The New England Journal of Medicine. 2015;**372**:241-248

[76] Howe CQ, Sullivan MD. The missing 'P' in pain management: How the current opioid epidemic highlights the need for psychiatric services in chronic pain care. General Hospital Psychiatry. 2014;**36**:99-104

[77] Workman EA, Hubbard JR, Felker BL. Comorbid psychiatric disorders and predictors of pain management program success in patients with chronic pain. Primary Care Companion to The Journal of Clinical Psychiatry. 2002;**4**:137-140

[78] Williams PT. The role of family physicians in the management of cancer patients. Journal of Cancer Education. 1994;**9**:67-72

[79] Klabunde CN et al. Primary care physicians and Cancer care. Journal of General Internal Medicine. 2009;**24**(9):1029-1036

[80] Harris MF, Harris E. Facing the challenges: General practice in 2020. The Medical Journal of Australia. 2006;**185**(2):122-124

[81] Barclay S. Controlling Cancer pain in primary care: The prescribing habits and knowledge base of general practitioners. Journal of Pain and Symptom Management. 2002;**23**:383-392

[82] Parkes CM. Home or hospital? Terminal care as seen by surviving spouses. Journal of the Royal College of General Practitioners. 1978;**28**:19-30

[83] Doyle D, Hanks G, MacDonald L. Oxford Textbook of Palliative Medicine. Oxford: Oxford University Press; 1998

[84] Davies AN et al. Dose titration to individualise treatment. European Journal of Pain. 2009;**13**:331-333

[85] Raphael J et al. Cancer pain: Part 2: Physical, interventional and complimentary therapies; management in the community; acute,

treatment-related and complex cancer pain: A perspective from the British pain society endorsed by the UK Association of Palliative Medicine and the Royal College of General Practitioners. Pain Medicine. 2010;**11**:872-896

Chapter 8

Breakthrough Cancer Pain

Xue-Bin Yan

Abstract

Breakthrough cancer pain has attracted more and more attentions recently because it has become the biggest obstacle to control cancer pain. Pain can occur at any stage of cancer. Despite the aggressive treatment, some patients still experience high-intensity pain in the short term, which is commonly referred to as breakthrough pain. Typical breakthrough pain has clinical features such as rapid onset and short duration, and it has uncontrollable and unpredictable characteristics, which impact the overall life quality of patients and the therapeutic effect of cancer pain. It has always been a puzzle and difficult in clinical treatment of breakthrough cancer pain. This paper aims to provide a more detailed review of the definition, assessment tools, classification and characteristics, epidemiology, and mechanism and treatment of breakthrough cancer pain, in order to facilitate the future development of this work in clinical treatment.

Keywords: breakthrough cancer pain, characteristics, mechanisms, therapy

1. Introduction

Pain is one of the most common clinical symptoms associated with malignant tumors. Thirty to forty percent of patients suffer from pain at the beginning of diagnosis [1]. In actively treated patients, this proportion is higher, accounting for 50%, and in advanced cancer, even up to 90% [2]. Although it can effectively control the background pain of most cancer patients according to the WHO three-step analgesic principle, it still suffers from cancer pain. Cancer patients, indeed, may suffer from intense pain spikes that break through the control of chronic pain. Uncontrollable and unpredictable characteristics of a complex manifestation of cancer pain, termed as breakthrough cancer pain (BTP), have always baffled the treatment and the adverse effects including diet, sleep, daily activities, relationships with others, aggravating depression and anxiety and will impact patients' quality of life. Therefore, the control of breakthrough cancer pain is still a very difficult problem for clinicians. In view of the current lack of research data on outbreak pain in China, this paper aims to provide a more detailed review of the breakthrough cancer pain, in order to facilitate the future development of this work in clinical treatment.

2. The definition of breakthrough cancer pain

Background pain in cancer patients manifests as a persistent state of pain (most commonly 12 hours or longer), usually controlled by long-term administration. According to the WHO three-step analgesia program, general background cancer pain can be adequately controlled in 70–90% of patients [3]. Despite good control of baseline pain, some patients have short-term, short-lived, intense pain episodes. This is called breakthrough cancer pain (BTP) [4].

The first definition of cancer pain is proposed by Portenoy and Hagen in 1989 as the following: BTP is a transient increase in pain, greater than moderate intensity, occurring on moderate- or lower-intensity baseline pain [5]. In the third edition of Oxford palliative medicine textbook, BTP is defined as a transient deterioration of pain experienced by patients with relatively stable and well-controlled baseline pain [6]. In 2009, the UK and Ireland Conservative Treatment Collaborative Committee (APM) put forward the following views on outbreak pain and concluded that as long as the following three conditions are met at the same time, it can be diagnosed as an BTP: (1) having background cancer pain, (2) the background cancer pain adequately controlled in the last week (NRS score ≤ 3 points), and (3) the pain temporarily acutely aggravated [7].

3. Evaluation tools for breakthrough cancer pain

For cancer patients, the intensity of pain should be assessed at each visit. The most common is the numerical score (NRS). The pain intensity level from 0 to 10 is evaluated as 0 indicating lack of pain (no pain) and 10 indicating the most extreme pain (the most imaginable pain). Visual analog scale (VAS) is also frequently used; patients use a 100 mm length digital scale to describe pain intensity (0, no pain; 100, the most powerful pain imaginable). The descriptive Likert scale (painless, mild pain, moderate pain, strong pain, severe pain) is the least accurate but is usually the most understandable for the patient.

But general tools may not be sufficient to adequately cover the complexity of BTP. Several specific features of BTP are reflected in background pain, treatment-related factors (including trigger events and predictability), and time factors. Key factors include relationship to background pain, time to last BTP, frequency, peak pain intensity, position, time from onset to maximum intensity, duration, cause, predictability, general remission, BTP relief, pain satisfaction with relief, the onset of pain relief, and satisfaction with the onset of pain relief. Other items completed by professionals include the etiology of BTP and the pathophysiology of BTP [8]. Understanding these factors is critical to being able to construct an effective analgesic strategy, which is the primary purpose of any pain assessment. The lack of BTP assessment tools may be related to the fact that some authors advocate the use of general pain tools without the need for a separate BTP assessment tool [9, 10]. Recently, a new evaluation tool was developed and validated for BTP (Webber's BAT tool). The assessment tool provides information about BTP and how the efficacy and toxicity of BTP drugs interfere with everyday life, and the reliability and effectiveness of testing in a group of patients is quite good [11].

Portenoy et al. used the Beck Depression Scale (BDI) questionnaire, the beck anxiety scale (BAI) questionnaire, and the baseline pain intensity measurement based on the VAS scale to assess the impact of BTP on quality of life. In 178 patients with well-controlled baseline pain, both groups were extracted and evaluated based on whether they had BTP. In 65% of patients, BTP is caused by cancer, and in other cases it is related to the treatment used. Baseline pain is more severe in patients with BTP. In addition, how pain affects mood, work, sleep, mobility, social relationships, and life satisfaction is also assessed. Each aspect is evaluated over a range of values from 0 to 10 (0, no effect; 10, overall impact). In the case of the BDI and BAI scales, the patient responded to 21 questions, ranging from 0 to 3 (0 for asymptomatic and 3 for highest symptom intensity) [12].

It is worth noting that BTP may have a negative impact on prognosis [13] and may also have an adverse effect on the duration of cancer treatment [14]. Accurate diagnosis of pain types and early introduction of appropriate treatments should be sought. Moreover, in the lack of exhaustive tools, successful BTP diagnosis (and management) is the result of the combination of adequate assessment, appropriate (tailored) treatment, and adequate reassessment.

4. Classification and characteristics of breakthrough cancer pain

Breakthrough cancer pain can be divided into sporadic pain (incidental pain), spontaneous or idiopathic pain, and discontinuation of drug withdrawal (end of dose). Mixing BTP can also be included as the fourth subtype [15]. Sporadic pain is a common type of BTP, with a shorter peak intensity and a shorter duration, more predictable, often caused directly after muscle or bone activity, such as getting up, turning over, going to toilets, coughs, etc. It can also be associated with contraction or spasm of visceral smooth muscle, such as bowel or bladder spasm, so patients are more willing to limit their activity to avoid triggering BTP, although the duration of pain is unpredictable even after cessation of activity. There is no obvious cause of self-explosive pain, and the duration of pain is more than 30 minutes. It is generally not directly related to regular analgesic treatment and has no significant correlation with physical activity [16]. In general, when there is sufficient analgesia for most of the day, three to four episodes per day are considered acceptable [17]. Insufficient analgesic drugs are relatively rare. It often occurs at the next point in the continuous analgesic treatment phase for 1–2 hours, and acute pain occurs on the basis of continuous pain treatment. APM believes that the analgesic drug dose-deficient outbreak is caused by insufficient control of the underlying cancer pain and that it is not a BTP [7].

BTP is characterized by a rapid onset, usually occurring in a matter of minutes or even seconds (average about 3 minutes), stronger than baseline pain, up to 7 points (NRS score), and very short duration (average 30 minutes) [1]. In a large study of 1412 patients, 80.6% of patients reported a significant negative impact of BTP on daily life. The average number of episodes was 2.4 per day with an average intensity of 7.4/10. In patients reporting a rapid onset of BTP, this is predictable in approximately half of the cases, while BTP with a gradual onset (>10 minutes) is less predictable. The average duration of an untreated episode of BTP was approximately 30 minutes [10]. These characteristics may change during the course of the disease. For example, patients who are receiving palliative care are older, have lower levels of Karnofsky, have fewer BTP episodes per day, and have slower BTP episodes than those assessed in the pain clinic or oncology ward. BTP is less predictable [18].

Davies et al. published the results of a multicenter clinical trial involving 1000 patients treated in 28 professional palliative care units in 13 European countries from 2008 to 2011. Patients were classified as eligible for trial according to a questionnaire on five questions. Forty-four percent of patients were induced by specific factors, 41.5% were idiopathic, and 14.5% were mixed. The results showed that specific factors caused by BTP patients' activity problems and basic daily activities were more frequent, while those with idiopathic pain were more common with changes in mood and sleep problems [18].

5. Epidemiology of breakthrough cancer pain

There are wide variations in the estimates of incidence reported in the literature, possibly due to the different backgrounds and implications of the definition of BTP. A multicenter study in the four Nordic countries in 201,135 surveyed the incidence of BTP in 320 patients with cancer pain by issuing questionnaires, all from palliative care centers or pain treatment centers. Of these, 83% had breakthrough cancer pain, in which 44% had sporadic outbreaks, 39% had spontaneous outbreaks, and 17% had both types of pain. On average, there were three outbreaks of pain every 24 hours. The longest interval was 2 times/week, and the shortest interval was 24 times a day. According to the degree of pain, 3% of patients were mild, 37% were moderate, and 60% were severe [8].

In some epidemiological studies, although not verified, the patient's background pain may be uncontrolled or not receiving opioids. For example, in more than half of patients with severe background pain, a different phenomenon than other patients was observed, and patients without BTP had higher background pain intensity. In other studies, most patients had uncontrolled background pain, who received non-opioid analgesics or weak opioids or were dissatisfied with pain management.

6. Mechanisms of breakthrough cancer pain

The pathogenesis of cancer pain is very complicated. The most common causes are malignant tumor compression and infiltration of pain-sensitive organ structures such as bones, muscle soft tissue, peripheral nerves, internal organs, and the others. There is also atrophy and cancer cachexia, or it may be the result of aggressive anticancer treatment, but the real cause in some patients is unclear [19].

The most common nociceptors associated with cancer pain are afferent nerves, which can transmit various noxious stimuli to the central nervous system through the periphery. Nociceptors mainly have two major functions: transduction of pain signals and transmission of pain signals. Various noxious stimuli can directly activate the nociceptors, transmitting the electrochemical nerve impulse signals generated by the afferent nerves to the central nervous system of the patient, and the patient has a feeling of pain. Cancer and immune cells in the tumor mass region release several neuroimmune mediators that interact with multiple receptors on peripheral nociceptive nerve terminals to promote abnormal discharge and hyperexcitability. In addition, tumors that grow near the peripheral nerve can impair the integrity of the nerve and induce neurological conditions associated with persistent pain, hyperalgesia, or allodynia. Both of these effects of the tumor on the peripheral nerves can lead to central sensitization, which further enhances the efficacy of nociceptive transmission through the spinal dorsal horn and the perception of BTP [20].

During the operation, tissue damage associated with damage to the surrounding small nerves can be caused. After tissue damage, inflammatory mediators and other substances (e.g., histamine, serotonin, nerve growth factor, bradykinin, leukotrienes, prostaglandins, norepinephrine, cytokines, etc.) are damaged at the wound site tissue and inflammatory cells, and sympathetic nerve endings are released. The released material can alter the excitability of nociceptors by phosphorylating and upregulating the cell membrane or upregulating ion channels in the nerve. This peripheral sensitization can explain the increased sensitivity of early postoperative clinical manifestations to mechanical stimulation of the wound site. However, postoperative pain cannot be explained only by peripheral mechanisms. Repetitive, detrimental input from sensitized C fibers causes activation of the signal cascade within the dorsal horn cells, thereby facilitating the response. Central sensitization may explain the increased sensitivity of noninvasive tissue around the wound to mechanical stimulation. Under these conditions, mechanical stimulation caused by exercise and cough may cause BTP [21].

Recent studies have found that specific nuclei located in the posterior thalamus are associated with pain-related networks. Related studies have found that the most effective inhibitors of noxious stimuli are β-endorphin, enkephalin, and dynorphin. The most common precursor of β-endorphin is proopiomelanocortin; the precursor of enkephalin and leucine enkephalin is mainly proenkephalin-A (pro-ENK); the precursor of dynorphin is enkephalin original B. B-Endorphin mainly binds to opioid receptors, and enkephalin mainly binds to opioid receptors, and dynorphin mainly binds to opioid κ receptors. The commonly used opioids, oxycodone and morphine sustained-release tablets, are combined with receptors and/or K receptors to mimic the action of endogenous opioid peptides to achieve analgesic treatment [22].

Visceral pain may be located in the visceral or distant body parts. Two types of nociceptors dominate the internal organs: high threshold receptors and intensity-encoded mechanoreceptors. In addition, the presence of "silent" nociceptors has been found. "Silent" nociceptors are activated in the event of tissue damage or inflammation and may contribute to the signaling of chronic visceral pain. High threshold nociceptors may be activated in acute pain states. For example, prolonged stimulation of the internal organs, such as inflammation, may sensitize high threshold nociceptors and activate "silent" nociceptors. Sensitized nociceptors may now also respond to harmless stimuli. Increased peripheral neuronal activity results in increased excitability in the visceral-somatic neurons in the spinal cord (central sensitization). For example, BTP caused by food intake can be explained by sensitization of visceral mechanoreceptors, and the increase in pain area is due to central sensitization [23].

Our team found that the activation of astrocytes in the dorsal horn of spinal cord and connexin 43 (Cx43) protein is involved in the process of bone pain in bone metastases in mice. The total amount of Cx43 protein and phosphorylation may be important factors affecting cancer outbreak pain factor. Gap 26 blocks the gap junction channel of the spinal dorsal horn, which can improve the pain behavior index of mice with cancerous outbreak pain and downregulate the expression of Cx43 protein, which can regulate the pain of cancerous outbreak. The spinal dorsal horn EAAT1 protein is involved in the pathogenesis of mouse basic cancer pain, and EAAT2 protein has an effect on the occurrence and maintenance of bone metastases. Activation of EAAT2 by Cef improves its pain behavioral metrics and regulates burst pain. Cx43 can affect the protein expression of EAATs but EAAT2 does not affect the expression of Cx43 protein. Spinal dorsal horn Cx43-EAATs may play a role in cancerous outbreaks [24].

7. Treatment of breakthrough cancer pain

Treatment with BTP includes medication, nerve block, nerve damage, TNES, palliative exposure to bone lesions, the use of bisphosphonates, and identification and prevention of factors that induce BTP (e.g., excessive physical labor, persistent cough, constipation). The NCCN guidelines for adult cancer pain [25] recommends the use of 10–15% of immediate-release opioids in total daily analgesics to treat BTP. If the number of outbreaks of pain per day exceeds 4 times, the amount of the basic analgesic drug is raised. Opioid analgesics have no ceiling effect. For severe refractory pain, high-dose opioid controlled-release preparations are often needed for analgesic treatment. Large doses are defined as daily doses of oxycodone sustained-release tablets (or equivalent doses of other opioid analgesics such as fentanyl transdermal patches or MS contin) up to 150 mg/d.

7.1 Drugs

Opioids are still the most important and effective drugs for the treatment of breakthrough cancer pain [26]. The main opioids currently used to treat BTP are morphine immediate-release tablets, oxycodone sustained-release tablets, fentanyl sublingual tablets (SLF), morphine sustained-release tablets and controlled-release tablets, fentanyl nasal spray (INFS), fentanyl transmucosal citrate (OTFC), morphine sulfate (injection), sufentanil injection (injection), and so on. The above various types of morphine agonists work in combination with secretory opioid receptors, which produce analgesic effects after agonizing the receptor.

Oral administration is the most common route of administration for cancerous outbreaks and is the recommended route of administration by the WHO. The NICE guidelines recommend immediate-release of morphine for BTP first-line first-aid drugs and do not provide fentanyl as a first-line rescue drug but morphine. The onset and duration of immediate-release tablets may not be suitable for the treatment of many BTP events [27]. Oxycodone sustained-release tablets can be used as a two-step drug or as a three-step analgesic drug, which can simultaneously agonize both receptors and K receptor opioid receptors, with high bioavailability and clinical good analgesic effect and less drug-related adverse reactions [22]; the analgesic intensity is about twice that of morphine immediate-release tablets. After oral administration, there will be two release phases, which provide early onset of rapid analgesia. The fast release phase and the subsequent sustained-release phase, through the rapid release phase to achieve the purpose of treating burst pain, do not require conversion of the dosage form; clinical application of oxycodone controlled-release tablets is more and more extensive.

In order to evaluate the efficacy of oral morphine and oral transmucosal fentanyl preparations to provide further insight into their relative merits as treatments for BTP, we conducted an analysis to compare the effects of fentanyl, morphine, and placebo on BTP indirectly (**Table 1**, **Figures 1–6**). The therapeutic effect was evaluated by the difference in pain intensity difference (PID) score. We found that all opioids provided better analgesic effects during the first hour after dosing, whereas fentanyl may provide a higher level of pain relief than oral morphine. Participants administered a transmucosal fentanyl showed lower pain intensity and higher pain relief at all time points than placebo or oral morphine, and the fentanyl achieved significant pain relief faster. But there is no significant difference between the various transmucosal fentanyl preparations. From the PID score, the analgesic effect of fentanyl is stronger than oral morphine. And improvements in pain relief were apparent within 30 minutes of treatment, with the PID being larger for the fentanyl preparations than for MSIR during this period. This is of potential importance because most BTP episodes occur within 30 minutes. However, there are few existing studies, especially regarding the comparison of fentanyl with oral morphine, which is a limitation of this mixed treatment. Moreover, the possibility of systematic differences between undetected data sources for heterogeneity analysis cannot be ruled out. In conclusion, although oral morphine is still an appropriate treatment option for BTP, oral transmucosal fentanyl may be more clinically advantageous in some patients.

The recently published guidelines support this approach and recommend the use of fast- or short-acting opioids to treat BTP, whose pharmacodynamics reflect the rapid onset and short duration of pain [28]. The Cochrane review reported the utility of seven different transmucosal fentanyl compared to oral opioids. Oral and nasal transmucosal fentanyls are an effective treatment for BTP [29]. The drugs such as fentanyl oral effervescent tablets and fentanyl sublingual tablets have also

DOI: http://dx.doi.org/10.5772/intechopen.84581

Fentanyl (F) and placebo/morphine PID (C)												
Study	5 minutes		10 minutes		15 minutes		30 minutes		45 minutes		60 minutes	
	F	C	F	C	F	C	F	C	F	C	F	C
INFS vs. placebo (HANS2009 [33])	N	N	2.58	1.22	N	N	N	N	N	N	4.57	2.46
INFS vs. placebo (RUSSELL2010 [34])	0.59	0.49	1.32	0.93	1.96	1.33	2.69	1.73	3.19	2.08	3.57	2.21
INFS vs. placebo (MORTEN2015 [35])	N	N	2.4	1.5	N	N	N	N	N	N	N	N
INFS vs. IRMS (FALLON2011 [36])	1	1	2.02	1.8	3.22	2.68	4.38	3.64	4.95	4.47	5.58	5
SFT vs. placebo (NAOHITO2015 [37])	N	N	N	N	2.43	2.06	4.11	3.39	N	N	5.58	4.52
SFT vs. placebo (RANCK2009 [38])	N	N	1.2	0.92	2.04	1.51	2.94	2.1	N	N	3.45	2.51
SFT vs. placebo (NOVOTNA2014 [39])	0.7	0.5	1.6	1.1	2.6	1.8	3.5	2.5	N	N	3.9	2.7
SFT vs. placebo (NAOHITO2015 [40])	N	N	N	N	N	N	3.18	2.7	N	N	N	N
OTFC vs. placebo (RAUCK2009 [41])	0.3	0.3	0.8	0.7	1.4	1.2	2.5	1.9	3	2.3	3.3	2.4
OTFC vs. IRMS (PAUL2001 [42])	N	N	N	N	1.86	1.46	2.88	2.4	3.55	3.03	4.03	3.57

Table 1.
META analysis data

Study or Subgroup	fentanyl Mean	fentanyl SD	fentanyl Total	placebo/morphine Mean	placebo/morphine SD	placebo/morphine Total	Weight	Std. Mean Difference IV, Random, 95% CI
FALLON2011	1	0.16	372	1	0.16	368	33.4%	0.00 [-0.14, 0.14]
NOVOTNA2014	0.7	0.05	436	0.5	0.08	218	33.3%	3.24 [3.00, 3.48]
RAUCK2010	0.3	0.06	394	0.3	0.06	197	33.4%	0.00 [-0.17, 0.17]
Total (95% CI)			**1202**			**783**	**100.0%**	**1.08 [-0.69, 2.85]**

Heterogeneity: Tau² = 2.44; Chi² = 579.76, df = 2 (P < 0.00001); I² = 100%
Test for overall effect: Z = 1.19 (P = 0.23)

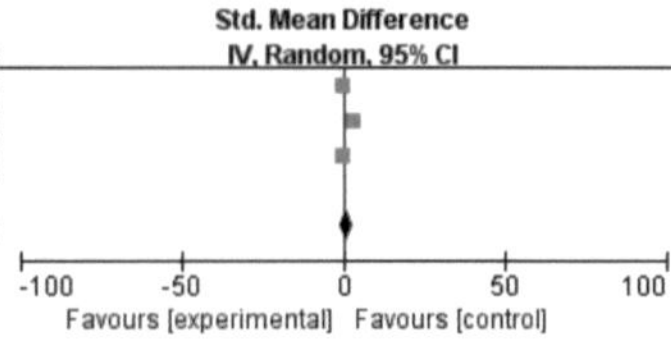

Figure 1.
Fentanyl versus placebo/morphine PID 5 minutes.

Study or Subgroup	fentanyl Mean	fentanyl SD	fentanyl Total	placebo/morphine Mean	placebo/morphine SD	placebo/morphine Total	Weight	Std. Mean Difference IV, Random, 95% CI
FALLON2011	2.02	0.15	372	1.8	0.17	368	14.6%	1.37 [1.21, 1.53]
Hans2009	2.58	0.13	111	1.22	0.12	110	13.1%	10.83 [9.78, 11.88]
MORTEN2015	2.4	2.29	15	1.5	1.52	15	13.9%	0.45 [-0.28, 1.18]
NOVOTNA2014	1.6	0.08	436	1.1	0.1	218	14.5%	5.73 [5.38, 6.08]
RANCK2009	1.2	0.14	393	0.92	0.15	168	14.6%	1.95 [1.74, 2.17]
RAUCK2010	0.8	0.07	394	0.7	0.05	197	14.6%	1.56 [1.37, 1.75]
RUSSELL2010	1.32	0.14	459	0.93	0.13	200	14.6%	2.84 [2.62, 3.07]
Total (95% CI)			**2180**			**1276**	**100.0%**	**3.44 [2.28, 4.61]**

Heterogeneity: Tau² = 2.40; Chi² = 846.69, df = 6 (P < 0.00001); I² = 99%
Test for overall effect: Z = 5.80 (P < 0.00001)

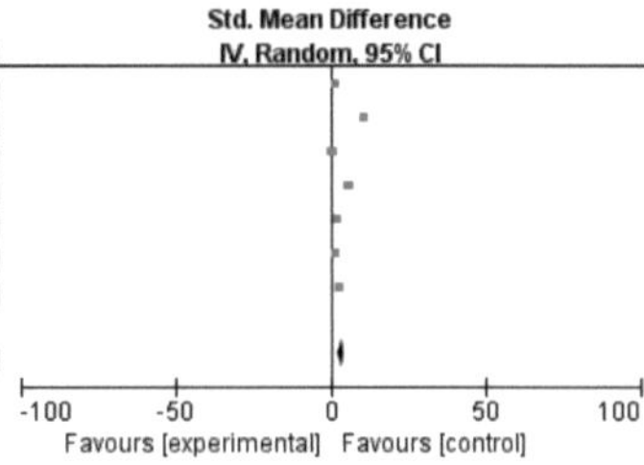

Figure 2.
Fentanyl versus placebo/morphine PID 10 minutes.

Study or Subgroup	fentanyl Mean	fentanyl SD	fentanyl Total	placebo/morphine Mean	placebo/morphine SD	placebo/morphine Total	Weight	Std. Mean Difference IV, Random, 95% CI
FALLON2011	3.22	0.21	373	2.68	0.16	368	14.4%	2.89 [2.68, 3.09]
NAOHITO2014	2.24	1.67	37	2.06	1.78	37	14.1%	0.10 [-0.35, 0.56]
NOVOTNA2014	2.6	0.09	436	1.8	0.15	218	14.2%	7.04 [6.62, 7.45]
PAUL2001	1.86	0.2	64	1.46	0.17	29	14.0%	2.07 [1.54, 2.61]
RANCK2009	2.04	0.17	393	1.51	0.22	168	14.4%	2.84 [2.59, 3.09]
RAUCK2010	1.4	0.1	394	1.2	0.1	197	14.4%	2.00 [1.79, 2.20]
RUSSELL2010	1.96	0.18	459	1.33	0.16	200	14.4%	3.61 [3.36, 3.87]
Total (95% CI)			**2156**			**1217**	**100.0%**	**2.94 [1.83, 4.04]**

Heterogeneity: Tau² = 2.19; Chi² = 637.45, df = 6 (P < 0.00001); I² = 99%
Test for overall effect: Z = 5.21 (P < 0.00001)

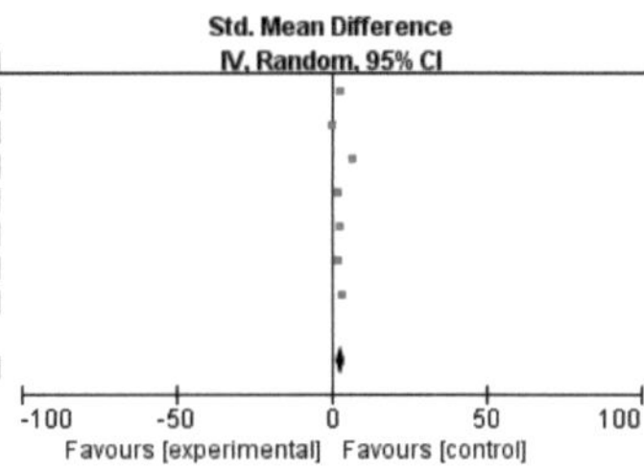

Figure 3.
Fentanyl versus placebo/morphine PID 15 minutes.

Study or Subgroup	fentanyl Mean	fentanyl SD	fentanyl Total	placebo/morphine Mean	placebo/morphine SD	placebo/morphine Total	Weight	Std. Mean Difference IV, Random, 95% CI
FALLON2011	4.38	3.64	368	3.64	0.23	368	12.6%	0.29 [0.14, 0.43]
NAOHITO2014	4.11	2.3	37	3.39	2.54	37	12.5%	0.29 [-0.16, 0.75]
NAOHITO2015	3.18	1.84	49	2.7	1.94	51	12.5%	0.25 [-0.14, 0.65]
NOVOTNA2014	3.5	0.1	436	2.5	0.16	218	12.5%	8.10 [7.63, 8.57]
PAUL2001	2.88	0.2	64	2.4	0.17	29	12.4%	2.49 [1.92, 3.06]
RANCK2009	2.94	0.17	393	2.1	0.27	168	12.5%	4.09 [3.79, 4.39]
RAUCK2010	2.5	0.1	394	1.9	0.13	197	12.5%	5.40 [5.05, 5.76]
RUSSELL2010	2.69	0.19	459	1.73	0.21	200	12.5%	4.89 [4.57, 5.20]
Total (95% CI)			**2200**			**1268**	**100.0%**	**3.22 [1.22, 5.23]**

Heterogeneity: Tau² = 8.33; Chi² = 2183.08, df = 7 (P < 0.00001); I² = 100%
Test for overall effect: Z = 3.15 (P = 0.002)

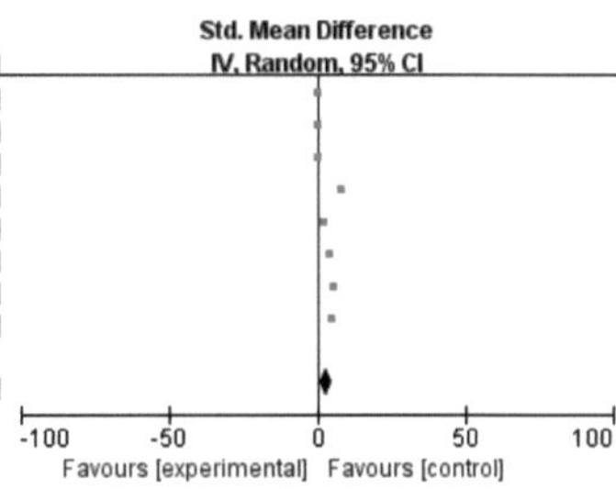

Figure 4.
Fentanyl versus placebo/morphine PID 30 minutes.

Study or Subgroup	fentanyl Mean	fentanyl SD	fentanyl Total	placebo/morphine Mean	placebo/morphine SD	placebo/morphine Total	Weight	Std. Mean Difference IV, Random, 95% CI
FALLON2011	4.95	0.27	372	4.47	0.23	368	26.0%	1.91 [1.74, 2.09]
PAUL2001	3.55	0.2	2	3.03	0.2	29	22.2%	2.53 [0.95, 4.12]
RAUCK2010	3	0.13	394	2.3	0.17	197	25.9%	4.84 [4.51, 5.16]
RUSSELL2010	3.19	0.22	459	2.08	0.24	200	25.9%	4.90 [4.59, 5.21]
Total (95% CI)			**1227**			**794**	**100.0%**	**3.58 [1.65, 5.51]**

Heterogeneity: Tau² = 3.71; Chi² = 414.74, df = 3 (P < 0.00001); I² = 99%
Test for overall effect: Z = 3.64 (P = 0.0003)

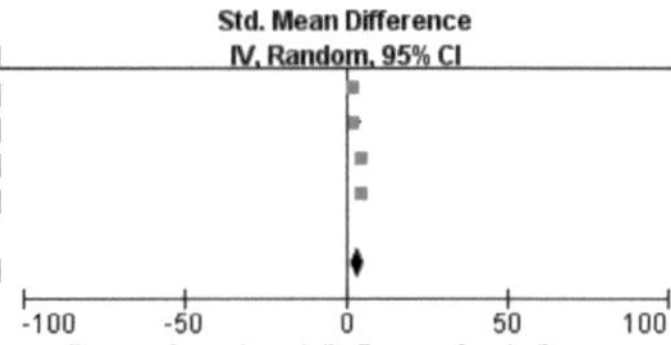

Figure 5.
Fentanyl versus placebo/morphine PID 45 minutes.

	fentanyl			placebo/morphine				Std. Mean Difference
Study or Subgroup	Mean	SD	Total	Mean	SD	Total	Weight	IV, Random, 95% CI
FALLON2011	5.58	0.28	272	5	0.24	368	14.4%	2.25 [2.05, 2.45]
Hans2009	4.57	0.17	111	2.46	0.23	110	13.9%	10.40 [9.39, 11.42]
NAOHITO2014	5.58	2.28	37	4.52	2.76	37	14.3%	0.41 [-0.05, 0.88]
NOVOTNA2014	3.8	0.11	436	2.7	0.17	218	14.3%	8.26 [7.78, 8.74]
RANCK2009	3.45	0.23	393	2.51	0.32	168	14.4%	3.61 [3.33, 3.89]
RAUCK2010	3.3	0.13	394	2.4	0.18	197	14.4%	6.05 [5.67, 6.44]
RUSSELL2010	3.57	0.24	459	2.21	0.24	200	14.4%	5.66 [5.31, 6.01]
Total (95% CI)			**2102**			**1298**	**100.0%**	**5.21 [3.33, 7.09]**

Heterogeneity: $Tau^2 = 6.38$; $Chi^2 = 1179.95$, df = 6 ($P < 0.00001$); $I^2 = 99\%$
Test for overall effect: $Z = 5.43$ ($P < 0.00001$)

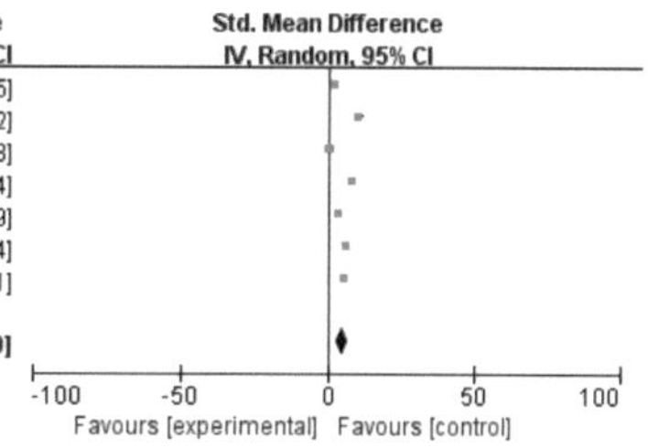

Figure 6.
Fentanyl versus placebo/morphine PID 60 minutes.

been approved for use in European and American countries. However, the state of oral mucosa, drug distribution, and oral infections will affect the absorption of drugs, thus affecting the analgesic effect of drugs. Fentanyl nasal spray (INFS) has been approved by the European Commission in 2009 and has been officially used in the clinic. It has been marketed globally and is mainly used for outbreak pain in cancer patients who maintain analgesic treatment with drugs such as oral opioids. Treatment: nasal mucosal sprays are suitable for those with oral mucosal damage or saliva dysfunction, but those with nasal mucosal bleeding or ulcers need to switch to other treatments [30].

Both morphine sulfate injection and sufentanil citrate injection can be administered intravenously. Intravenous use of opioids has a fast onset and a positive effect [31, 32]. However, it is necessary to evaluate the pain every 15 minutes, and should be alert to the acute side effects of drugs such as respiratory depression [32], vomiting, dizziness, acute urinary retention, etc., especially acute respiratory depression, severe cases can be directly life-threatening, so opioid veins The application should be performed in a ward with emergency conditions or in an emergency ward, and an opiate rescuer naloxone is prepared at the bedside.

Individualized doses and modes of administration can also be tailored to the condition, and stable morphine is delivered to the human body via intravenous (PCIA), epidural (PCEA), and subcutaneous (PCPA).

7.2 Cell therapy

Cell treatment is to return autologous cells cultured in vitro to patients. Through these cells with biological micro-pump function, they can continue to secrete analgesic substances to relieve pain or improve pain thresholds, such as serotonin, norepinephrine, dynorphin, enkephalin, neurotrophic factor, etc., to achieve the purpose of relieving cancer pain or improving the pain threshold of patients. The most extensive and intensive research is the analgesic effect of adrenal chromaffin cells, sympathetic ganglion cells, and some neurotumor cells.

7.3 Gene therapy

Gene therapy refers to a method of achieving analgesic effects by altering gene expression in a patient. It can be divided into in vivo pathways and in vitro pathways. In vitro route refers to the removal of target cells from the body or the adoption of cell lines and the in vitro introduction of therapeutic genes into the body for therapeutic purposes. In vivo route refers to the direct introduction of therapeutic genes into the body. In pain research, there are two main aspects of gene therapy, namely, by upregulating anti-pain gene expression and downregulating pain gene expression, specifically interfering with the biological behavior of pain for therapeutic purposes.

7.4 Interventional neuroradiologic therapy

Nerve block and nerve damage are one of the main treatments for cancer pain by blocking the pain transmission pathway. The current clinical damage treatment is damage to peripheral nerves, nerve roots, celiac plexus, subarachnoid space, and pituitary gland. Before the operation, physical examination and imaging methods were used to fully determine the pain range of the patient, and the nerves to be controlled were determined. Under the guidance of CT, the target nerve was destroyed by means of anhydrous alcohol, chemotherapy drugs such as doxorubicin, or physical ablation. Analgesic effect, with positive effect, fast onset, and little effect on other organ functions, has unique advantages for outbreak pain and intractable cancer pain that are ineffective for medical treatment. Currently, nerve blockers or lesions often have anesthesiologists, or the implementation of pain specialists in specialist hospitals has extremely high requirements for the operation of doctors in the positioning of nerves and imaging; otherwise it is likely to cause serious consequences.

8. Summary

Breakthrough cancer pain is a type of problem that clinicians urgently need to solve. There is currently no recognized definition and classification system for cancer BTP, and there are no well-proven BTP assessment tools that pose significant challenges to clinical management. Although breakthrough cancer pain has common clinical features, there are significant differences between individuals, which require clinicians to emphasize the importance of individualized, multidisciplinary analgesic programs on the basis of comprehensive treatment. In short, the current overall treatment effect of breakthrough cancer pain is not good; it is worthy of our attention.

Author details

Xue-Bin Yan
The Third Xiang-Ya Hospital of Central South University, Changsha, China

*Address all correspondence to: yanxb999@126.com

References

[1] Xavier GB, Federico M, Francisco M, et al. Breakthrough cancer pain: Prevalence and characteristics in patients in Catalonia, Spain. Journal of Pain and Symptom Management. 2002;**24**(1):45-52

[2] Lesage P, Portenoy RK. Trends in cancer pain management. Cancer Control. 1999;**6**(2):136-145

[3] World Health Organization. Cancer Pain Relief: With a Guide to Opioid Availability. 2nd ed. Geneva: World Health Organization; 1996. http://www.who.int/iris/handle/10665/37896

[4] Portenoy RK, Hagen NA. Breakthrough pain: Definition, prevalence and characteristics. Pain. 1990;**41**(3):273-281

[5] Portenoy RK, Hagen NA. Breakthrough pain: Definition and management. Oncology. 1989;**3**(8 Suppl):25-29

[6] Portenoy R, Forbes K, Lussier D, et al. Difficult pain problems: An integrated approach. In: Oxford Textbook of Palliative Medicine. Vol. 3. Oxford University Press (OUP); 2004. pp. 438-458. ISBN: 978-0-199-65609-7

[7] Davies AN, Dickman A, Reid C, et al. The management of cancer-related breakthrough pain: Recommendations of a task group of the Science Committee of the Association for Palliative Medicine of Great Britain and Ireland. European Journal of Pain. 2009;**13**(4):331-338

[8] Mercadante S, Marchetti P, Cuomo A, et al. Breakthrough pain and its treatment: Critical review and recommendations of IOPS (Italian oncologic pain survey) expert group. Supportive Care in Cancer. 2016;**24**(2):961-968

[9] Andrew ND. Cancer-related breakthrough pain. British Journal of Hospital Medicine. 2006;**67**(8):414-416

[10] Payne R. Recognition and diagnosis of breakthrough pain. Pain Medicine. 2007;**8**(suppl 1):S3-S7

[11] Webber K, Davies AN, Zeppetella G, et al. Development and validation of the breakthrough pain assessment tool (BAT) in cancer patients. Journal of Pain and Symptom Management. 2014;**48**(4):619-631

[12] Portenoy RK, Payne D, Jacobsen P. Breakthrough pain: Characteristics and impact in patients with cancer pain. Pain. 1999;**81**(1-2):129-134

[13] Bruera E, Schoeller T, Wenk R, et al. A prospective multicenter assessment of the Edmonton staging system for cancer pain. Journal of Pain and Symptom Management. 1995;**10**(5):348-355

[14] Hwang SS, Chang VT, Kasimis B. Cancer breakthrough pain characteristics and responses to treatment at a VA medical center. Pain. 2003;**101**(1-2):55-64

[15] Gutgsell T, Walsh D, Zhukovsky DS, et al. A prospective study of the pathophysiology and clinical characteristics of pain in a palliative medicine population. American Journal of Hospice & Palliative Medicine. 2003;**20**(2):140-148

[16] Porta-Sales J. Breakthrough cancer pain and current treatment options. European Journal of Pain Supplements. 2010;**4**(3):181-185

[17] Mercadante S. Breakthrough pain in cancer patients: Prevalence, mechanisms and treatment options. Current Opinion in Anaesthesiology. 2015;**28**(5):559-564

[18] Davies A, Buchanan A, Zeppetella G, et al. Breakthrough cancer pain: An observational study of 1000 European oncology patients. Journal of Pain and Symptom Management. 2013;**46**(5):619-628

[19] Svendsen KB, Andersen S, Arnason S, et al. Breakthrough pain in malignant and non-malignant diseases: A review of prevalence, characteristics and mechanisms. European Journal of Pain. 2005;**9**(2):195-206

[20] Schmidt BL, Hamamoto DT, Simone DA, et al. Mechanism of cancer pain. Molecular Interventions. 2010;**10**(3):164

[21] Jandhyala R, Fullarton JR, Bennett MI. Efficacy of rapid-onset oral fentanyl formulations vs. oral morphine for cancer-related breakthrough pain: A meta-analysis of comparative trials. Journal of Pain and Symptom Management. 2013;**46**(4):573-580

[22] Cheng Y, Yu S-y. Mechanism of cancer pain and the analgesia mechanism of common opiate drugs. Drug Evaluation. 2012;**3**:6-9

[23] Cervero F, Jänig W. Visceral nociceptors: A new world order? Trends in Neurosciences. 1992;**15**(10):374-378

[24] Li X, Jiang S, Yang H, et al. Breakthrough cancer pain is associated with spinal gap junction activation via regulation of connexin 43 in a mouse model. Frontiers in Cellular Neuroscience. 2017;**11**:207

[25] Kim H L, Puymon M R, Qin M, et al. NCCN Clinical Practice Guidelines in Oncology™. 2014

[26] Mercadante S. Opioid titration in cancer pain: A critical review. European Journal of Pain. 2007;**11**(8):823-830

[27] Zeppetella G. Evidence-based treatment of cancer-related breakthrough pain with opioids. Journal of the National Comprehensive Cancer Network. 2013;**11**(suppl 1): S-37-S-43

[28] Caraceni A, Bertetto O, Labianca R, et al. Episodic (breakthrough) pain prevalence in a population of cancer pain patients. Comparison of clinical diagnoses with the QUDEI—Italian questionnaire for intense episodic pain. Journal of Pain and Symptom Management. 2012;**43**(5):833-841

[29] Zeppetella G, Davies AN. Opioids for the management of breakthrough pain in cancer patients. Cochrane Database of Systematic Reviews. 2013;**10**:CD004311

[30] Mercadante S, Villari P, Ferrera P, et al. Rapid titration with intravenous morphine for severe cancer pain and immediate oral conversion. Cancer. 2002;**95**(1):203-208

[31] Soares LGL, Martins ML, Uchoa R. Intravenous fentanyl for cancer pain: A "fast titration" protocol for the emergency room. Journal of Pain and Symptom Management. 2003;**26**(3):876-881

[32] Elsner F, Sabatowski R, Radbruch L. Emergency pain treatment-ambulatory intravenous morphine titration in a patient with cancer pain. Anästhesiologie Intensivmedizin Notfallmedizin Schmerztherapie. 2000;**35**(7):462-464

[33] Kress HG, Orońska A, Kaczmarek Z, et al. Efficacy and tolerability of intranasal fentanyl spray 50 to 200 μg for breakthrough pain in patients with cancer: A phase III, multinational, randomized, double-blind, placebo-controlled, crossover trial with a 10-month, open-label extension treatment period. Clinical Therapeutics. 2009;**31**(6):1177-1191

[34] Portenoy RK, Burton AW, Gabrail N, et al. A multicenter, placebo-controlled, double-blind, multiple-crossover study of fentanyl pectin nasal spray (FPNS) in the treatment of breakthrough cancer pain. Pain. 2010;**151**(3):617-624

[35] Thronæs M, Popper L, Eeg M, et al. Efficacy and tolerability of intranasal fentanyl spray in cancer patients with breakthrough pain. Clinical Therapeutics. 2015;**37**(3):585-596

[36] Fallon M, Reale C, Davies A, et al. Efficacy and safety of fentanyl pectin nasal spray compared with immediate-release morphine sulfate tablets in the treatment of breakthrough cancer pain: A multicenter, randomized, controlled, double-blind, double-dummy multiple-crossover study. The Journal of Supportive Oncology. 2011;**9**(6):224-231

[37] Shimoyama N, Gomyo I, Katakami N, et al. Efficacy and safety of sublingual fentanyl orally disintegrating tablet at doses determined by titration for the treatment of breakthrough pain in Japanese cancer patients: A multicenter, randomized, placebo-controlled, double-blind phase III trial. International Journal of Clinical Oncology. 2015;**20**(1):198-206

[38] Rauck RL, Tark M, Reyes E, et al. Efficacy and long-term tolerability of sublingual fentanyl orally disintegrating tablet in the treatment of breakthrough cancer pain. Current Medical Research and Opinion. 2009;**25**(12):2877-2885

[39] Novotna S, Valentova K, Fricova J, et al. A randomized, placebo-controlled study of a new sublingual formulation of fentanyl citrate (fentanyl ethypharm) for breakthrough pain in opioid-treated patients with cancer. Clinical Therapeutics. 2014;**36**(3):357-367

[40] Naohito S, Ikuo G, Osamu T, et al. Efficacy and safety of sublingual fentanyl orally disintegrating tablet at doses determined from oral morphine rescue doses in the treatment of breakthrough cancer pain. Japanese Journal of Clinical Oncology. 2015;**45**(2):189-196

[41] Rauck R, North J, Gever L, et al. Fentanyl buccal soluble film (FBSF) for breakthrough pain in patients with cancer: A randomized, double-blind, placebo-controlled study. Annals of Oncology. 2009;**21**(6):1308-1314

[42] Coluzzi PH, Schwartzberg L, Conroy JD Jr, et al. Breakthrough cancer pain: A randomized trial comparing oral transmucosal fentanyl citrate (OTFC®) and morphine sulfate immediate release (MSIR®). Pain. 2001;**91**(1-2):123-130

Section 4

Non-Pharmacological Approaches

Chapter 9

Wireless Neuromodulation: From Bench to Bedside

Laura Tyler Perryman

Abstract

Spinal cord stimulation (SCS), as a neuromodulation therapy, has rapidly evolved over the past few decades to become the treatment of choice for many chronic pain syndromes. However, many equipment-related limitations such as the bulk of the equipment, an implantable pulse generator (IPG), the limited therapeutic stimulation frequency utilized, and the potential adverse events have restricted SCS applications. Recently, advanced nanotechnology and minimally invasive surgical techniques have shown promising options to expand the indications due to reduced surgical trauma/hospital time/costs. We describe the basis for nanotechnology neuromodulation and the preliminary experience with wireless SCS in the treatment of chronic pain conditions. The equipment utilizes a miniature stimulator with microelectronics, percutaneously placed at the appropriate stimulation target, with wireless control to provide the desired stimulation, and then moderated by the clinician and the patient. The wireless device reduces the bulk of the SCS equipment to a single electrode (with embedded sensors), using the new improved neural-electric interface. This wireless neuromodulation (WNM) has been clinically used in several chronic pain conditions, including failed back surgery syndrome, facial pain, chronic regional pain syndrome, and postherpetic neuralgia, with encouraging outcome, without the complications of a traditional SCS resulting from the IPG or its accessories.

Keywords: neuromodulation, wireless, nanotechnology, chronic pain, spinal cord stimulation

1. Introduction

Therapeutic modulation of excitable neural tissues in the body by electrical stimulation has become an important intervention to manage chronic disabling conditions like pain, involuntary movements, extrapyramidal syndromes, chronic peripheral vascular disease, and cardiac arrhythmias [1–9]. Devices are being implanted to deliver stimulatory signals to the target tissue, record vital signs or action potentials, perform electric cardiac pacing, and control drug release, as well as interface with auditory systems for assisted hearing or even image formation for visual prosthesis. All these systems utilize a subcutaneous battery-operated implanted pulse generator (IPG) to provide power.

Spinal cord stimulation (SCS) has been utilized for over five decades to provide therapeutically effective pain relief from chronic conditions like failed back surgery syndrome (FBSS), regional pain syndromes, and neuralgias, reducing the need for opioids. Several measurable outcomes like pain scores, disability scores, and quality

IntechOpen

of life scales have shown consistent improvement with SCS in patients with back pain and leg pain [1–3].

Outcomes following SCS therapy have demonstrated superior results compared to conservative medical treatment for patients with FBSS in several studies [2, 4], and SCS was also shown to be more cost-effective over the long term due to a decrease in follow-up visits, diagnostic tests, and overall consumption of healthcare facilities [4, 5]. Historically, on the other hand, SCS has not been devoid of complications and limitations in its conventional form utilizing an IPG, since the device options have had a long history of severe adverse events primarily related to the IPG [6, 7]. A large percentage of patients, reportedly as high as 50%, have failed the trial period utilizing conventional SCS devices [6–8], while additional failures came from equipment complications caused by the migration/fracture of the electrodes as well as IPG failures and complications in recharging or reimplantation. Postsurgical complications like infection, hemorrhage, and painful operative wounds were frequently seen associated with IPG and its extension wires. Additionally, SCS in its conventional form is incapable of reaching some anatomical locations to provide targeted therapeutic localized pain relief [6, 8–12].

Several modifications have been introduced to the SCS equipment over the past few years, which have reduced adverse events while promoting the efficacy of the modality, thereby increasing the number of clinical indications [13]. Percutaneous techniques, smaller compact batteries, rechargeable batteries, increased life of the IPG, and improved anchoring methods are some of these modifications currently in use. Part of the refinement also comes from the advancements in the technology of nanomaterials and wireless power transfer techniques.

2. Nanoelectrodes and wireless technology for neuromodulation

An advancement in this field is the new miniature pulse generator (mini PG) with wireless access (WPG) utilizing a dipole antenna for electric field coupling. This is accomplished with "microwaves", which are very short wavelength pulsed electromagnetic waves at gigahertz (GHz) frequencies. This device (Stimwave Technologies, Florida, USA), instead of using lower frequencies of 100 – 500 kHz of the inductive range operational in most of the present-day implanted medical devices, is powered by a radiative electric field coupling through tissues at microwave frequencies that enable smaller-sized implants to be placed at a significant tissue depth through a percutaneous technique. It also affords minimal power loss, since the higher frequency allows a much better energy transfer to a smaller implant [14]. The principle behind the frequency changes in relation to the wavelength was elaborated earlier by Feynman: "If you build a corresponding circuit on a small scale, its natural frequency goes up, since the wave length goes down as the scale; but the skin depth only decreases with the square root of the scale ratio, and so resistive problems are of increasing difficulty. Possibly we can beat resistance through the use of superconductivity if the frequency is not too high, or by other tricks [15]."

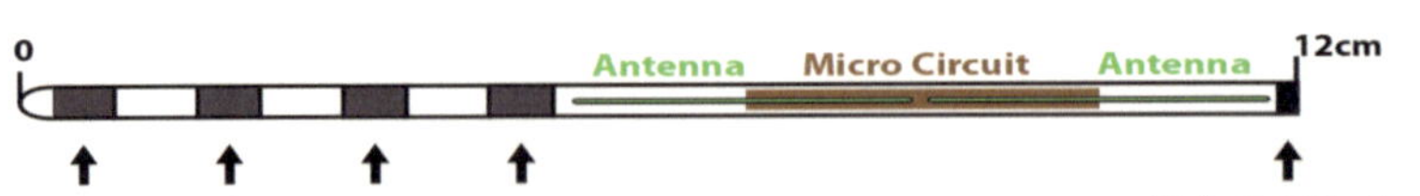

Figure 1.
MRI compatible electrode with nanostimulator and microcircuit to contact wireless pulse generator. This is the only implantable component required for WSCS.

The micro-implant WPG is capable of delivering clinically appropriate stimulation with dimensions of 800–1350 μm diameter, a significantly miniature size compared to the conventional SCS-IPG. This is equal to the size of a standard lead body that also incorporates the nanoelectronics within the device itself. It also can be integrated with a variety of lead types carrying four or eight contacts, either in a percutaneous or a paddle-type electrode, and the receiver wire has circuits in the stimulator device internally with wireless access (**Figure 1**).

3. The implantable wireless lead or the implantable neural stimulator (INS)

The INS has an enclosure housing the stimulating electrode array, designed to apply electrical pulses to the target tissue and antenna-1 and configured to receive electric energy input from an external antenna-2 through electrical radiative coupling. The antenna-2, physically separated from the INS lead, is connected to the antenna-1 by electric circuits configured to generate electrical pulses for stimulating the neural tissue (**Figure 1**).

4. The nanoelectronic substrate of the miniature wireless pulse generator

The INS is without any power source and stays in contact with the excitable neural tissue with passive components capable of receiving an external input signal at a frequency between 300 MHz and 8 GHz. A controller module, positioned in proximity to the patient body, to generate the input signals, sends them to the antenna-2; the latter transmits the input signal to the first dipole antenna placed within the INS through electrical radiative coupling, and antenna-1 extracts the stimulus feedback signal from signals received by the antenna-2 to adjust the parameters of the input signals based on the stimulus feedback.

The electrical pulses from the activated stimulating electrode, however, result in zero net charge within the patient's body. The electrodes can be selectively marked as a stimulating return electrode or an inactive one. It can have one capacitor in series with one or more electrodes.

At present, several therapeutic intra-body electrical stimulation techniques are available to manage neuropathic pain. However, they utilize a bulky, heavy, subcutaneous IPG connected to the implantable wired leads and have many failures or adverse events like mechanical dislodgement, impingement of the lead extension cables, and infection, along with IPG-related discomfort, pain, and irritation. The lead configuration includes cylindrical percutaneous or paddle leads. Cylinders are usually 1.3 mm in diameter and contain several circular electrodes, which are used for trial testing, later followed by permanent placement by minimally invasive, percutaneous approach. Paddles contain electrodes with a wider surface area directionally targeted for control over neural excitation and require invasive surgical procedures like laminectomy or laminotomy.

INS is designed to be placed in the patient through an introducer or a needle with electrodes (**Figure 2**) that include a semicylindrical array of electrodes/contacts made up of platinum, or platinum-iridium, or gallium-nitride, or titanium-nitride, or iridium-oxide or similar combinations. The contacts can be 2–16 in number having a length of 1 to 6 mm and 0.4 to 3 mm in width. They are spaced 1 to 6 mm apart with a combined surface area of 0.8 to 60 mm^2. The lead can also be a paddle type, deliverable through a 14-gauge needle. The enclosure has an external

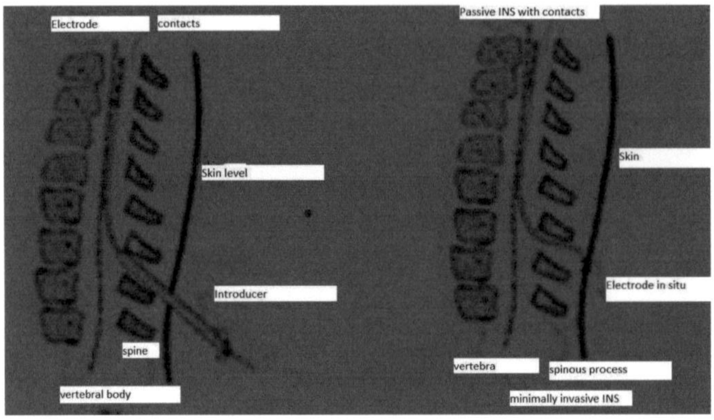

Figure 2.
Minimally invasive approach to place the wireless implantable neural stimulator in the spinal epidural space.

biocompatible coating of polymethyl methacrylate (PMMA), polydimethylsiloxane (PDMS), perylene, polyurethane, polytetrafluoroethylene (PTFE), polycarbonate, or a silicone elastomer.

The antenna-1 within the INS enclosure has 2 to 8 contacts, configured to couple with each other as well as the circuit, and these contacts are located proximally relative to the electrode inside the enclosure. These contacts are 1 to 6 mm in length, 1 to 2.5 mm in width, and spaced 30 to 80 mm apart. One antenna is constructed as a conductive trace contained on the circuits and can be fabricated as a conductive wire connected to the circuits, which are flexible with a bend radius of 0.5 mm and located proximal in the enclosure with a waveform conditioning circuit.

5. Remote control of power or polarity selection for a neural stimulator

The dipole antenna receives input signals containing polarity assignment information and electrical energy, the former designating the polarities for the electrode contacts. The circuits are configured to control an electrode interface so that these electrode contacts have polarities designed by the polarity assignment information to create electrical pulses from the electrical energy contained in the input signal. These electrical pulses reach the contacts according to the polarities assigned.

6. The remote radiofrequency power system with a low-profile transmitting antenna

The antenna for this wireless system includes a metal signal layer with radiating surface, a feed port, a wave guide surrounding the antenna, and a configuration to guide electromagnetic (EM) energy transmitted from the radiating surface in a direction away from the antenna. It also has a controller module connected to the feed port to drive the antenna to transmit EM energy from the radiating surface, while the antenna, wave guide, and controller module are configured to match a reception characteristic of an implantable device, so that the latter can produce electrical pulses of sufficient amplitude to stimulate the target neural tissue utilizing the EM energy received from the antenna-2, located up to 10 cm away.

Adverse events related to the IPG, due to excessive absorption of EM energy, include burning of tissue, creation of undesirable blood clots, and skin irritation

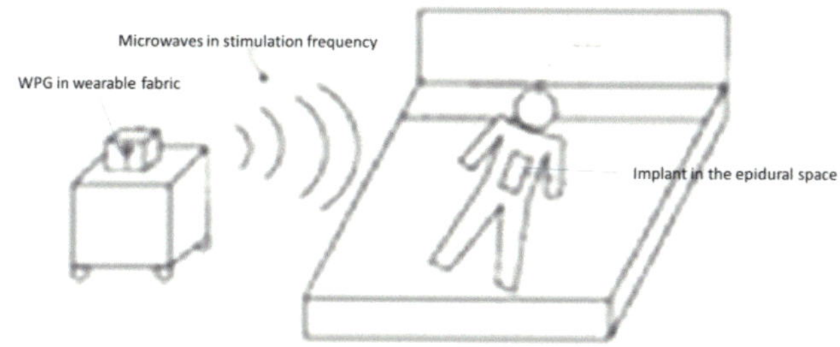

Figure 3.
Remote access by wireless antenna (experimental setting).

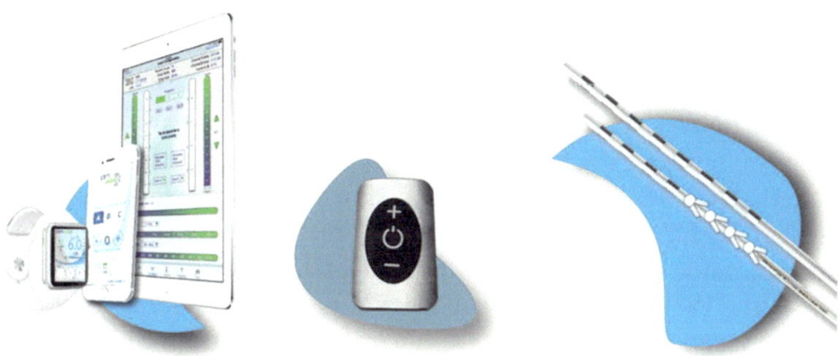

Figure 4.
Neurostimulator receiver. The contacts on the electrodes are managed by independently integrated, circuits that are application specific. The circuitry system within the device produces charge-balanced waveforms.

because of adhesions between the implant and tissues. A wireless device, on the other hand, has the antenna located outside the body with a controller module connecting the implantable device with the antenna (**Figures 3** and **4**).

The antenna has a dielectric lens filling the wave guide, protruding outward from an opening of the wave guide to narrow the transmitted EM energy and direct it away from the transmitting surface. It also has a return loss cutoff frequency associated with the wave guide; the dielectric lens lowers the return loss of cutoff frequency. The antenna operates within 500 MHz to 4 GHz frequency band.

7. Wireless energy supply

The INS receives energy by a wireless method, which includes radiating EM energy from the surface on an antenna located up to 10 cm away, inside the patient, so that the implanted device creates appropriate electrical pulses to stimulate the target neural tissue, using the received EM energy, even during sleep. The radiating surface of the antenna can be placed 1 to 6 feet away from the INS and can be adjusted to increase the EM energy provided to the latter (**Figure 3**). The interface is facilitated by a link between the programmable module and the controller module so that the stimulation pulses created at the implantable device are transmitted as data-encoded parameters from the programming module to the controller module, thus effectively stimulating the neural tissue.

A dipole antenna receiver intercepts the high-frequency microwave EM energy coming from outside the body to produce an oscillating electric field. Frequencies in the range of GHz were found to be more energy efficient [16]. Typically, the antenna within the device lumen can be anywhere from 2 to 8cm long and can be modified depending upon the indications and the depth at which the device is implanted, since the EM field energy is dissipated across the tissue layers of the skin, fat, muscle, blood vessels, and bone. The deeper the placement, the longer the antenna should be to receive adequate power. Each contact on the electrodes is provided with independent power, a part of an "application-specific" integrated circuit; the embedded circuitry within the device enables production of charge-balanced waveforms. This is managed by internalized addressing systems within the device (**Figure 4**). It is important to note that microwave fields are safe, since these high frequencies fail to activate cell membranes and thus nervous tissue damage is unlikely.

8. Wireless pulse generator (WPG)

The WPG employs standard cellular phone technology, with an average pulse output power of up to 1 W, depending upon the stimulation parameters and according to the requirements of the target tissue. A radiofrequency (RF) transmitter placed inside the WPG encodes stimulus waveforms into the signal according to the program settings. A microprocessor inside this transmitter controls the data communications and settings (**Figures 3** and **4**). Clinicians as well as patients communicate with the WPG via a controller that uses Bluetooth technology (**Figure 5**) and also can be accessed by a software application (app) on a mobile phone [14].

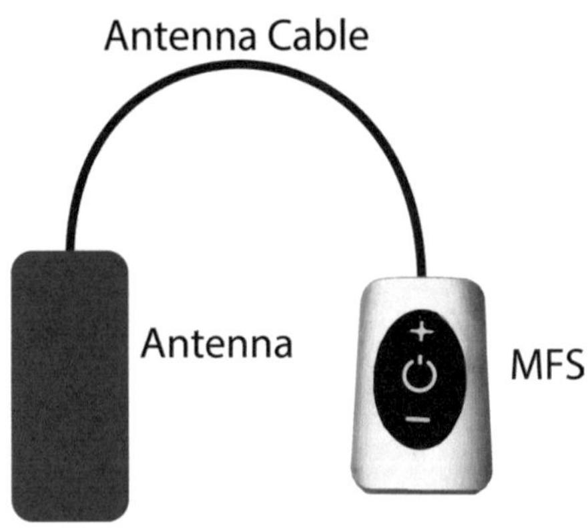

Figure 5.
External wireless pulse generator.

9. Discussion

The traditional SCS (TSCS) system has electrodes in a catheter enclosure attached to a long extension cable(s) that connects the electrodes to an IPG that is placed inside the patient's body, inheriting the complications due to failure or malfunction of any of these components. Efforts have been ongoing to reduce the bulk of the implanted material and yet improve the efficiency of the system. Reduction in size has a challenge from the battery life expectancy with the conventional energy settings. Thus, TSCS equipment requires implantation of electrodes, extension cables, and the battery inside the body, requiring multiple incisions along with long segment tunnels under the skin, producing considerable tissue trauma with pain and hemorrhage.

The wireless SCS system with nanotechnology has been clinically used for SCS, dorsal root ganglia (DRG) stimulation, and peripheral nerve stimulation (PNS) throughout Europe and the USA for several years, and multiple trials have shown encouraging results. The capabilities of this system enabled its utility to be tested in a variety of chronic pain syndromes. Poon et al. [16, 17] demonstrated that in a biological media, the operating frequency for wireless-powered devices was in GHz range as opposed to the MHz, which could have potential advantages. At this frequency range, the size reduction of the receiver has been demonstrated in the subsequent studies by Tyler Perryman et al., while the tissue depth relationship to the energy transmission were further elaborated [17, 18]. Tyler Perryman et al. conducted studies in animals and verified the tissue depths at which the wireless stimulation could achieve effective current density [18]. The dipole antenna of the wireless system (at 915 MHz) could energize the stimulators implanted at a depth of 12 cm in porcine models, especially efficient with a 4.3 cm antenna. Successful stimulation has been observed to provide significant pain relief in patients with back and leg pain with FBSS [19, 20], post herpetic neuralgia [21], refractory craniofacial pain [22], occipital neuralgia [23], and CRPS [24]. Patients undergo implantation of the INS with integrated microcircuits enabling coupling with a pulse generator, while the wireless pulse generator circuit excludes surgical implantation of the IPG, thus eliminating complications related to multiple surgical incisions and interventions for failed IPG or its extension cables. Consequently, there is reduced operating time, minimal consumables, and increased comfort to the patient. In the long run, this should decrease the costs of SCS and reduce overall healthcare budget in neuromodulation.

10. Financial implications and economic benefits with the wireless neuromodulation technology

Every innovation carries financial burden, and there are economic repercussions as the inventions arrive into the clinical practice. For easy understanding, traditional SCS has a structure as follows:

1. Electrodes + connection cables + implantable pulse generator inside the patient body
2. External controller (for the patient as well as the clinician)

Conversely, wireless neuromodulation with nanotechnology utilizes only implantable stimulating electrodes and an implantable receiver placed in a micro-incision pocket. Because of the reduced bulk of the implants, wireless technology has much more to offer other than the costs alone. It reduces surgical trauma, operating time, con-sumables, anesthesia, complications secondary to multiple incisions/tissue trauma, and hospital visits.

11. Costs involved with nanotechnology wireless SCS

The initial implantation of the wireless stimulator	18,000 Euros
IPG costs:	Zero (0)
Annual maintenance of the neuromodulation cost	1500 Euros/3

Compared to the wireless neuromodulation, TSCS was reported to be more expensive (**Table 1**). There have been limited reports on the costs and long-term maintenance

	Author	Journal	Year	No. of patients	Cost
1.	Manca et al. [25]	European J Pain	2008	52	CAD 19,486, Euro 12,653
2.	Kumar et al. [10]	J Neurosurg Spine	2006	160	CAD 23,205
3.	Kumar and Bishop [26]	J Neurosurg Spine	2009	197	CAD 21,595, USD 32,882
4.	Hornberger et al. [27]	Clin J Pain	2008	NA	USD 26,005 (nonrechargeable)
					USD 35,109 (rechargeable)
5.	Babu et al. [28]	Neuromodulation	2013	4536	USD 30,200 (percutaneous)
				4536	USD 29,963 (paddle electrodes)
6.	Annemans et al. [29]	J LTE Med Implants	2014	Model	UK£ 15,056 (HF SCS)

Table 1.
Literature on TSCS cost.

Procedure	TSCS USD*	TSCS CAD*	TSCS UKS*	Stimwave WSCS
Implantation	32,882	21,595	15,081	€18,000
Complication cost	9649	5191	576	NA
Revision cost	5450		5339 (lead)	€2500
IPG cost	**13,150**	**10,591**	**7243**	**0**
Maintenance	**5071 (4 years)**	**3539 (4 years)**	**NA**	**1500 (3 years)**

HF SCS therapy was similar to TSCS in its costs and complications. USD, US dollar; CAD*, Canadian dollar; UKS*, United Kingdom Sterling Pound.*

Table 2.
Reported costs of traditional SCS (TSCS) and the wireless SCS (WSCS).

		European experience [30]	American experience [31]
1.	Repositioning of electrode	€360	$2700
2.	Replacement	€1530	$5450
3.	Reimplantation following infection	€6192	$19,600

Table 3.
Costs for lead revision/repositioning in TSCS.

of TSCS in the literature. Detailed report on follow-up costs, complications, and replacement charges for reimplantation has not been forthcoming. However, the natural course of TSCS with its multiple implant components leading to their inherent complications could be expected as reported in a few of the studies (**Tables 1–3**). Wireless neuromodulation is evolving, and only limited experience has been reported so far. However, large-scale multicenter studies have been initiated to improve our understanding about the efficacy and acceptable long-term results in the form of improved quality of life, reduced complications, reduction in healthcare costs, and better cosmetic results.

12. Conclusions

Nanoelectronics have contributed to the development of miniature implants for therapeutic purposes, and wireless technology coupled with mini WPG appears to enhance the quality of neuromodulation in the field of functional neurosurgery and pain management therapies. Wireless neuromodulation, so far applied as SCS, DRG, and PNS, has provided efficient pain relief in cases of FBSS, neuralgic pain, CRPS, and facial pain syndromes. The results observed in small case series or case illustrations are comparable to traditional SCS methods and devoid of many of the complications of TSCS, primarily related to IPG/battery accessories. Further wireless neuromodulation experience may demonstrate improved quality of life associated with significant reduction in cost as well as reduction in complications, with improved cosmetic and functional results.

Copyright information

Authors hold the following patents. Information in the chapter includes material from the patent applications.

1. US9409029B2. Remote RF power system with low profile transmitting antenna
2. US9254393B2. Wearable antenna assembly
3. US9220897B2. Implantable lead
4. US9199089B2. Remote control of power or polarity selection for a neural stimulator
5. US8849412B2. Microwave field stimulator
6. US8903502B2. Methods and devices for modulating excitable tissue of the exiting spinal nerves
7. US9409030B2. Neural stimulator system
8. US15228715. Remote rf power system with low profile transmitting antenna
9. US9522270B2. Circuit for an implantable device

Author has copyrights on the publications referenced [18, 19, 22, 23].

Author details

Laura Tyler Perryman
Stimwave Technologies, Inc., Pompano Beach, Florida, USA

*Address all correspondence to: laura@stimwave.com

References

[1] Turner JA, Loeser JD, Bell KG. Spinal cord stimulation for chronic low back pain: A systematic literature synthesis. Neurosurgery. 1995;**37**:1088-1096

[2] Kumar K, Taylor RS, Jacques L, et al. The effects of spinal cord stimulation in neuropathic pain are sustained: A 24-month follow-up of the prospective randomized controlled multicenter trial of the effectiveness of spinal cord stimulation. Neurosurgery. 2008;**63**:762-770

[3] Kapural L, Yu C, Doust M, et al. Novel 10-kHz high-frequency therapy (HF10 therapy) is superior to traditional low-frequency spinal cord stimulation for the treatment of chronic back and leg pain the SENZA-RCT randomized controlled trial. Anesthesiology. 2015;**123**:851-860

[4] Deer TR, Mekhail N, Provenzano D, et al. The appropriate use of neurostimulation of the spinal cord and peripheral nervous system for the treatment of chronic pain and ischemic diseases: The neuromodulation appropriateness consensus committee. Neuromodulation. 2014;**17**:515-550

[5] Mekhail NA, Aeschbach A, Stanton-Hicks M. Cost benefit analysis of neurostimulation for chronic pain. The Clinical Journal of Pain. 2004;**20**:462-468

[6] Turner JA, Loeser JD, Deyo RA, Sanders SB. Spinal cord stimulation for patients with failed back surgery syndrome or complex regional pain syndrome: A systematic review of effectiveness and complications. Pain. 2004;**108**:137-147

[7] Mekhail NA, Mathews M, Nageeb F, Guirguis M, et al. Retrospective review of 707 cases of spinal cord stimulation: Indications and complications. Pain Practice. 2011;**11**:148-153

[8] Cameron T. Safety and efficacy of spinal cord stimulation for the treatment of chronic pain: A 20-year literature review. Journal of Neurosurgery. 2004;**100**:254-267

[9] Krishna K, Jefferson RW, Gupta S. Complications of spinal cord stimulation, suggestions to improve outcome, and financial impact. Journal of Neurosurgery. 2006;**5**:191-203

[10] Kumar K, Hunter G, Demeria D. Spinal cord stimulation in treatment of chronic benign pain: Challenges in treatment planning and present status, a 22-year experience. Neurosurgery. 2006;**58**:481-496

[11] North RB, Kidd DH, Zahurak M, et al. Spinal cord stimulation for chronic, intractable pain: Experience over two decades. Neurosurgery 1993;**32**:384-394; discussion 394-395.

[12] Pineda A. Complications of dorsal column stimulation. Journal of Neurosurgery. 1978;**48**:64-68

[13] Slavin KV. Spinal stimulations for pain: Future applications. Neurotherapeutics. 2014;**11**:535-542

[14] Yearwood TL, Perryman LT. Peripheral neurostimulation with a microsize wireless stimulator. In: Slavin KV, editor. Stimulation of the Peripheral Nervous System. The Neuromodulation Frontier. Progress in Neurological Surgery. Basel, Switzerland: Karger Publishing; 2016. pp. 168-191

[15] Feynman RP. There's plenty of room at the bottom. CalTech, Pasedena CA: Presentation to the American Physical Society; 1959

[16] Poon AS, O'Driscoll S, Meng TH. Optimal operating frequency in wireless power transmission for implantable devices. In: Conf Proc IEEE Eng Med

Biol Soc; Lyon, France. 2007. pp. 5674-5679

[17] Poon A, O'Driscoll, Meng TH. Optimal frequency for wireless power transmission into dispersive tissue. IEEE Transactions on Antennas and Propagation. 2010;**58**:1739-1750

[18] Tyler Perryman L, Larson P, Glaser J. Tissue depth study for a fully implantable, remotely powered and programmable wireless neural stimulator. International Journal of Nano Studies and Technology. 2016;**S2**(001):1-6

[19] Weiner RL, Yeung A, Garcia CM, Perryman LT, Speck B. Treatment of FBSS low back pain with a novel percutaneous DRG wireless stimulator: Pilot and feasibility study. Pain Medicine. 2016;**17**:1911-1916

[20] Billet B, Wynendaele R, Vanquathem N. Wireless neuromodulation by a minimally invasive technique for chronic refractory pain. Report of preliminary observations. Medical Research Archives. 2017;**5**:1-8

[21] Billet B, Wynendaele R, Vanquathem N. A novel minimally invasive wireless technology for neuromodulation via percutaneous intercostal nerve stimulation (PNS) for post-herpetic neuralgia: A case report with short term follow up. Pain Practice. 2018;**3**:374-379

[22] Weiner RL, Garcia CM, Vanquathem N. A novel miniature wireless neurostimulator in the management of chronic craniofacial pain: Preliminary results from a prospective pilot study. Scandinavian Journal of Pain. 2017:350-354

[23] Perryman LT, Speck B, Weiner RL. A novel wireless minimally invasive neuromodulation device for the treatment of chronic intractable occipital neuralgia: Case illustrations. Journal of Neurology & Stroke. 2017;**6**:00213

[24] Herschkowitz D, Kubias J. Wireless peripheral nerve stimulation for complex regional pain syndrome type I of the upper extremity: A case illustration introducing a novel technology. Scandinavian Journal of Pain. July 2018:555-560

[25] Manca A, Kumar K, Taylor RS, Jacques L, Eldabe S, Meglio M, et al. Quality of life, resource consumption and costs of spinal cord stimulation versus conventional medical management in neuropathic pain patients with failed back surgery syndrome (PROCESS trial). European Journal of Pain. 2008;**12**:1047-1058

[26] Kumar K, Bishop S. Financial impact of spinal cord stimulation on the health care budget: A comparative analysis of costs in Canada and the United States. Journal of Neurosurgery: Spine. 2009;**10**:564-573

[27] Hornberger J, Kumar K, Verhulst E, Clark MA, Hernandez J. Rechargeable spinal cord stimulation versus non-rechargeable system for patient with failed back surgery syndrome: A cost consequences analysis. The Clinical Journal of Pain. 2008;**24**:244-252

[28] Babu R, Hazzard MA, Huang KT, Ugiliweneza B, Patil CG, Boakye M, et al. Outcomes of percutaneous and paddle lead implantation for spinal cord stimulation: A comparative analysis of complications, reoperation rates, and health-care costs. Neuromodulation. 2013;**16**:418-427

[29] Annemans L, Van Buyten JP, Smith T, Al-Kaisy A. Cost effectiveness of a novel 10 kHz high-frequency spinal cord stimulation system in patients with failed back surgery syndrome (FBSS). Journal of Long-Term Effects of Medical Implants. 2014;**24**:173-183

[30] Kemler MA, Furnee CA. Economic evaluation of spinal cord stimulation for chronic reflex sympathetic dystrophy. Neurology. 2002;**59**:1203-1209

[31] Bell GK, Kidd D, North RB. Cost-effectiveness analysis of spinal cord stimulation in treatment of failed back surgery syndrome. Journal of Pain and Symptom Management. 1997;**13**:286-295

Chapter 10

myoActivation: A Structured Process for Chronic Pain Resolution

Gillian Lauder, Nicholas West and Greg Siren

"The good physician treats the disease; the great physician treats the patient who has the disease".

Sir William Osler, 1849–1919

Abstract

Chronic pain is a significant burden in all societies. The myofascial origins of chronic pain are often unrecognized but play a major role in chronic pain generation. Myofascial release has been shown to be effective and can augment the limited number of therapeutic tools available to manage chronic pain. However, there is no standardized approach that allows for comparative analysis of this technique. *myoActivation*® is a unique therapeutic system, which targets active myofascial trigger points, fascia in tension, and scars in patients with chronic pain. Targets for intervention are determined through obtaining a history of lifetime trauma and a structured, reproducible posture, and movement assessment. Catenated cycles of movement tests, palpation, and needling are used to achieve the goal of pain resolution through restoration of soft tissue integrity. This chapter describes the distinctive features of *myoActivation* from the important key elements of the patient's clinical history, through to the aftercare instructions. Relevant evidence for each component will be presented. Case studies will be used to illustrate some important concepts and the effectiveness of *myoActivation*. This chapter is relevant to all clinicians that manage people living with chronic pain.

Keywords: pain, chronic pain, paediatric pain, mobility dysfunction, fascia, myofascial trigger points, timeline of lifetime trauma, physical trauma, scars, palpation, catenated cycles, structured assessment, non-pharmaceutical, pain management

1. Introduction

Pain is defined by the International Association for the Study of Pain (IASP) as "an unpleasant sensory and emotional experience associated with actual or potential tissue damage or described in terms of such damage" [1]. Pain is a highly subjective sensation influenced by: degree of tissue damage, response to medications, diet, age, sex, genetics, cultural background, and psychosocial factors including attention, emotion, cognition, beliefs, expectations, and socioeconomic status (**Figure 1**).

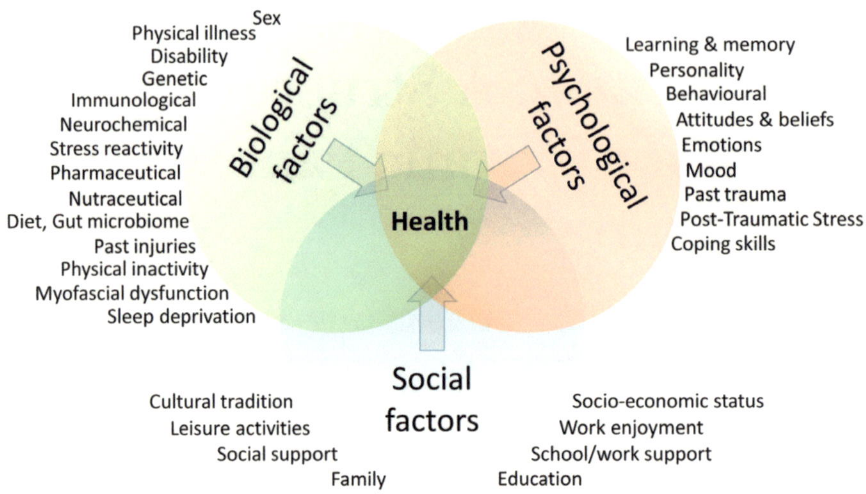

Figure 1.
The biopsychosocial contributors to chronic pain.

Pain is a sensory output from the brain when the brain is on alert. In acute pain, this sensory output is important to protect the organism from further harm during the healing phase, and, is usually associated with a nociceptive stimulus.

Chronic pain is quite different; although it is typically considered to refer to pain lasting longer than 3 months, such a time limit seems to be reductive, and it more properly refers to "pain that extends beyond the expected period of healing" [2]. The overall prevalence of chronic pain conditions is estimated to be in the order of 35–51% of the adult population [3] and the incidence of widespread chronic pain estimated to be 10–15% [4]. Chronic pain occurs across the lifespan, including children [5] and the elderly [6]. The frequency of visits to physicians, emergency departments, and other healthcare providers is significantly increased in the presence of chronic pain [7]. Currently, the burden of chronic pain has a huge impact on quality of life in the lives of people with chronic pain [8, 9]. The economic burden of chronic pain in terms of healthcare costs is substantial, but pales in significance compared to the costs of lost productivity due to job redundancy and sick days [9].

1.1 Background

Chronic pain is a complex biopsychosocial phenomenon that requires a multidisciplinary approach to management. This usually includes return to physical function [10], graded return to work/school, medications to help with pain, mood and sleep, as well as non-pharmacological techniques to address the psychosocial components of pain [9, 11, 12]. The weakest link in this therapeutic process is the pharmacological approach, especially the overreliance on the use of *opioid* medications. The prescription of opioids for chronic non-cancer pain increased fourfold in USA from the early 1990s up to 2011 [13, 14]. Opioids contribute only modest relief of chronic pain. They have limited effects on improvement in function but cause significant opioid side effects [15]. Opioid substance abuse and opioid-related death are major issues associated with prescription of opioids for chronic pain. Review of opioid-related deaths demonstrates that the majority had a diagnosis of chronic pain in their last year of life [16]. Prescription of opioid medications has gradually decreased since 2011, but the opioid-related overdose death rate continues to rise exponentially [17]. This current opioid crisis constitutes a critical public health issue in USA and Canada [13]. Even though the prescription of opioid drugs does not appear to be causally related to overdose deaths, it is clear that their prescription is one pathway to long-term use: 5.3% of opioid naïve adults prescribed opioids will still be on opioids 1 year later [18]. Increased numbers of opioids prescribed on the first prescription predicts a lower likelihood of opioid discontinuation [18]. It is notable that 20% of children with chronic musculoskeletal pain are prescribed opioids [19].

Up to 22.5% of chronic pain patients develop their chronic pain condition after surgery [20]. *Persistent postsurgical pain* (*PPSP*) represents a significant clinical problem, occurring after 10–50% of surgeries and resulting in severe chronic pain in 2–10% of these patients [21]. PPSP is considered to be primarily neuropathic (nerve damage during surgery) where the incidence depends on various perioperative factors, including genetic predisposition, preoperative anxiety, depression, preoperative pain, the extent of the surgical insult, surgical technique, length of surgery, and the quality of acute postoperative pain management [21, 22]. In 27% of patients receiving chronic opioid therapy, treatment for pain after surgery was the reason for opioid initiation [23]. There is 5.9–6.5% incidence of new persistent opioid use after surgery, not only after major surgery but also after minor surgical procedures [24].

Multiple traumas have a cumulative effect on chronic pain [25], independent of post-traumatic distress disorder symptoms [26]. Increased risk of physical ill-health is associated with exposure to a single traumatic event but accrues as more events are experienced [27]. It is not clear what characteristics of past traumatic experiences (type, duration, severity, earlier onset) influence the strength of the relationship between accumulative traumatic events and subsequent medical conditions [28]. Contemporary clinical history taking often neglects distant trauma as significant contributor to a chronic pain issue presenting many years later.

Chronic pain occurs from various combined sources, including nociceptive, inflammatory, neuropathic, myofascial, as well as peripheral and central sensitisation. *Musculoskeletal* (*MSK*) conditions are a predominant source of chronic pain worldwide [29]. The clinical and etiological characteristics of myofascial pain have been poorly investigated. The subsequent lack of evidence has led to undertraining of health care professionals, and poor recognition of the clinical importance of *myofascial pain syndromes* (a group of painful conditions that affect muscles and connective tissues) [30, 31].

Myofascial pain syndromes are characterized by pain, *myofascial trigger points* (*MTPs*) (palpable nodules in taut bands of muscle fibres), referred pain, coupled pain, and autonomic changes. Chemical changes within the muscle may also lead to peripheral sensitization. MTPs can generate continual nociceptive traffic to induce central sensitization, cortical re-organization, and alterations in descending inhibitory pain pathways [32–36]. MTPs are associated with muscles in sustained contraction causing limited movement across joints [37]. The MSK system is symmetrical; a muscle in sustained contraction on one side will cause compensatory MSK issues to occur on the other. Therefore, a patient with MSK imbalance may proceed to have many different myofascial areas affected from one previous injury or insult. It is important to note that *palpable pain points* (*PPPs*) exist, not only in skeletal muscle, but also in fascia and scars.

One of the components of MSK pain is *coupled pain*, which is distinct from referred pain. Referred pain is pain perceived at a location other than the site of the painful stimulus or origin of pain. Referred pain results from neuronal stimulation within a dermatome (a localized area of skin that has its sensation via a single nerve, from a single nerve root of the spinal cord). In coupled pain, the source of pain is distant, not dermatomal, from the localized area of pain. Examples include shoulder pain or knee pain originating from strained ipsilateral external oblique muscle, or lower quadrant abdominal pain originating from an ipsilateral quadratus lumborum muscle in sustained contraction [38–40]. This distant site has no direct muscular or neurological connection, yet the coupled pain is resolved by restoration of the originating tissue to a normal anatomical state [41].

Myofascial release can be effective but lacks a standardized approach and therefore prevents good quality comparative analysis.

Given the societal burden of pain and overuse of opioid medications, it is clear that clinicians require a different and more effective model of assessment and treatment that minimizes opioid prescriptions and realizes myofascial components of pain [19, 42]. This chapter will outline the importance of surgical scars and myofascial dysfunction as other important determinants of a chronic pain presentation. *myoActivation* is one component of the multimodal approach to patient care that helps to accurately determine and treat the myofascial components of chronic pain without the need for prescription medications.

1.2 Aim

The aim of this chapter is to describe a system of standardized assessment and treatment for chronic pain called *myoActivation*®. We will comprehensively describe the distinctive features of this system, from the patient's clinical history to after-care management. We will present evidence for the scientific background and individual component techniques of *myoActivation*, where it exists, and outline future approaches for gathering evidence of the effectiveness and efficiency of the *myoActivation* treatment programme as a whole.

This chapter is practically orientated to enable clinicians to understand what *myoActivation* means. Three case studies will illustrate the effectiveness of *myoActivation*. Then, the next steps in the development and evaluation of *myoActivation* will be discussed. Barriers to integrative care (including alternative therapies) are awareness, availability, accessibility, and affordability [43]; these will be discussed in relation to *myoActivation* as well as the need to establish a firm basis of clinical evidence for this treatment system.

Finally, we must emphasize that *myoActivation* should be seen as one component of multidisciplinary care, i.e., part of a multimodal approach to care, which includes focus on eventual return to physical function and work/school, improving recovery from opioid dependency, weaning prescription drug use as well treating the psychosocial components of pain.

1.3 *myoActivation* overview

myoActivation is a unique structured system of assessment and treatment designed to reduce myofascial components of chronic pain. A key principle of *myoActivation* is to understand that the site of pain is often not the source of pain [38–41, 44]. For example, spasm of the quadratus lumborum muscle mimics appendicitis and low back pain may originate from the abdominal wall musculature [38, 39, 45]. Myofascial pain is characterised by the presence of myofascial trigger points. Myofascial trigger points develop in response to many different insults such as trauma, injury, surgery, repetitive microtrauma, poor posture, muscle overuse, or overload [46, 47]. Myofascial trigger points that cause pain can originate in scars, skeletal muscle, and/or fascia.

The *myoActivation* assessment is distinguished by recognition of the importance of lifetime trauma and the mechanisms of any injuries identified. Postural observations during systematized, ordered, movement tests identify the true origin of pain in soft tissues. The most painful or restricted movement on core tests distinguishes the most important tissues to treat first. Careful inspection and palpation of these tissues identifies the myofascial source of pain. Treatment entails refined trigger point injections, using micro-aliquots of physiological saline, to restore anatomic integrity to injured tissues. Fine gauge hypodermic needles are inserted into trigger points that compromise function of muscle, ligament, tendon, subcutaneous fascia, scar tissue, and the peripheral nerves of the skin. After each individual myofascial area is treated, movement tests are repeated to demonstrate immediate change and direct the clinician to the next most important target area. Several cycles occur during each *myoActivation* session. The purpose of these catenated cycles (see **Figure 6**) is to help unravel multiple sources that contribute to the full myofascial pain presentation.

Immediate treatment responses occur, which include reduction in pain, increased flexibility, and improved fluidity of movement. After-care instructions require the patient to change posture frequently but to refrain from exertional activity for 5 days following every *myoActivation* session. To understand how this technique might be useful in everyday care of patients with chronic pain, it is important to understand the essential components of myofascial pain (skeletal muscle in sustained contraction, scars, fascial lines of tension, and the interstitial space).

2. Scientific background

2.1 Skeletal muscle in sustained contraction

Myofascial pain syndrome is characterized by multisite pain, referred pain, coupled pain, and peripheral and central sensitisations. A component of myofascial pain is due to MTPs associated with muscles in sustained contraction causing limitation of movement across joints [37]. The mechanisms of myofascial pain have been reviewed by Jafri [31] and Shah et al. [48].

A 2007 review identified 19 different descriptions of diagnostic criteria for myofascial trigger points and associated pain but found lack of consensus or standard definition [49].

A trigger point is a hyperirritable spot in fascia or surrounding skeletal muscle. Muscular trigger points are associated with palpable nodules in taut bands of muscle fibres. Compression of a trigger point may elicit local tenderness, referred pain, coupled pain, autonomic symptoms, or a local twitch response. The *local twitch response (LTR)* is recognized as a spinal reflex [50]. An LTR when the MTP is needled or activated is considered a positive response to intervention [51].

Microdialysis techniques demonstrate unique biochemical changes in the region of trigger points, which include low pH, increased concentrations of bradykinin, calcitonin gene-related peptide, substance P, tumour necrosis factor (TNF), interleukins, serotonin, and norepinephrine. These are also associated with decreased local blood flow, reduced oxygen content, and increased reactive oxygen species. These nociceptive neuropeptides and inflammatory markers may be the source of peripheral nociception potentially initiating and maintaining central sensitization in myofascial pain syndrome [48, 52, 53].

The veracity of myofascial trigger points representing true pathologic entities have been questioned and debated [54]. However, leading experts in myofascial techniques consider this to be a biased view [55].

A systematic MSK exam can distinguish patients with MTPs and chronic pain from subjects with no pain [56]. One of the main problems with medical community acceptance of MTPs has been the lack of objective imaging techniques to corroborate examination findings and to assess treatment outcomes [57]. Imaging techniques that have been reported to establish the presence of muscle MTPs include: *magnetic resonance elastography* (MRE) [58], and *sonoelastography* (SEG) (**Figure 2**) [59]. MRE couples MRI with cyclic shear waves to assess tissue stiffness in myofascial taut bands. Stiffness in taut bands was found to be 50% greater than adjacent normal muscle tissue. SEG is a non-invasive method that combines

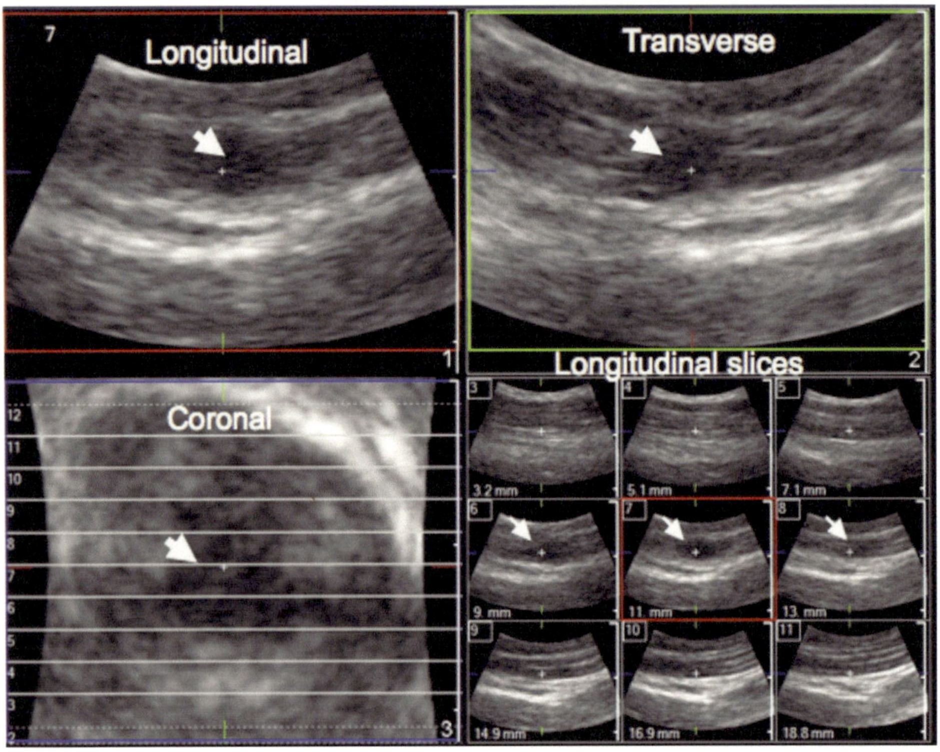

Figure 2.
Sonography of muscle trigger points (reproduced from Sikdar et al. [59], with permission from Elsevier).

ultrasound with simultaneously applied external vibration to distinguish ultrasound colour variance with tissue stiffness. Muscle trigger points identified as palpable painful nodules in muscle appear as focal, elliptical shaped, hypoechogenic areas. Localized regions of low entropy in symptomatic muscle make the tissue macroscopically more heterogeneous than a normal muscle that has relatively uniform echotexture. Texture analysis of SEG images can distinguish between painful muscle trigger points compared to normal muscle [60, 61].

2.1.1 Muscle activation

Muscle activation is the term used to describe when a muscle in sustained contraction is restored to a normal relaxed state, through manipulative therapies or needling techniques [62]. When a needling technique is used, there is no difference in outcomes between dry needling compared to a liquid injectate (such as lidocaine) [63–65]. Muscle activation is associated with reduction in pain, and improved flexibility, fluidity and range of movement. There is no consensus on the most effective needling techniques for different pain presentations [66]. Elicitation of an LTR has classically been required for effective muscle activation [51]. Recent work disputes that an LTR is necessary, but acknowledges more research is required [67]. Decreased spontaneous electrical activity and acetylcholine levels are seen at active myofascial trigger points after dry needling in rats [68].

Vascular, chemical, endocrine, neural, and central changes have been demonstrated following needling techniques [68–86]. Interestingly, dry needling also appears to be associated with activation of diffuse noxious inhibitory control reducing pain sensitivity in remote areas to the site of needling. This may be mediated through endogenous opioid mechanisms [69, 79–84].

There are a number of papers in support of the treatment effects, beyond the placebo effect, of myofascial release [51, 62, 66, 87–99]. Recent reviews have concluded that better quality studies with standardized interventions and outcomes are required to show that myofascial release is an effective intervention in the different types of myofascial pain syndromes [100–102]. Despite this, it is clear that myofascial trigger points in skin, fascia, and muscles play an important role in myofascial chronic pain presentations.

MTPs and their referral patterns have been eloquently outlined in two volumes by Travell and Simons, the first volume for the upper body and the second for the lower half of the body [46, 47]. Unfortunately, the publication of these volumes did not translate into everyday use in common clinical practice due to a number of factors: lack of basic scientific evidence around the aetiology of MTPs, no gold standard to identify clinical MTPs, failure to include reproducible assessment and examination of MTPs in medical curricula, complexity and diagnostic uncertainty from the interaction of more than one MTP on perceived pain, co-occurrence of myofascial pain with other disorders such as arthritis, and under-recognition of myofascial components in chronic pain [30].

2.2 Skin and the impact of scars

The skin is one of the largest organs in the body and is naturally exposed to external stimuli. The skin provides a crucial interface between the body and its environment. Skin has different functions and connections, which include connections to the nervous system through the autonomic nervous system and the locomotor apparatus [103]. The autonomic nervous system constitutes the most important connection between the skin, the fascia, and the body [39]. There is continual nervous activity, in afferent and efferent mode, between the skin and central nervous system to maintain normal homeostasis [39, 104].

There is an independent central emotional connection principally between the anterior cingulate cortex and the skin whereby a sympathetic electrical signal can be detected in the skin in response to viewing emotionally charged images [105]. The skin is also a primary site of small fibre nociceptive endings [106]. It is not difficult to speculate that any restriction or impact on the skin, like a scar, will have an impact on normal homeostasis and function and hold emotional memory [107, 108].

2.2.1 Scars

When the skin is breached by surgery or injury, a healing process occurs. There are four stages to healing: haemostasis, inflammation, proliferation, and remodelling [109]. The remodelling process can take many years and depends on the size and nature of the initial wound. During remodelling, type 3 collagen is replaced by a stronger type 1 collagen, but not in an ordered manner. Scar tissue is therefore strong but not as elastic or flexible as normal tissue [109]. There is an increase in nerves and neuropeptides in scar tissue especially hypertrophic scars [110]. In patients asked to move actively, electrical activity from a scarred area is higher than that from normal tissue in the same patient doing the same movement [111].

Mechanoreceptors and mechanosensitive nociceptors in scarred areas sense an alteration from normal and send non-physiological signals creating a pathological reflex arc [39]. Scars can limit normal movement and flexibility of skin, and underlying fascia and muscles. For example, an ankle scar will alter the gait dynamics through maldistribution of myofascial loads [39]. Patients with scars in the abdominal region often have low back pain related to impaired mobility of the soft tissues [111, 112]. Scars also have an impact on the distribution of forces that pass through the body following motor vehicle accident (MVA) or injury [39]. It has also been suggested that the skin can keep a memory of trauma [107, 108]. It is clinically important to consider this when releasing scars associated with a particular emotional traumatic event. More research is required to ascertain the characteristics of scars that make a significant contribution to a chronic pain presentation.

2.2.2 Scar release

Scar release can be achieved with soft tissue mobilization techniques or subcision [107, 111, 113]. *Subcision*, or microneedling, also known as percutaneous collagen induction therapy, is a minimally invasive minor surgical procedure used for treating depressed cutaneous scars and wrinkles. Subcision is performed using a hypodermic needle inserted through a puncture in the skin surface [114] or dermaroller. First described in 1995 [115], subcision is a safe, and effective microneedling technique used as an aesthetic treatment for several different dermatological conditions including scars, rhytids, and striae [114, 116, 117]. Microneedling has been shown to induce new collagen formation via platelet and neutrophil release of growth factors (TGFβ, platelet derived growth factor, connective tissue growth factor, connective tissue activating protein), resulting in increased production of collagen, elastin, and glycosaminoglycans [118]. The penetration of a needle through skin has been shown to produce other physiological effects such as activation of the diffuse noxious inhibitory control systems [119], as well as oxytocin mediated peripheral stimulation that inhibits c-fibre discharge to suppress experimental behavioural nociception in rats [120].

Currently, the immediate relief of chronic pain following needling of surgical scars is limited to case reports [110], and to date, there is insufficient evidence to advise on the right time to treat scars after surgery [121]. It will be seen later that scar identification and release is an integral part of *myoActivation* therapy for chronic pain.

2.3 Fascial lines of tension

Fascia is described as "dense irregular connective tissue, this tissue surrounds and connects every muscle, even the tiniest myofibril, and every single organ of the body. It forms a true continuity throughout our whole body" [122, 123]. Fascia has traditionally been named according to the region in which it invests, for example, thoracolumbar fascia or the iliotibial band. This regional focus is considered to be a barrier to the understanding the whole-body interconnectivity of fascia [124]. Fascia has both loose and hard fibrous connective tissue components. Loose fascia functions to help slide and glide between structures and dense fascia exerts a tensile strength in tissues like tendons. Fascia is a complex structure. It contains cells (fibroblasts, fasciocytes, myofibroblasts, and telocytes), an extracellular matrix (fibres, hyaluronan, and water), nerve elements (proprioceptors, interoceptors, and nociceptors), and a system of microchannels (the primovascular system) [125]. The contractile elements may contribute to spasms, dysfunction, and pain [39]. The fasciocytes produce hyaluronan in response to shear stresses [125]. The fascial fibroblasts produce collagen in response to load and stretching. Telocytes are probably important in regeneration [126]. Fascia is rich in proprioceptors and is an essential integrative component in the locomotor apparatus in assessment and control of human posture and movement organization [70]. Fascia has been nicknamed our organ of form [39, 127, 128]. Techniques are currently being developed to improve imaging of fascia [129].

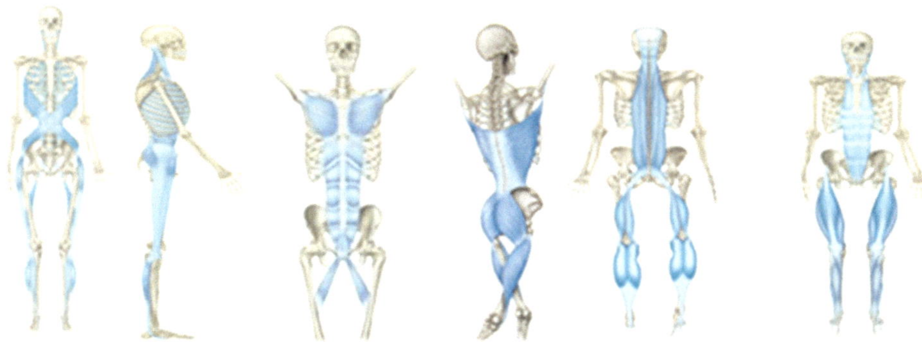

Figure 3.
Proposed myofascial chains (reproduced from Wilke et al. [136], with permission from Elsevier).

Fascia flexibility is reduced following injury and subsequent immobility; this worsens with time and persists even with restoration of movement [130]. Stretching, however, reduces thickness of inflammatory lesions, reduces migration of neutrophils, and increases concentration of pro-resolving mediators (resolvins) [130–134]. It is becoming increasingly clear that fascia has an extremely important role to play in molecular biology, functional anatomy, exercise, sport science, repair mechanisms, as well as therapeutic modalities [135]. As *myoActivation* is associated with improvements in flexibility and posture, it may well be that one of its effects is mediated through fascial mechanisms that enable movement and stretch in a more normal anatomical manner.

Biotensegrity is a structural design concept that defines the relationship between parts of an organism and the mechanical system that integrates them into a functional unit. Humans are described as tension-dependent organisms with myofascial chains (**Figure 3**) [136]. These myofascial chains enable three-dimensional movement while continually providing information on balance, stability, and mobility. These chains often have an opposing chain to help achieve this balance within the MSK system; for example, a posterior myofascial chain pairs with an anterior myofascial chain.

These chains may well help to explain how some pain presentations at distant sites, and how myofascial release at distant sites (or opposite sides of the body) resolve coupled pain presentations. For example, release of the external oblique muscle in sustained contraction will help shoulder pain, release of tension around the coccyx will help with neck pain, and/or release of the gastrocnemius/soleus muscles in sustained contraction relieves occipital headaches.

2.4 The interstitial space

The interstitial space is a major fluid compartment present in many parts of the body. It contains dynamically compressible and distensible sinuses through which interstitial fluid flows around the body. It is distinct from, but drains into, the lymphatic system. In the average human, up to 15 L of extracellular fluid are normally housed in the extracellular interstitial space. *Interstitial fluid* (ISF) and flow is an important element of normal tissue function; it bathes and surrounds cells, delivers nutrients, and removes metabolic waste [137]. ISF also affects cell signalling, differentiation, remodelling, and migration (giving directional cues to cells) [138]. The ISF only flows under conditions of low hydraulic resistance. Blockage of these channels in pigs induces hyperalgesia [139]. Release of tight tissues, following *myoActivation*, may help to restore interstitial fluid flow and promote the delivery of nutrients and removal of metabolic waste of surrounding tissues.

More research is required to determine exactly which component (muscle, biomechanics, the interstitium, fascia, skin, scars or a combination of these) is the major contributor to a chronic pain presentation. The rest of this chapter will outline the specific details of the basics of *myoActivation*, which provides the much-needed standardized process to correctly identify and treat MTPs in priority order, to reduce chronic pain.

3. *myoActivation*: detailed methods

3.1 Clinical history

As with all chronic pain presentations, it is important to define the clinical problem, the main site of perceived pain, with its transition over time, as well as the goals of treatment for the patient. The focus of a *myoActivation* history frames the clinical problem as the *Timeline of Lifetime Trauma* (TiLT) and the mechanisms of any injuries reported. TiLT requires careful questioning to determine if there have been any motor vehicle accidents, fractures, sprains, falls, tailbone injury, major surgery, minor surgery, burns, bites, or other scars (e.g., chicken pox or acne). The associated healing process of any scar is essential to determine their significance in the pain presentation. Infection during a healing process or injuries and scars sustained at a young age appear to have significant impact. Recreational and occupational activities with any associated injuries are important components that need to be asked. An important enquiry in the *myoActivation* history is to ask the patient what they consider to be their greatest physical trauma. All these details will be synthesized with the subsequent examination findings to help determine the true source of pain.

3.1.1 Investigations

Routine imaging investigations are typically not useful to guide *myoActivation* treatment. However, reports on imaging studies that are provided with a referral or by the patient should be reviewed and acknowledged in the encounter documentation.

3.1.2 Examination

Optimally, the patient has as much skin exposed as possible to allow easier evaluation of postural asymmetries, fascial lines of tension, skin creases, and forgotten scars. Initially, the patient is asked to identify the location of their perceived pain; this point helps direct the examination and is used as an index for subsequent treatment effect. Where the patient identifies the perceived origin of pain is rarely the tissue that is responsible for the true origin of pain. Then, core Biomechanical Assessment and Symmetry Evaluation (BASE) tests are administered (**Figure 4**). In execution of all tests, the clinician is always looking for postural asymmetries.

3.1.3 Balance

The first BASE test is balance. The talus has no muscular attachments and functions as a ball and socket joint around which the skeleton sways depending on the distribution of myofascial forces (**Figure 5**). The centre of the body mass is normally located anterior to the S2 vertebrae in humans. In an erect stance where there is no significant anatomical postural distortion, the centre of mass or gravity will be evenly distributed between the feet and over each plantar surface. Therefore, if one

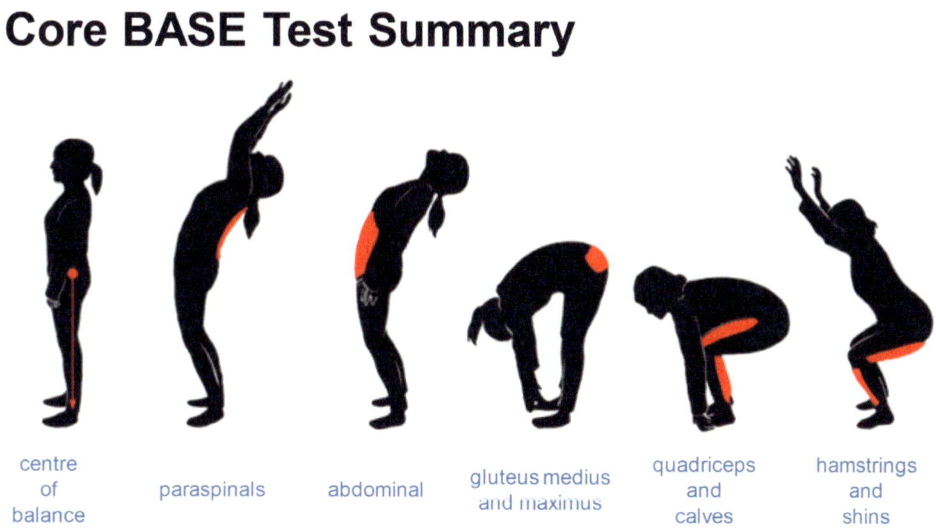

Figure 4.
The core biomechanical assessment and symmetry evaluation (BASE) tests.

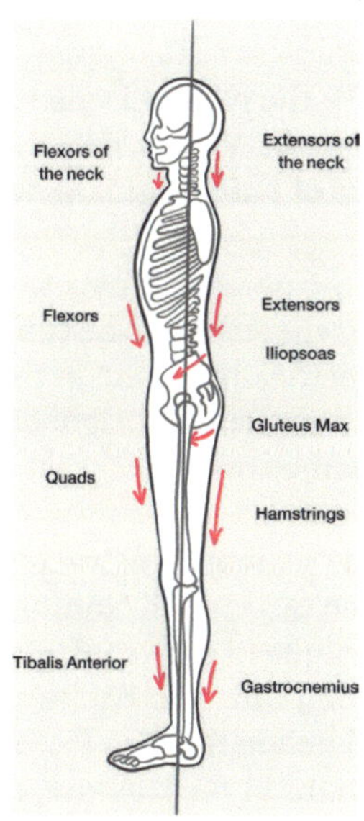

Figure 5.
Muscle groups that play a part in balancing the upright skeleton.

foot feels heavier than the other, then there is a shift of the centre of mass or gravity towards that side of the body. For example, if weight is perceived to be more on the right foot, then there is likely contracted musculature in the right leg "pulling" the pelvis to the right and shifting the centre of mass to the right. At this time, the patient is asked to report about the distribution of weight on their feet (i.e., right or left predominance, towards heels or balls, outside of feet or inside).

At the time of the balance test, the clinician observes postural and position between the right and left sides reviewing; feet (e.g., pronated, elevated little toe, clawed toes), knees (e.g., hyperextended or hyperflexed), level of the hips, shoulder height, any pelvic rotation or tilt, as well as any tilt of the torso or the head. No abnormality detected (NAD) should also be documented.

This will be the first time the clinician touches the patient and a verbal consent prior to examination of any asymmetries is pertinent.

Then, the remaining five core BASE movement tests are performed. These tests are used to screen a patient's body for the true origin of pain. BASE tests compartmentalize the true origin of pain to a defined anatomical region. The objective in having the patient perform these BASE tests is to identify the most painful or restrictive BASE test. The most painful or restrictive BASE test identifies the tissues that are the most significant current contributor to perceived pain. There is a simple elegance to this construct in that each test defines a specific muscle group or body area. The most painful or restrictive test generally provides a clear indication of a starting point for treatment when a patient has multiple sites of pain or widespread pain. Even though the individual BASE tests are common human movements, the coordinated use of these movement tests to define anatomical areas that are the true origin of pain is unique. Administering these core BASE tests is quick, reproducible, and consistent. This is the distinctive feature of *myoActivation*, which will enable future reliable comparative research.

- *Extension arms raised* (*EAR*): the patient is instructed to bend backwards from the hips with his/her arms overhead. Wherever pain is perceived by the patient in this posture, the true source of pain originates in the paraspinal muscles.

- *Extension arms down* (*EAD*): the patient is instructed to arch backwards from the hips with his/her arms down. Wherever pain is perceived by the patient in this posture, the true source of pain originates in the abdominal muscles.

- *Flexion arms down* (*FAD*): the patient is instructed to flex forward with straight knees and bend forward to wherever he/she can reach comfortably. The patient is questioned in regards specifically to pain in the low back. If pain is perceived in the low back in this posture, the true origin of pain is in the medial gluteus medius and/or gluteus maximus muscles.

- *Squat arms down* (*SAD*): the patient is instructed to squat with their arms by their side to where he/she can crouch comfortably. If a patient has a very restricted squat, their technique in performing the squat can be improved by instructing them to drive their buttocks backwards. A deeper squat will invariably result due to increased pelvic rotation from this manoeuver. Wherever pain is perceived by the patient in this posture, the true origin of pain is in the quadriceps or calf muscles. If the pain is perceived to be in the upper leg, then the quadriceps will be the pain source. If in the lower leg, then the gastrocnemius and/or soleus will be the source.

- *Squat arms raised* (*SAR*): the patient is instructed to squat with his/her arms overhead to where he/she can crouch comfortably. Wherever pain is perceived by the patient in this posture, the true origin of pain is in the hamstrings or tissues overlying the shin. If the pain is perceived to be in the upper leg, then the hamstrings will be the pain source. If the pain report is the lower leg, then the medial tibial fascia or soft tissues will be the source.

In performing these core BASE tests, the patient will subconsciously accomplish the required movements through accommodation of his/her previous injuries and joint restrictions. Deviations from normal symmetry often indicate tissue abnormalities. Common postural deviations seen in the performance of core BASE tests include: shifting of the pelvis, lifting of heels or toes, medial deviation of knees, shoulder girdle rotation, or asymmetry.

The most restricted or painful of the five movement core BASE tests is the guide to a starting point for treatment.

If EAR and EAD or SAD and SAR seem to be equivalent/comparable in causing pain or restriction, then the clinician needs to review lateral muscles and tissues. For example, comparable EAR and EAD requires testing of the quadratus lumborum muscles or the three lateral abdominal wall muscles (external oblique, internal oblique, and transversus abdominis = triceps abdominis). Comparable SAD and SAR requires testing of the tensor fascia lata, vastus lateralis, and the adductor muscles (see **Table 1** for specific muscles).

Once core BASE tests are complete, there are 55 regional BASE tests used in *myoActivation* to assess pain in the head, face, neck, shoulders, and limbs/extremities. It is beyond the scope of this chapter to outline all these regional tests.

3.1.4 Palpation

The technique of palpation develops with experience, but is not difficult to learn. A rolling motion is used, applied using both thumbs or index fingertips simultaneously, on symmetrical tissues to compare right and left sides. Differences between right and left may be apparent by the patient's physical reaction, patient's verbal report, and/or by sensory feedback to the examiner from digital pressure.

The goal in palpation of soft tissues is to identify increased density, which is painful to the patient and feels different to the clinician when comparing the same tissue on the other side. In most instances, when increased density of a soft tissue is identified, the patient will express or react to the noticeable increase in discomfort or pain associated with palpation of the abnormal tissue. When there are conflicting results between the results of BASE tests and findings from palpation, the palpation findings are more important as the indicator of the true source of pain. Where a patient has a high pain threshold, they may not feel discomfort with palpation. The clinician may need to rely on clinical experience to identify the palpable sensation of normal tissue density to identify points in the soft tissues that are outside of the normal range for distortion with fingertip pressure.

Code	BASE test	Tissues commonly responsible
BAL	Balance	
EAR	Extension arms raised	paraspinal muscles
EAD	Extension arms down	triceps abdominis/rectus abdominis
FAD	Flexion arms down	gluteus maximus/gluteus medius
SAD	Squat arms down—upper leg pain Squat arms down—lower leg pain	quadriceps gastrocnemius/soleus
SAR	Squat arms raised—upper leg pain Squat arms raised—lower leg pain Squat arms raised—back pain	hamstrings medial tibial fascia quadratus femoris
	Comparable EAD/EAR	triceps abdominis/quadratus lumborum
	Comparable SAD/SAR	vastus lateralis/tensor fascia lata adductor magnus/adductor longus

Table 1.
Specific muscles associated with BASE tests.

3.1.5 Synthesis

At this time, it is helpful to stop and consider the: history of the presenting complaint, TiLT, most painful or restrictive BASE tests, identified postural anomalies, and notable findings on palpation. This deliberation serves to connect all these factors to discern the relevant myofascial components of the pain presentation. Reviewing the cascade of chronological events that have altered the normal anatomical form will help to untangle the multiple sources associated with the presenting chronic pain complaint. With experience, pattern recognition will be part of this process for common conditions like low back pain.

3.1.6 Consent

Written consent should be obtained after informing the patient of associated risks.

3.1.7 Contraindications to needling treatment

Contraindications to a needling-based treatment include current anticoagulant use, immunocompromised state, needle aversion (trypanophobia), or presyncope.

3.1.8 Treatment anticipation

Patients may be anxious due to needle aversion and anticipation of pain from an unfamiliar procedure. Offering to provide a trial of a single needle insertion usually allows the patient to realize that the actual discomfort is less than the anticipated pain of the needling technique. Use of non-pharmacological and pharmacological techniques to minimise pain of injection and anxiety are essential [140–143].

3.1.9 Choosing a starting point

Once patients are comfortable with the process, start in the area directed by the most painful or restricted core BASE test. In anxious patients, consider an easily tolerated point first. This may be a treatment area that they cannot visualize or a less sensitive body area such as the gluteus medius. In patients who seem skeptical or uncertain, begin treatment closer to their perceived source of pain. Alternatively, start at a site that is guaranteed to make a significant difference in pain and/or flexibility, such as releasing any scar that is in a tissue area directed by the most restrictive or painful core BASE test, i.e., considered to have some association with the presenting problem.

3.1.10 Scars

Scars have significant biomechanical consequences in movement and in the transmission of forces following a subsequent injury. Abdominal incisions are major contributors to pain, pain at distant site, and disturbances in function of internal organs [144, 145]. Inspection of scars for guttering or tethering with movements helps to determine their significance. Scars with a very high potential of significance are associated with Caesarean-section procedures, surgical drains, bone grafts, burns, fasciotomies, chicken pox, and penetrating wounds. Scars with moderate potential of significance include any incisional or excisional surgical scar, especially in the feet. Other important scars include immunization scars, or scars from glass cuts, animal bites, and cystic acne.

Scars can be released by a series of needle insertions through scar tissue. Release of normal skin adjacent to the scar and palpably dense myofascial tissues surrounding the scar will also contribute to reduction of scar-related tension. Wide scars can be released in a zigzag pattern of needle insertions through the scar tissue. Release of myofascial tension following scar release is proportional to the degree of the "biting" sensation felt while undermining the scar. With experience, it will become apparent that some scars hold emotions related to the traumatic event when the scar occurred [108]. Release of traumatic scars can induce some remarkable, involuntary patient emotional responses. Patients need to be pre-warned about this possible experience. The patient may maintain composure during the clinical encounter, but subsequently report that the emotional release occurred minutes or hours after the treatment.

3.1.11 Needling MTPs technique

Palpation of the targeted tissue, based on the core BASE tests, will provide the clinician with the relevant tissue to release. It is important to release this tissue at the most painful palpable pain point. Skin antisepsis prior to needling will be dictated by the clinician's institutional policy. Needle selection depends on the site to be treated but usually requires a 30-gauge 25 mm or a 25-gauge 50 mm hollow-bore needle connected to a syringe of 0.9% normal saline.

Common responses to trigger point activation (release) reported by patients include pain reduction, pain resolution, movement of the pain from the original site, pain with needle insertion, "biting" (especially with significant scars), burning (presumed blood flow into a released muscle), muscle twitch, muscle relaxation, release of tension, or shooting pain down a limb (not related to needling of an adjacent nerve). All these sensations are positive therapeutic symptoms and merit acknowledgement. In the uncommon instance where needling results in a muscle spasm, additional needle insertions are indicated to activate more trigger points.

3.1.12 Tips and tricks to help with tolerating needling techniques

Breathing techniques and other appropriate non-pharmacological techniques should also be utilized to distract from the needling process [140–142]. At all times, the clinician must observe the patient for any signs of potential light-headedness/presyncope.

3.1.13 Catenated cycles

Catenated cycles (**Figure 6**) are repeated sequences of BASE testing, palpation, and needling in each session to unravel the multiple sites of anatomical distortion contributing to chronic pain. This is an important process as chronic pain, particularly when it has been persistent for years or decades, results from multiple sites or contributors to the pain pattern. Catenated cycles assist in identifying the various contributing tissues to the larger pain pattern. Each cycle usually identifies the next new and different most painful or restrictive BASE test resulting in a new area of treatment. Poor results from *myoActivation* will result from only performing an initial series of BASE tests to find a starting point for treatment and then needling many tissues without undertaking the catenated cycles.

Catenated cycles demonstrate to the clinician some or all of the following visible changes in patient movement: increase in joint range, greater range of motion, increase in speed of movement, increase in ease, smoothness, or fluidity of movement. This provides immediate feedback on treatment.

For the patient, catenated cycles will demonstrate some or all of the following subjective changes in post-treatment movement: reduction in overall perceived pain at rest and/or in movement, reduction or a diffusion in the area of pain, shift in pain location, perception of pain only at end range rather than throughout the range, or a

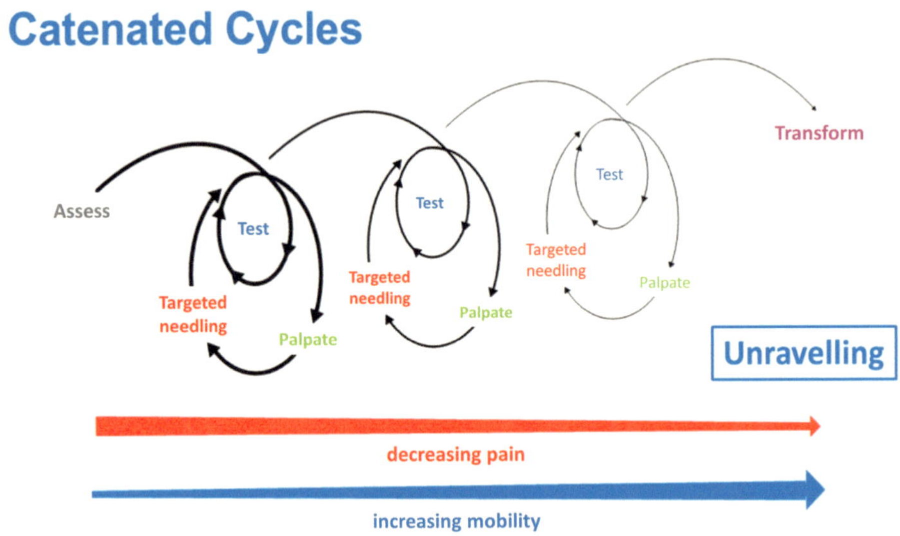

Figure 6.
Catenated cycles, unravelling pain.

different pain focus altogether at a different location that only becomes perceptible when the initial painful site has been treated. Another advantage of the catenated cycles is that the patient has to get up and move after each treatment, which distracts from any pain resulting from the treatment process.

3.1.14 When to stop

It is optimal to end sessions at a successful end-point. These might include resolution of pain, reduction in pain, improved flexibility, increased fluidity of movement, positive postural changes, or change in the weight distribution of the feet to being more grounded (even plantar weight distribution). Otherwise, the decision during treatment to stop further needle insertions is a clinical judgement that is dictated primarily by the patient's ability to tolerate the procedure. Fatigue and feeling overwhelmed are not uncommon responses especially during the first treatment session. Despite receiving written consent, it is always advisable to request ongoing verbal consent at the appropriate times to ensure the patient is agreeable with ongoing care. An important principle is not to do too much at each session.

3.1.15 Risks

In general, there are very few significant risks associated with *myoActivation*. Most common are bruising and short-term muscle pain. The most significant, but extremely rare complication is potential for a pneumothorax. All clinicians needling in the neck and thoracic region must be aware of the preventative strategies, and the symptoms and signs of pneumothorax. Written information should be supplied to patients detailing: what symptoms to notice, and the contact numbers for help and an algorithm of appropriate actions if these symptoms occur once the patient has left a clinical area.

Potential side effects of *myoActivation* include: sweating, light-headedness/presyncope, pain from needle insertion, hematoma, muscle spasm, nausea, vomiting, syncope, post-treatment muscle pain [146], pneumothorax, infection, and failure to respond.

3.1.16 myoActivation after-care

Instructions following treatment are directed to promote recovery of treated tissues and prevent symptom regression. Patients are advised to move regularly, with frequent changes in posture (every 10–15 minutes) while awake in the first 24–48 hours after each treatment. They are also advised to avoid myofascial loading, repetitive exertion, and prolonged postures for 5 days. After this time, they can start graduated activity. The post-treatment response will be an individualized experience for each patient. Multiple factors will govern the outcome resulting from treatment including: degree of sedentary activity in daily life, physical demands in the workplace, patient age, genetically determined responsiveness of soft tissues, and the psychosocial factors related to chronic pain.

3.1.17 Number of sessions

It is optimal to schedule 2–3 sessions, 1 or 2 weeks apart, to minimize the need to do too much at each session, minimize pain following therapy and to help determine responsiveness. After three sessions, the clinician can determine if there is sufficient positive response to continue. There is a wide range in numbers of sessions required in positive responders.

3.1.18 Concurrent therapy

Chronic pain is a complex biopsychosocial problem. *myoActivation* is just one component of a multidisciplinary care. Most patients benefit from concurrent treatment in collaboration with other health professionals knowledgeable in treatment of patients living with chronic pain.

4. Case studies

Three cases are presented. Patients 1 and 2 were seen by a family physician with a focused practice in chronic pain exclusively employing *myoActivation.* Patient 3 received care from a paediatric pain physician. Assessment and treatment for all cases primarily involved application of the *myoActivation* methodology.

4.1 A 31-year-old male with right sciatic and low back pain

A 31-year-old labourer was referred by his family physician for management of back and right lower extremity pain. He was not using regular prescription analgesia medications, but used occasional ibuprofen and marijuana. He had been dealing with intermittent lower back pain since he was 15.

Eight months prior to this assessment, he "pinched a nerve on the left side of this body" while lifting a granite countertop. He was off work for 1 month, participated in a return to work program, and was judged fit for work. He did not feel ready to return to physical labour and took 3 months off. At the end of this period (2 months before this visit), he experienced a pinching sensation in the right buttock while sitting. The symptoms progressed to "sciatic pain" in his upper back radiating to the right knee. These symptoms dissipated but he presented with episodic excruciating pain in the right upper buttock radiating down the right leg. The pain was precipitated by standing, going up stairs, or starting to walk. He had no symptoms of motor weakness, saddle numbness or urinary dysfunction.

TiLT revealed a laceration to the right upper lip from a shovel at age 6 requiring stitches, multiple sutured lacerations on hands from work as a chef and a chicken pox scar on right upper lip. He sustained a right ankle injury from a snowboarding injury aged 15. He had snowboarded for 21 years prior to his work-related back injury but felt that he would never be able to snowboard again.

Past medical history included a 12-year history of depression with frequent suicidal ideation. Current antidepressant medications include bupropion and escitalopram.

Standing posture findings	
Pain focus	No pain at rest while standing
Postural assessment	Feet, no abnormality detected (NAD)
	Knees level, hips level
	No pelvic rotation or tilt, no torso shift
	Left shoulder elevated
	Head NAD
Plantar weight distribution	Equal weight on feet, lateral edges, central

BASE testing	
Extension arms raised	Normal range of motion (ROM), pain low back
Extension arms down	Normal ROM with no pain
Flexion arms down	Limited ROM, pain low back, right more than left
Squat arms down	Normal ROM with no pain
Squat arms raised	Normal ROM with no pain

Worst BASE test in terms of limited ROM and pain was flexion arms down.

Treatment	
Trigger point injections	Right gluteus maximus at origin
Post-treatment assessment	Normal ROM in flexion arms down
Patient quotes	"I am not feeling any pain. It feels nice."

On the principle of not doing too much especially on the first visit, it was deemed appropriate to stop at this time. Over the course of the next 28 days, the patient was seen three times to manage ever diminishing right-sided back and leg pains. Right-sided jaw and neck pains became more prominent in the patient's symptomatology with resolution of his back pain. *myoActivation* principles and process were followed using core and regional BASE tests to resolve these issues as well.

On visit 5, 51 days after initial assessment, the patient stated he was doing really well. Nothing was really troubling him although he was a bit stiff after snowboarding 2 days previously. He remarked his hamstrings were tight, but he was working on stretching them every day and doing some yoga. He did, however, snowboard for a half-day and then a full day. He told himself he would go easy, but was able to snowboard without limitation. He reported that to have the confidence in his body and be able to snowboard was important for him as it was very meditative and his escape. His also reported that his mood had significantly improved. No treatment was necessary on this visit and the patient was discharged.

4.2 A 42-year-old female with fibromyalgia and chronic fatigue syndrome

4.2.1 Visit 1

A 42-year-old hospital kitchen worker was referred by her family physician for fibromyalgia and chronic fatigue syndrome. She had been receiving out-patient care (assessment, investigations (MRIs, X-rays, bone scan) and therapy) through a hospital-based complex chronic diseases programme. She had completed an online programme for pain self-management strategies at a local university, which she found tremendously helpful.

The patient described the onset of pain symptoms 15 years previously following a tooth extraction with subsequent infection. She had a pain and fatigue crisis 3 years previously from which she was unable to get out of bed for 4 months. She reported that currently she has had widespread symptoms including; gastrointestinal upset, brain fog, left temporomandibular joint dysfunction, nerve issues, right-sided migraines, central posterior neck pain, and bilateral scapular pain, left greater than right. A diagnosis of fibromyalgia and chronic fatigue syndrome was made 2 months prior to this visit. She is on long-term disability.

TiLT revealed that at age 10, she had been launched over the handle bars of her bicycle breaking an upper front tooth. Again, at age 10, she fell onto her tailbone requiring her to sit on a donut for a prolonged time after injury. At age 11, she rode a bike that was too big for her and injured her right knee from repetitive movement. She had bilateral knee scars from childhood injuries, right forearm burns from cooking, and a scar from a cut in the mid back from an exploding soda bottle, aged 12.

Past medical history revealed that she had had previous surgeries including dental and a lower segment C-section (LSCS). The patient reported post traumatic stress disorder related to severe pain during her LSCS due to inadequate analgesia from her epidural. Other relevant past medical issues included Hashimoto's thyroiditis, postural orthostatic tachycardia syndrome, irritable bowel syndrome, and fibromyalgia.

Current medications	Synthroid, naltrexone, acetaminophen with codeine

Standing posture findings	
Pain focus	Left scapula
Postural assessment	Feet NAD
	Knees level, hips level
	No pelvic rotation or tilt, no torso shift
	Right shoulder elevated
	Head NAD
Plantar weight distribution	More weight on left foot, medial sides, heels

4.2.1.1 Catenated cycle 1

The TiLT identified a significant tailbone injury in childhood. Clinical experience has demonstrated that tethering of soft tissues overlying the coccyx results in a significant biomechanical distortion. Therefore, in this case the first test indicated is sacrococcygeal palpation.

BASE testing	
Palpation findings	**Exquisitely tender in midline over coccyx**
Treatment	**Fascia over coccyx**

4.2.1.2 Catenated cycle 2

BASE testing	
Extension arms raised	Severe ROM limitation with left shoulder pain
Extension arms down	Moderate ROM limitation, left shoulder pain
Flexion arms down	Moderate ROM limitation with pain lower back
Squat arms down	Moderate ROM limitation with pain calves
Squat arms raised	Severe ROM limitation with pain thighs
Palpation findings	**Palpable pain points C5-T11, left more than right**
Treatment	**Bilateral paraspinals from C6 to T12**

4.2.1.3 Catenated Cycle 3 and Cycle 4

BASE testing	
Extension arms raised	Severe ROM limitation with left shoulder pain
Extension arms down	Moderate ROM limitation, left shoulder pain
Flexion arms down	Moderate ROM limitation with pain lower back
Squat arms down	Moderate ROM limitation with pain calves
Squat arms raised	Severe ROM limitation with pain thighs
Palpation findings	**Palpable pain points C5-T11, left more than right**
Treatment	**Bilateral paraspinals from C6 to T12**
Extension arms raised	Mild ROM limitation with left shoulder pain
Extension arms down	Moderate ROM limitation with left shoulder pain
Flexion arms down	Moderate ROM limitation with pain lower back
Squat arms down	Moderate ROM limitation with pain calves
Squat arms raised	Moderate ROM limitation with pain thighs
Straight arm pinch	Limited range in left shoulder

The straight-arm pinch BASE test specifically assesses restriction in scapular mobility from sustained contraction of the ipsilateral serratus anterior muscle.

Palpation findings	**Palpable densities overlying left ribs 4–6 between anterior and posterior axillary lines**
Treatment	**Left serratus anterior**

4.2.1.4 Post-treatment assessment

Decreased lower back pain and left posterior shoulder pain. Increased ease and range in flexion arms down, extension arm raised, extension arms down, and straight-arm pinch.

4.2.1.5 Patient quotes

"That's crazy!" "I feel so light!"

4.2.2 Visit 2 (7 days after visit 1)

The patient reported she had had a rough week, with soreness and pain for about 5 days, especially from the injection over the coccyx. She felt her pain pattern was different. She felt lighter but was still feeling brain fog. The left shoulder blade felt stiff but not painful.

Standing posture findings	
Pain focus	Head pressure
Postural assessment	Feet NAD
	Knees' level, hips' level
	No pelvic rotation or tilt, no torso shift
	Shoulders' level
	Head NAD
Plantar weight distribution	Equal weight on feet, medial sides, heels

4.2.2.1 Catenated cycle 1

BASE testing	
Extension arms raised	Mild ROM limitation with pain lower back
Extension arms down	Moderate ROM limitation with pain lower back
Flexion arms down	Normal ROM with no pain
Squat arms down	Normal ROM with no pain
Squat arms raised	Normal ROM with no pain
Treatment	**C-section scar**

4.2.2.2 Post-treatment assessment

Decreased brain fog. Increased ease in ambulation.

4.2.3 Visit 3 (14 days after visit 1)

She has not had any pain in her neck or shoulder. Right knee was biggest problem.

Standing posture findings	
Pain focus standing	No pain at rest while standing
Postural assessment	Feet NAD
	Knees' level, hips' level
	No pelvic rotation or tilt, no torso shift
	Shoulders' level
	Head NAD
Plantar weight distribution	Equal weight on feet, central, balls of feet

4.2.3.1 Catenated cycle 1

BASE testing	
Extension arms raised	Moderate ROM limitation with fatigue in right lower back
Extension arms down	Severe ROM limitation with fatigue in right lower back and neck
Flexion arms down	Limited ROM with pain in low back
Squat arms down	Normal ROM with no pain
Squat arms raised	Normal ROM with no pain
Palpation findings	**Palpable tender density in right external oblique muscle medial to anterior superior iliac spine (ASIS)**
Treatment	**Right external oblique**

4.2.3.2 Catenated cycle 2

BASE testing	
Right lateral arch	Mild ROM limitation with right low back pain
Left lateral arch	Mild ROM limitation with hip tension

[The lateral arch BASE test specifically assesses restriction in pelvic mobility from sustained contraction of the ipsilateral iliopsoas muscle].

Palpation findings	**Exquisite tenderness to light palpation of the right iliopsoas tendon in the femoral triangle**
Treatment	**Right iliopsoas**

4.2.3.3 Post-treatment assessment

Decreased lower back and flank pain. Increased ease in ambulation, extension arms raised, extension arms down, and lateral arches.

4.2.4 Visit 4 (50 days after visit 1)

She had a lot more mobility since the last visit with no significant pain other than the right knee. She had not had a migraine in several weeks.

Standing posture findings	
Pain focus standing	Right knee
Plantar weight distribution	Equal weight on feet, medial sides, heels

4.2.4.1 Catenated cycle 1

BASE testing	
Extension arms raised	Moderate ROM limitation, pain in quadriceps
Extension arms down	Moderate ROM limitation, pain in right knee
Flexion arms down	Normal ROM with no pain
Squat arms down	Normal ROM with no pain
Squat arms raised	Normal ROM with no pain
Palpation findings	**Palpable tenderness and density in right external oblique inferomedial to ASIS**
Treatment	**Right external oblique**

4.2.4.2 Post-treatment assessment

Decreased right knee pain. Increased range in extension arms raised, extension arms down, and lateral arch BASE tests as well as ease in ambulation.

4.2.5 Follow-up (294 days after visit 1)

The patient reported significant improvement in all her symptoms. Previous blinding aura migraines occurring 2–3/week were now reduced to mild aura migraines 1–2/month. She had full resolution of her neck pain at the base of her skull (pain previously scored at 7–10/10), her coccygeal pain (previously 2–4/10), and hip pain (previously 6–8/10). She reported significant reductions in her left scapular pain (previously 6–8/10, now 2–6/10) and right knee pain (previously 4–7/10, now 2–4/10). She was also experiencing improved cognitive function, improved focus and reduced sensitivity to light and sound.

4.3 Paediatric case study: low back pain

A 4-year-old girl was referred to a paediatric complex pain clinic by her neurosurgeon with a 2-year history of low back pain. Her mother reported that her daughter's pain started approximately 1 month following lumbosacral dermal sinus tract surgery. There had been no obvious pain prior to surgery. Her pain was focused in the midline from level of T12 to sacrum. The pain was variable but worse towards end of day, early evening, and night-time. The pain was associated with her being "cranky and irritable". Relief was gained with heat, necessitating many hours per day in a warm bath. The pain was aggravated by swimming, sitting and cold weather, but there were no issues with walking. The pain was not relieved by acetaminophen or ibuprofen. There were no scoliosis, no motor deficits, and no urinary or bladder issues.

In the past medical history, there had been no motor vehicle accidents, no fractures or other trauma, no falls on the coccyx/tailbone, and no other surgeries. The only scar was that related to her dermal sinus surgery. In response to the question "What has been her greatest physical trauma?" the answer was her dermal sinus surgery with a minor delayed healing of a part of the wound. The child was born at term by normal spontaneous vaginal delivery following a normal pregnancy. There were no other health issues, no allergies, and no current medications.

The lumbosacral dermal sinus tract excision surgery was uncomplicated, followed by an uneventful recovery and discharge from hospital 3 days postoperatively. Recent investigations included blood work, X-rays, and an MRI of the spine: all reported to be normal. Neurological, neurosurgical, and orthopaedic consultations revealed no abnormality to explain her ongoing pain.

The child was 22 kg and very active and clingy to her mother. She was reluctant to be examined, but interestingly was keen to participate in the core BASE tests as long as she was copying her mum. Pain site was as reported in the history.

Standing posture findings	
Pain focus	Low back
Postural assessment	Hips level, shoulders level
Plantar weight distribution	Patient unable to differentiate

BASE testing	
Extension arms raised	Mildly ROM with pain low back
Extension arms down	Normal ROM with no pain
Flexion arms down	Limited ROM with pain low back, right greater than left
Squat arms down	Normal ROM with no pain
Squat arms raised	Normal ROM with no pain

The worst BASE test in terms of limited ROM and pain was EAR and FAD.

It was not possible to determine the weight distribution on the feet. The core BASE tests that appeared to be most restricted were EAR and FAD; the most painful of these was EAR. The child was able to perform the other core BASE tests with no apparent difficulty. The surgical scar over her sacral area was well healed, but the mid portion of it had a 2-cm wider part that had presumably been the site of the reported delayed healing. There was no tenderness over the coccyx.

The examination revealed no obvious abnormality other than the scar in the midline and a right paraspinal muscle in sustained contraction.

The child was started on magnesium bisglycinate, vitamin K2, and vitamin D3. Three weeks later, scar release and right paraspinal release were performed under general anaesthesia. At follow-up, 4 months after initial assessment, the child was pain free and active in dance.

5. Discussion

5.1 How does myoActivation work?

myoActivation is a process that enables the clinician to connect or link the patient's TiLT with the myofascial findings on examination. The targeted myofascial activations appear to restore the biomechanical, neuroendocrine, and autonomic balance to reduce chronic pain. Research is required to determine which components of the myofascial system are really important in making the observed changes seen following *myoActivation*.

5.2 What makes myoActivation different?

A distinctive and foundational principle of *myoActivation* is that the perceived site of pain is often not the source of pain. *myoActivation* constitutes a paradigm shift in how to take a pain history and examine a patient with chronic pain.

The history focuses on a TiLT, including surgery, motor vehicle accidents, fractures, scars, and injuries. It highlights the importance of scars as contributors to chronic pain, especially scars inflicted at a young age or associated with poor healing. It relies on excellent clinical acumen to observe postural abnormalities and skeletal asymmetries, and to locate palpable painful points that help guide therapy as illustrated in the cases presented.

Standard structured BASE tests are used to distinguish significant fascial or muscle trigger point contributors to chronic pain. This structured assessment and treatment is reproducible and therefore a unique framework to perform comparative research. A synthesis of pertinent findings connects the dots that link the patient's TiLT with the myofascial findings, looking at the patient as a whole biomechanical structure and not as segmented symptomatic parts.

Needling is performed with hollow bore needles, with a cutting tip, which is utilized to target and release scars, fascia in tension and PPPs in muscles; therefore, it is not the same as classical intramuscular stimulation (IMS), traditional Chinese acupuncture, western medicine acupuncture, prolotherapy, or dry needling targeted at the site of pain. Immediate changes occur such as decreased pain, improved flexibility and improved fluidity of movement, which are easily demonstrated with the repetition of BASE tests.

Even if a needling technique is not used, for example in children or in individuals with needle aversion, the *myoActivation* TiLT, assessment, and examination can be used to determine if there is a myofascial component to chronic pain and direct patients to non-needling therapies such as physiotherapy and massage.

myoActivation uses catenated cycles of intervention and reassessment of baseline tests to unravel the important muscle groups and fascial tensions contributing to the particular pain problem, then repeats baseline tests to highlight the next biomechanically significant tissue in tension. It typically requires 2–5 *myoActivation* sessions to get to the treatment goal of improved flexibility and reduced pain or resolution of pain.

myoActivation can be used to reduce pain in different pain populations for a variety of different pain conditions. It can cause an emotional release, fatigue, sense of lightness, or well-being at the time of *myoActivation*. It restores hope to patients as it provides an answer to the cause of years of pain. It provides a tool in the toolbox for clinicians, which is low cost, effective, and does not require specialized equipment or imaging. It can be easily incorporated into primary care practice and, therefore, not subject to tertiary care waitlists. However, to be effective, it does need to be applied by an appropriately trained clinician.

myoActivation as an effective tool means the clinician does not have to rely on pharmaceutical analgesic agents for myofascial pain. Pain resolution and its effects on improved function, and ultimately mood, enables weaning of established analgesia medications, including opioid medications.

5.3 What is the future of myoActivation?

With its low cost and no requirement for resource-intensive clinical investigations, *myoActivation* has the potential to support the movement for "winding back the harms of too much medicine" [147]. However, for that to happen, we need to develop programmes of research and training and to address the barriers of awareness, availability, and accessibility [43].

Demonstrating a firm evidence base for the perceived benefits of *myoActivation* will ultimately require prospective research studies, including multi-centre clinical trials [148]. Many questions remain about mechanism of action, specific approaches in different populations, benefits of integration with other therapeutic techniques, timing of *myoActivation,* and integration with other management techniques. In the meantime, we must rely on patient voices, case studies, audit through patient registries (where *myoActivation* has been delivered by accredited personnel), population–based, case-controlled studies [149] and N-of-1 studies, especially considering the diversity of chronic pain presentations in the population [150].

Clinicians will need to be trained in the art of determining palpable pain points and to learn *myoActivation* before they can fully incorporate this process into their everyday practice. A core group of *myoActivation* faculty, led by Dr. Siren, is developing a programme for training and dissemination of *myoActivation.* Assessment and treatment strategies often begin as local initiatives and are developed into widely accepted standards for care; for example, Managing Emergencies in Paediatric Anaesthesia started in one centre in the UK [151], but is now an internationally recognized course teaching a standard approach worldwide [152, 153]. Other examples include Advanced Cardiac Life Support and Advanced Paediatric Life Support [154].

6. Conclusion

In the face of the burden of chronic pain, including its economic impact, it is imperative to establish new and effective tools to minimize the impacts of this condition. Early intervention is key to success in managing chronic pain. This requires that a tool be available, accessible, and affordable to community clinicians. The current opioid crisis and limited therapeutic effectiveness of many pharmaceutical agents in chronic pain necessitate a different approach.

This chapter has described the core assessment and therapeutic process of a novel technique to manage myofascial components of chronic pain. *myoActivation* is structured and reproducible, with a high benefit to risk ratio. It can be applied to many different chronic pain presentations and different age groups.

Clinicians will need to be trained to successfully incorporate core and regional components of *myoActivation* into their practice. We hope that this chapter will be an incentive for clinicians to learn more about this system of care. It is clear from experience that this is an effective approach and brings a much-needed tool into the toolbox for chronic pain, which, so far, has evaded an efficacious therapeutic modality.

> *"In departing from any settled opinion or belief, the variation, the change, the break with custom may come gradually; and the way is usually prepared; but the final break is made, as a rule, by some one individual, [...] who sees with his own eyes, and with an instinct or genius for truth, escapes from the routine in which his fellows live."*
>
> *Sir William Osler, 1849–1919.*

Acknowledgements

The authors would like to thank Mark Ansermino, Patrick Yu, and Barbara Eddy for their insightful comments on a draft of this chapter and Shona Massey for the artwork in **Figure 5**.

Disclosures

Dr. G. Siren is the inventor of *myoActivation*. He trademarked *myoActivation* principally to ensure that a structured assessment and process is followed and maintained.

Dr. G. Lauder and Mr. N. West have no disclosures.

Author details

Gillian Lauder[1], Nicholas West[2] and Greg Siren[3]*

1 BC Children's Hospital, Vancouver, BC, Canada

2 University of British Columbia, Vancouver, BC, Canada

3 The myo Clinic, Victoria, BC, Canada

*Address all correspondence to: greg.siren@myoclinic.ca

References

[1] International Association for the Study of Pain. IASP Terminology [Internet]. 2018. Available from: http://www.iasp-pain.org/Education/Content.aspx?ItemNumber=1698#Pain

[2] Turk D, Okifuji A. Pain terms and taxonomies. In: Fishman S, Ballantyne J, Rathmell JP, editors. Bonica's Management of Pain. 4th ed. Philadelphia, PA: Lippincott Williams & Wilkins; 2010. pp. 13-23

[3] Fayaz A, Croft P, Langford RM, Donaldson LJ, Jones GT. Prevalence of chronic pain in the UK: A systematic review and meta-analysis of population studies. BMJ Open. 2016;**6**(6):e010364

[4] Mansfield KE, Sim J, Jordan JL, Jordan KP. A systematic review and meta-analysis of the prevalence of chronic widespread pain in the general population. Pain. 2016;**157**(1):55-64

[5] King S, Chambers CT, Huguet A, MacNevin RC, McGrath PJ, Parker L, et al. The epidemiology of chronic pain in children and adolescents revisited: A systematic review. Pain. 2011;**152**(12):2729-2738

[6] Larsson C, Hansson EE, Sundquist K, Jakobsson U. Chronic pain in older adults: Prevalence, incidence, and risk factors. Scandinavian Journal of Rheumatology. 2017;**46**(4):317-325

[7] Mann EG, Johnson A, VanDenKerkhof EG. Frequency and characteristics of healthcare visits associated with chronic pain: Results from a population-based Canadian study. Canadian Journal of Anaesthesia. 2016;**63**(4):411-441

[8] Breivik H, Collett B, Ventafridda V, Cohen R, Gallacher D. Survey of chronic pain in Europe: Prevalence, impact on daily life, and treatment. European Journal of Pain. 2006;**10**(4):287-333

[9] Tick H, Nielsen A, Pelletier KR, Bonakdar R, Simmons S, Glick R, et al. Evidence-based nonpharmacologic strategies for comprehensive pain care. EXPLORE. 2018;**14**(3):177-211

[10] Booth J, Moseley GL, Schiltenwolf M, Cashin A, Davies M, Hübscher M. Exercise for chronic musculoskeletal pain: A biopsychosocial approach. Musculoskeletal Care. 2017;**15**(4):413-421

[11] Jensen MP. Psychosocial approaches to pain management: An organizational framework. Pain. 2011;**152**(4):717-725

[12] Becker WC, Dorflinger L, Edmond SN, Islam L, Heapy AA, Fraenkel L. Barriers and facilitators to use of non-pharmacological treatments in chronic pain. BMC Family Practice. 2017;**18**(1):41

[13] Geissert P, Hallvik S, Van Otterloo J, O'Kane N, Alley L, Carson J, et al. High-risk prescribing and opioid overdose: Prospects for prescription drug monitoring program-based proactive alerts. Pain. 2018;**159**(1):150-156

[14] Volkow N, Benveniste H, McLellan AT. Use and misuse of opioids in chronic pain. Annual Review of Medicine. 2018;**69**:451-465

[15] Noble M, Tregear SJ, Treadwell JR, Schoelles K. Long-term opioid therapy for chronic noncancer pain: A systematic review and meta-analysis of efficacy and safety. Journal of Pain and Symptom Management. 2008;**35**(2):214-228

[16] Olfson M, Wall M, Wang S, Crystal S, Blanco C. Service use preceding opioid-related fatality. The American Journal of Psychiatry. 2018;**175**(6):538-544

[17] Hedegaard H, Warner M, Miniño AM. Drug overdose deaths in the

United States, 1999-2016. NCHS Data Brief. 2017;(294):1-8. https://www.cdc.gov/nchs/data/databriefs/db294.pdf (accessed 5/feb/2019)

[18] Shah A, Hayes CJ, Martin BC. Factors influencing long-term opioid use among opioid naive patients: An examination of initial prescription characteristics and pain etiologies. The Journal of Pain. 2017;**18**(11):1374-1383

[19] Gmuca S, Xiao R, Weiss PF, Sherry DD, Knight AM, Gerber JS. Opioid prescribing and polypharmacy in children with chronic musculoskeletal pain. Pain Medicine. 2018. DOI: 10.1093/pm/pny116

[20] Crombie IK, Davies HT, Macrae WA. Cut and thrust: Antecedent surgery and trauma among patients attending a chronic pain clinic. Pain. 1998;**76**(1-2):167-171

[21] Kehlet H, Jensen TS, Woolf CJ. Persistent postsurgical pain: Risk factors and prevention. Lancet (London, England). 2006;**367**(9522):1618-1625

[22] Macrae WA. Chronic post-surgical pain: 10 years on. British Journal of Anaesthesia. 2008;**101**(1):77-86

[23] Callinan CE, Neuman MD, Lacy KE, Gabison C, Ashburn MA. The initiation of chronic opioids: A survey of chronic pain patients. The Journal of Pain. 2017;**18**(4):360-365

[24] Brummett CM, Waljee JF, Goesling J, Moser S, Lin P, Englesbe MJ, et al. New persistent opioid use after minor and major surgical procedures in US adults. JAMA Surgery. 2017;**152**(6):e170504

[25] Sledjeski EM, Speisman B, Dierker LC. Does number of lifetime traumas explain the relationship between PTSD and chronic medical conditions? Answers from the National Comorbidity Survey-Replication (NCS-R). Journal of Behavioral Medicine. 2008;**31**(4):341-349

[26] Cloitre M, Cohen LR, Edelman RE, Han H. Posttraumatic stress disorder and extent of trauma exposure as correlates of medical problems and perceived health among women with childhood abuse. Women & Health. 2001;**34**(3):1-17

[27] Scott KM, Koenen KC, Aguilar-Gaxiola S, Alonso J, Angermeyer MC, Benjet C, et al. Associations between lifetime traumatic events and subsequent chronic physical conditions: A cross-national, cross-sectional study. PLoS One. 2013;**8**(11):e80573

[28] Schilling EA, Aseltine RH, Gore S. The impact of cumulative childhood adversity on young adult mental health: Measures, models, and interpretations. Social Science & Medicine. 2008;**66**(5):1140-1151

[29] Croft P, Blyth F, van der Windt D. Chronic Pain Epidemiology: From Aetiology to Public Health. Oxford: Oxford University Press; 2010

[30] Simons DG. Review of enigmatic MTrPs as a common cause of enigmatic musculoskeletal pain and dysfunction. Journal of Electromyography and Kinesiology. 2004;**14**(1):95-107

[31] Jafri MS. Mechanisms of myofascial pain. International Scholarly Research Notices. 2014;**2014**:16. Article ID 523924. DOI: 10.1155/2014/523924

[32] Gerwin RD. Diagnosis of myofascial pain syndrome. Physical Medicine and Rehabilitation Clinics of North America. 2014;**25**(2):341-355

[33] Botelho LM, Morales-Quezada L, Rozisky JR, Brietzke AP, Torres ILS, Deitos A, et al. A framework for understanding the relationship between descending pain modulation, motor corticospinal, and neuroplasticity regulation systems in chronic myofascial pain. Frontiers in Human Neuroscience. 2016;**10**:308

[34] Botelho L, Angoleri L, Zortea M, Deitos A, Brietzke A, Torres ILS, et al. Insights about the neuroplasticity state on the effect of intramuscular electrical stimulation in pain and disability associated with chronic myofascial pain syndrome (MPS): A double-blind, randomized, sham-controlled trial. Frontiers in Human Neuroscience. 2018;**12**:388

[35] Thibaut A, Zeng D, Caumo W, Liu J, Fregni F. Corticospinal excitability as a biomarker of myofascial pain syndrome. Pain Reports. 2017;**2**(3):e594

[36] Thapa T, Graven-Nielsen T, Chipchase LS, Schabrun SM. Disruption of cortical synaptic homeostasis in individuals with chronic low back pain. Clinical Neurophysiology. 2018;**129**(5):1090-1096

[37] Akamatsu FE, Yendo TM, Rhode C, Itezerote AM, Hojaij F, Andrade M, et al. Anatomical basis of the myofascial trigger points of the gluteus maximus muscle. BioMed Research International. 2017;**2017**:4821968

[38] Roldan CJ, Hu N. Myofascial pain syndromes in the emergency department: What are we missing? The Journal of Emergency Medicine. 2015;**49**(6):1004-1010

[39] Bordoni B, Zanier E. Skin, fascias, and scars: Symptoms and systemic connections. Journal of Multidisciplinary Healthcare. 2013;7:11-24

[40] Bordoni B, Zanier E. Clinical and symptomatological reflections: The fascial system. Journal of Multidisciplinary Healthcare. 2014;7:401-411

[41] Wainner RS, Whitman JM, Cleland JA, Flynn TW. Regional interdependence: A musculoskeletal examination model whose time has come. The Journal of Orthopaedic and Sports Physical Therapy. 2007;**37**(11):658-660

[42] Qaseem A, Wilt TJ, McLean RM, Forciea MA, Clinical Guidelines Committee of the American College of Physicians. Noninvasive treatments for acute, subacute, and chronic low Back pain: A clinical practice guideline from the American College of Physicians. Annals of Internal Medicine. 2017;**166**(7):514-530

[43] Burke A, Nahin RL, Stussman BJ. Limited health knowledge as a reason for non-use of four common complementary health practices. PLoS One. 2015;**10**(6):e0129336

[44] Gerwin RD, Dommerholt J, Shah JP. An expansion of Simons' integrated hypothesis of trigger point formation. Current Pain and Headache Reports. 2004;**8**(6):468-475

[45] Bordoni B, Zanier E. Cranial nerves XIII and XIV: Nerves in the shadows. Journal of Multidisciplinary Healthcare. 2013;**6**:87-91

[46] Travell J, Simons D. Myofascial Pain and Dysfunction: The Trigger Point Manual. 2nd ed. Vol. I. Baltimore: Williams and Wilkins; 1999

[47] Travell J, Simons D. Myofascial Pain and Dysfunction: The Trigger Point Manual. 1st ed. Vol. II. Baltimore: Williams and Wilkins; 1992

[48] Shah JP, Thaker N, Heimur J, Aredo JV, Sikdar S, Gerber L. Myofascial trigger points then and now: A historical and scientific perspective. PM & R : The Journal of Injury, Function, and Rehabilitation. 2015;7(7):746-761

[49] Tough EA, White AR, Richards S, Campbell J. Variability of criteria used to diagnose myofascial trigger point pain syndrome—Evidence from a review of the literature. The Clinical Journal of Pain;**23**(3):278-286

[50] Hong C-Z, Torigoe Y, Yu J. The localized twitch responses in responsive taut bands of rabbit skeletal muscle fibers are related to the reflexes at spinal cord level. Journal of Musculoskeletal Pain. 1995;**3**(1):15-33

[51] Tekin L, Akarsu S, Durmuş O, Cakar E, Dinçer U, Kıralp MZ. The effect of dry needling in the treatment of myofascial pain syndrome: A randomized double-blinded placebo-controlled trial. Clinical Rheumatology. 2013;**32**(3):309-315

[52] Mense S. The pathogenesis of muscle pain. Current Pain and Headache Reports. 2003;**7**(6):419-425

[53] Mense S, Gerwin RD. Muscle Pain: Understanding the Mechanisms. Berlin, Heidelberg: Springer-Verlag; 2010

[54] Quintner JL, Bove GM, Cohen ML. A critical evaluation of the trigger point phenomenon. Rheumatology (Oxford, England). 2015;**54**(3):392-399

[55] Dommerholt J, Gerwin RD. A critical evaluation of Quintner et al: Missing the point. Journal of Bodywork and Movement Therapies. 2015;**19**(2):193-204

[56] Gerber LH, Sikdar S, Armstrong K, Diao G, Heimur J, Kopecky J, et al. A systematic comparison between subjects with no pain and pain associated with active myofascial trigger points. PM & R: The Journal of Injury, Function, and Rehabilitation. 2013;**5**(11):931-938

[57] Vulfsons S, Ratmansky M, Kalichman L. Trigger point needling: Techniques and outcome. Current Pain and Headache Reports. 2012;**16**(5):407-412

[58] Chen Q, Bensamoun S, Basford JR, Thompson JM, An K-N. Identification and quantification of myofascial taut bands with magnetic resonance elastography. Archives of Physical Medicine and Rehabilitation. 2007;**88**(12):1658-1661

[59] Sikdar S, Shah JP, Gebreab T, Yen R-H, Gilliams E, Danoff J, et al. Novel applications of ultrasound technology to visualize and characterize myofascial trigger points and surrounding soft tissue. Archives of Physical Medicine and Rehabilitation. 2009;**90**(11):1829-1838

[60] Turo D, Otto P, Shah JP, Heimur J, Gebreab T, Zaazhoa M, et al. Ultrasonic characterization of the upper trapezius muscle in patients with chronic neck pain. Ultrasonic Imaging. 2013;**35**(2):173-187

[61] Ballyns JJ, Turo D, Otto P, Shah JP, Hammond J, Gebreab T, et al. Office-based elastographic technique for quantifying mechanical properties of skeletal muscle. Journal of Ultrasound in Medicine. 2012;**31**(8):1209-1219

[62] Llamas-Ramos R, Pecos-Martín D, Gallego-Izquierdo T, Llamas-Ramos I, Plaza-Manzano G, Ortega-Santiago R, et al. Comparison of the short-term outcomes between trigger point dry needling and trigger point manual therapy for the management of chronic mechanical neck pain: A randomized clinical trial. The Journal of Orthopaedic and Sports Physical Therapy. 2014;**44**(11):852-861

[63] Ay S, Evcik D, Tur BS. Comparison of injection methods in myofascial pain syndrome: A randomized controlled trial. Clinical Rheumatology. 2010;**29**(1):19-23

[64] Cummings TM, White AR. Needling therapies in the management of myofascial trigger point pain: A systematic review. Archives of Physical Medicine and Rehabilitation. 2001;**82**(7):986-992

[65] Rodríguez-Mansilla J, González-Sánchez B, De Toro García Á, Valera-Donoso E, Garrido-Ardila EM, Jiménez-Palomares M, et al. Effectiveness of dry needling on reducing pain intensity in patients with myofascial pain syndrome: A meta-analysis. Journal of Traditional Chinese Medicine = Chung i tsa Chih Ying wen pan. 2016;**36**(1):1-13

[66] Boyles R, Fowler R, Ramsey D, Burrows E. Effectiveness of trigger point dry needling for multiple body regions: A systematic review. The

Journal of Manual & Manipulative Therapy. 2015;**23**(5):276-293

[67] Perreault T, Dunning J, Butts R. The local twitch response during trigger point dry needling: Is it necessary for successful outcomes? Journal of Bodywork and Movement Therapies. 2017;**21**(4):940-947

[68] Liu Q-G, Liu L, Huang Q-M, Nguyen T-T, Ma Y-T, Zhao J-M. Decreased spontaneous electrical activity and acetylcholine at myofascial trigger spots after dry needling treatment: A pilot study. Evidence-based Complementary and Alternative Medicine. 2017;**2017**:3938191

[69] Tsai C-T, Hsieh L-F, Kuan T-S, Kao M-J, Chou L-W, Hong C-Z. Remote effects of dry needling on the irritability of the myofascial trigger point in the upper trapezius muscle. American Journal of Physical Medicine & Rehabilitation. 2010;**89**(2):133-140

[70] Langevin HM, Bouffard NA, Badger GJ, Churchill DL, Howe AK. Subcutaneous tissue fibroblast cytoskeletal remodeling induced by acupuncture: Evidence for a mechanotransduction-based mechanism. Journal of Cellular Physiology. 2006;**207**(3):767-774

[71] Langevin HM, Sherman KJ. Pathophysiological model for chronic low back pain integrating connective tissue and nervous system mechanisms. Medical Hypotheses. 2007;**68**(1):74-80

[72] Shah JP, Phillips TM, Danoff JV, Gerber LH. An in vivo microanalytical technique for measuring the local biochemical milieu of human skeletal muscle. Journal of Applied Physiology. 2005;**99**(5):1977-1984

[73] Shah JP, Danoff JV, Desai MJ, Parikh S, Nakamura LY, Phillips TM, et al. Biochemicals associated with pain and inflammation are elevated in sites near to and remote from active myofascial trigger points. Archives of Physical Medicine and Rehabilitation. 2008;**89**(1):16-23

[74] Larsson R, Oberg PA, Larsson SE. Changes of trapezius muscle blood flow and electromyography in chronic neck pain due to trapezius myalgia. Pain. 1999;**79**(1):45-50

[75] Lee S-H, Chen C-C, Lee C-S, Lin T-C, Chan R-C. Effects of needle electrical intramuscular stimulation on shoulder and cervical myofascial pain syndrome and microcirculation. Journal of the Chinese Medical Association. 2008;**71**(4):200-206

[76] Ahsin S, Saleem S, Bhatti AM, Iles RK, Aslam M. Clinical and endocrinological changes after electro-acupuncture treatment in patients with osteoarthritis of the knee. Pain. 2009;**147**(1-3):60-66

[77] Napadow V, Webb JM, Pearson N, Hammerschlag R. Neurobiological correlates of acupuncture: November 17-18, 2005. Journal of Alternative and Complementary Medicine. 2006;**12**(9):931-935

[78] Cagnie B, Barbe T, De Ridder E, Van Oosterwijck J, Cools A, Danneels L. The influence of dry needling of the trapezius muscle on muscle blood flow and oxygenation. Journal of Manipulative and Physiological Therapeutics. 2012;**35**(9):685-691

[79] Graven-Nielsen T, Arendt-Nielsen L. Peripheral and central sensitization in musculoskeletal pain disorders: An experimental approach. Current Rheumatology Reports. 2002;**4**(4):313-321

[80] Reinert A, Treede R, Bromm B. The pain inhibiting pain effect: An electrophysiological study in humans. Brain Research. 2000;**862**(1-2):103-110

[81] Srbely JZ, Dickey JP, Lee D, Lowerison M. Dry needle stimulation of myofascial trigger points evokes segmental anti-nociceptive effects. Journal of Rehabilitation Medicine. 2010;**42**(5):463-468

[82] Hsieh Y-L, Chou L-W, Joe Y-S, Hong C-Z. Spinal cord mechanism involving the remote effects of dry needling on the irritability of myofascial trigger spots in rabbit skeletal muscle. Archives of Physical Medicine and Rehabilitation. 2011;**92**(7):1098-1105

[83] Mejuto-Vázquez MJ, Salom-Moreno J, Ortega-Santiago R, Truyols-Domínguez S, Fernández-de-Las-Peñas C. Short-term changes in neck pain, widespread pressure pain sensitivity, and cervical range of motion after the application of trigger point dry needling in patients with acute mechanical neck pain: A randomized clinical trial. The Journal of Orthopaedic and Sports Physical Therapy. 2014;**44**(4):252-260

[84] Hsieh Y-L, Hong C-Z, Liu S-Y, Chou L-W, Yang C-C. Acupuncture at distant myofascial trigger spots enhances endogenous opioids in rabbits: A possible mechanism for managing myofascial pain. Acupuncture in Medicine. 2016;**34**(4):302-309

[85] Langevin HM, Churchill DL, Cipolla MJ. Mechanical signaling through connective tissue: A mechanism for the therapeutic effect of acupuncture. The FASEB Journal. 2001;**15**(12):2275-2282

[86] Langevin HM, Bouffard NA, Badger GJ, Iatridis JC, Howe AK. Dynamic fibroblast cytoskeletal response to subcutaneous tissue stretch ex vivo and in vivo. American Journal of Physiology. Cell Physiology. 2005;**288**(3):C747-C756

[87] E Silva DCCM, de Andrade Alexandre DJ, Silva JG. Immediate effect of myofascial release on range of motion, pain and biceps and rectus femoris muscle activity after total knee replacement. Journal of Bodywork and Movement Therapies. 2018;**22**(4):930-936

[88] Hu H-T, Gao H, Ma R-J, Zhao X-F, Tian H-F, Li L. Is dry needling effective for low back pain?: A systematic review and PRISMA-compliant meta-analysis. Medicine (Baltimore). 2018;**97**(26):e11225

[89] Arguisuelas Martinez MD, Lisón Párraga JF, Zuriaga DS, Martinez-Hurtado I, Fernández JD. Myofascial release improves pain and disability in non-specific chronic low back pain: A randomized clinical trial. Journal of Bodywork and Movement Therapies. 2018;**22**(4):857

[90] Cerezo-Téllez E, Torres-Lacomba M, Fuentes-Gallardo I, Perez-Muñoz M, Mayoral-Del-Moral O, Lluch-Girbés E, et al. Effectiveness of dry needling for chronic nonspecific neck pain: A randomized, single-blinded, clinical trial. Pain. 2016;**157**(9):1905-1917

[91] Cerezo-Téllez E, Lacomba MT, Fuentes-Gallardo I, Mayoral Del Moral O, Rodrigo-Medina B, Gutiérrez Ortega C. Dry needling of the trapezius muscle in office workers with neck pain: A randomized clinical trial. The Journal of Manual & Manipulative Therapy. 2016;**24**(4):223-232

[92] Pecos-Martín D, Montañez-Aguilera FJ, Gallego-Izquierdo T, Urraca-Gesto A, Gómez-Conesa A, Romero-Franco N, et al. Effectiveness of dry needling on the lower trapezius in patients with mechanical neck pain: A randomized controlled trial. Archives of Physical Medicine and Rehabilitation. 2015;**96**(5):775-781

[93] France S, Bown J, Nowosilskyj M, Mott M, Rand S, Walters J. Evidence for the use of dry needling and physiotherapy in the management of cervicogenic or tension-type headache: A systematic review. Cephalalgia. 2014;**34**(12):994-1003

[94] Mayoral O, Salvat I, Martín MT, Martín S, Santiago J, Cotarelo J, et al. Efficacy of myofascial trigger point dry needling in the prevention of pain after total knee arthroplasty: A randomized, double-blinded, placebo-controlled trial. Evidence-based Complementary and Alternative Medicine. 2013;**2013**:694941

[95] Kietrys DM, Palombaro KM, Azzaretto E, Hubler R, Schaller B, Schlussel JM, et al. Effectiveness of dry needling for upper-quarter myofascial pain: A systematic review and meta-analysis. The Journal of Orthopaedic and Sports Physical Therapy. 2013;**43**(9):620-634

[96] Gerber LH, Shah J, Rosenberger W, Armstrong K, Turo D, Otto P, et al. Dry needling alters trigger points in the upper trapezius muscle and reduces pain in subjects with chronic myofascial pain. PM & R: The Journal of Injury, Function, and Rehabilitation. 2015;**7**(7):711-718

[97] Liu L, Huang Q-M, Liu Q-G, Ye G, Bo C-Z, Chen M-J, et al. Effectiveness of dry needling for myofascial trigger points associated with neck and shoulder pain: A systematic review and meta-analysis. Archives of Physical Medicine and Rehabilitation. 2015;**96**(5):944-955

[98] Arguisuelas MD, Lisón JF, Sánchez-Zuriaga D, Martínez-Hurtado I, Doménech-Fernández J. Effects of myofascial release in nonspecific chronic low back pain: A randomized clinical trial. Spine (Phila Pa 1976). 2017;**42**(9):627-634

[99] Liu L, Huang Q-M, Liu Q-G, Thitham N, Li L-H, Ma Y-T, et al. Evidence for dry needling in the management of myofascial trigger points associated with low back pain: A systematic review and meta-analysis. Archives of Physical Medicine and Rehabilitation. 2018;**99**(1):144-152.e2

[100] Canadian Agency for Drugs and Technologies in Health. Dry Needling and Injection for Musculoskeletal and Joint Disorders: A Review of the Clinical Effectiveness, Cost-Effectiveness, and Guidelines [Internet]. CADTH Rapid Response Reports. 2016. Available from: https://www.ncbi.nlm.nih.gov/pubmedhealth/PMH0089724/

[101] Gattie E, Cleland JA, Snodgrass S. The effectiveness of trigger point dry needling for musculoskeletal conditions by physical therapists: A systematic review and meta-analysis. The Journal of Orthopaedic and Sports Physical Therapy. 2017;**47**(3):133-149

[102] Starkweather A. The evidence on dry needling for pain management. Topics in Pain Management. 2018;**34**(4):1-9

[103] Jang SH, Seo JP, Ahn SH, Lee MY. Comparison of cortical activation patterns by somatosensory stimulation on the palm and dorsum of the hand. Somatosensory & Motor Research. 2013;**30**(3):109-113

[104] Mondelli M, Aretini A, Ballerini M, Vecchiarelli B, Rossi A. Sympathetic skin response. Glabella stimulation may be more useful than peripheral nerve stimulation in clinical practice. Autonomic Neuroscience. 2011;**164**(1-2):101-104

[105] Henderson LA, Stathis A, James C, Brown R, McDonald S, Macefield VG. Real-time imaging of cortical areas involved in the generation of increases in skin sympathetic nerve activity when viewing emotionally charged images. NeuroImage. 2012;**62**(1):30-40

[106] Dalsgaard CJ, Rydh M, Haegerstrand A. Cutaneous innervation in man visualized with protein gene product 9.5 (PGP 9.5) antibodies. Histochemistry. 1989;**92**(5):385-390

[107] Minasny B. Understanding the process of fascial unwinding. International Journal of Therapeutic Massage & Bodywork. 2009;**2**(3):10-17

[108] Tozzi P. Does fascia hold memories? Journal of Bodywork and Movement Therapies. 2014;**18**(2):259-265

[109] Bran GM, Goessler UR, Hormann K, Riedel F, Sadick H. Keloids: Current concepts of pathogenesis (review). International Journal of Molecular Medicine. 2009;**24**(3):283-293

[110] Scott JR, Muangman P, Gibran NS. Making sense of hypertrophic scar: A role for nerves. Wound Repair and Regeneration. 2007;**15**(Suppl 1):S27-S31

[111] Valouchová P, Lewit K. Surface electromyography of abdominal and back muscles in patients with active scars. Journal of Bodywork and Movement Therapies. 2009;**13**(3):262-267

[112] Kobesova A, Morris CE, Lewit K, Safarova M. Twenty-year-old pathogenic "active" postsurgical scar: A case study of a patient with persistent right lower quadrant pain. Journal of Manipulative and Physiological Therapeutics. 2007;**30**(3):234-238

[113] Wasserman JB, Abraham K, Massery M, Chu J, Farrow A, Marcoux BC. Soft tissue mobilization techniques are effective in treating chronic pain following cesarean section. Journal of Women's Health Physical Therapy. 2018;**1**. DOI: 10.1097/JWH.0000000000000103

[114] Alster TS, Graham PM. Microneedling: A review and practical guide. Dermatologic Surgery. 2018;**44**(3):397-404

[115] Orentreich DS, Orentreich N. Subcutaneous incisionless (subcision) surgery for the correction of depressed scars and wrinkles. Dermatologic Surgery. 1995;**21**(6):543-549

[116] Ramaut L, Hoeksema H, Pirayesh A, Stillaert F, Monstrey S. Microneedling: Where do we stand now? A systematic review of the literature. Journal of Plastic, Reconstructive & Aesthetic Surgery. 2018;**71**(1):1-14

[117] Hou A, Cohen B, Haimovic A, Elbuluk N. Microneedling: A comprehensive review. Dermatologic Surgery. 2017;**43**(3):321-339

[118] Nair P, Arora T. Microneedling using Dermaroller a means of collagen induction therapy. Gujarat Medical Journal. 2014;**69**(1):24-27

[119] Liu X, Zhu B, Zhang SX. Relationship between electroacupuncture analgesia and descending pain inhibitory mechanism of nucleus raphe magnus. Pain. 1986;**24**(3):383-396

[120] González-Hernández A, Manzano-García A, Martínez-Lorenzana G, Tello-García IA, Carranza M, Arámburo C, et al. Peripheral oxytocin receptors inhibit the nociceptive input signal to spinal dorsal horn wide-dynamic-range neurons. Pain. 2017;**158**(11):2117-2128

[121] Chung MK, LaRiccia PJ. Successful integrative medicine assessment and treatment of chronic pain associated with breast surgery: A report of 3 cases. Holistic Nursing Practice. 2017;**31**(1):21-29

[122] Schleip R. Fascial plasticity – A new neurobiological explanation: Part 1. Journal of Bodywork and Movement Therapies. 2003;**7**(1):11-19

[123] Schleip R. Fascial plasticity—A new neurobiological explanation part 2. Journal of Bodywork and Movement Therapies. 2003;**7**(2):104-116

[124] Benjamin M. The fascia of the limbs and back—A review. Journal of Anatomy. 2009;**214**(1):1-18

[125] Stecco C, Fede C, Macchi V, Porzionato A, Petrelli L, Biz C, et al. The fasciacytes: A new cell devoted to fascial gliding regulation. Clinical Anatomy. 2018;**31**(5):667-676

[126] Bei Y, Wang F, Yang C, Xiao J. Telocytes in regenerative medicine. Journal of Cellular and Molecular Medicine. 2015;**19**(7):1441-1454

[127] Varela F, Frenk S. The organ of form: Towards a theory of biological shape. Journal of Social and Biological Systems. 1987;**10**(1):73-83

[128] van der Wal J. The architecture of the connective tissue in the musculoskeletal system—An often overlooked functional parameter as to proprioception in the locomotor apparatus. International Journal of Therapeutic Massage & Bodywork. 2009;**2**(4):9-23

[129] Steinke H, Wiersbicki D, Speckert M-L, Merkwitz C, Wolfskämpf T, Wolf B. Periodic acid-Schiff (PAS) reaction and plastination in whole body slices. A novel technique to identify fascial tissue structures. Annals of Anatomy. 2018;**216**:29-35

[130] Langevin HM, Bishop J, Maple R, Badger GJ, Fox JR. Effect of stretching on thoracolumbar fascia injury and movement restriction in a porcine model. American Journal of Physical Medicine & Rehabilitation. 2018;**97**(3):187-191

[131] Serhan CN, Levy BD. Resolvins in inflammation: Emergence of the pro-resolving superfamily of mediators. The Journal of Clinical Investigation. 2018;**128**(7):2657-2669

[132] Berrueta L, Muskaj I, Olenich S, Butler T, Badger GJ, Colas RA, et al. Stretching impacts inflammation resolution in connective tissue. Journal of Cellular Physiology. 2016;**231**(7):1621-1627

[133] Xiong Y, Berrueta L, Urso K, Olenich S, Muskaj I, Badger GJ, et al. Stretching reduces skin thickness and improves subcutaneous tissue mobility in a murine model of systemic sclerosis. Frontiers in Immunology. 2017;**8**:124

[134] Bae H-I, Kim D-Y, Sung Y-H. Effects of a static stretch using a load on low back pain patients with shortened tensor fascia lata. Journal of Exercise Rehabilitation. 2017;**13**(2):227-231

[135] Avila Gonzalez CA, Driscoll M, Schleip R, Wearing S, Jacobson E, Findley T, et al. Frontiers in fascia research. Journal of Bodywork and Movement Therapies. 2018;**22**(4):873-880

[136] Wilke J, Krause F, Vogt L, Banzer W. What is evidence-based about myofascial chains: A systematic review. Archives of Physical Medicine and Rehabilitation. 2016;**97**(3):454-461

[137] Zhang W-B, Tian Y-Y, Li H, Tian J-H, Luo M-F, Xu F-L, et al. A discovery of low hydraulic resistance channel along meridians. Journal of Acupuncture and Meridian Studies. 2008;**1**(1):20-28

[138] Rutkowski JM, Swartz MA. A driving force for change: Interstitial flow as a morphoregulator. Trends in Cell Biology. 2007;**17**(1):44-50

[139] Zhang W-B, Xu Y-H, Tian Y-Y, Li H, Wang G-J, Huang T, et al. Induction of Hyperalgesia in pigs through blocking low hydraulic resistance channels and reduction of the resistance through acupuncture: A mechanism of action of acupuncture. Evidence-based Complementary and Alternative Medicine. 2013;**2013**:654645

[140] Balanyuk I, Ledonne G, Provenzano M, Bianco R, Meroni C, Ferri P, et al. Distraction technique for pain reduction in peripheral venous catheterization: Randomized, controlled trial. Acta Bio-Medica. 2018;**89**(4–S):55-63

[141] Taddio A, McMurtry CM, Shah V, Riddell RP, Chambers CT, Noel M, et al. Reducing pain during vaccine injections: Clinical practice guideline. CMAJ. 2015;**187**(13):975-982

[142] Birnie KA, Chambers CT, Taddio A, McMurtry CM, Noel M, Pillai Riddell R, et al. Psychological interventions for vaccine injections in children and adolescents: Systematic review of randomized and quasi-randomized controlled trials. The Clinical Journal of Pain. 2015;**31**(10 Suppl):S72-S89

[143] Yılmaz D, Güneş ÜY. The effect on pain of three different nonpharmacological methods in peripheral intravenous catheterisation in adults. Journal of Clinical Nursing. 2018;**27**(5-6):1073-1080

[144] Courtney CA, Duffy K, Serpell MG, O'Dwyer PJ. Outcome of patients with severe chronic pain following repair of groin hernia. The British Journal of Surgery. 2002;**89**(10):1310-1314

[145] Awonuga AO, Fletcher NM, Saed GM, Diamond MP. Postoperative adhesion development following cesarean and open intra-abdominal gynecological operations: A review. Reproductive Sciences. 2011;**18**(12):1166-1185

[146] Martín-Pintado-Zugasti A, Rodríguez-Fernández ÁL, Fernandez-Carnero J. Postneedling soreness after deep dry needling of a latent myofascial trigger point in the upper trapezius muscle: Characteristics, sex differences and associated factors. Journal of Back and Musculoskeletal Rehabilitation. 2016;**29**(2):301-308

[147] Moynihan R, Glasziou P, Woloshin S, Schwartz L, Santa J, Godlee F. Winding back the harms of too much medicine. BMJ. 2013;**346**:f1271

[148] BMJ. What is GRADE? [Internet]. BMJ Best Practice. 2018. Available from: https://bestpractice.bmj.com/info/toolkit/learn-ebm/what-is-grade/

[149] Izquierdo JN, Schoenbach VJ. The potential and limitations of data from population-based state cancer registries. American Journal of Public Health. 2000;**90**(5):695-698

[150] Schork NJ. Personalized medicine: Time for one-person trials. Nature. 2015;**520**(7549):609-611

[151] Molyneux M, Lauder G. A national collaborative simulation project: Paediatric anaesthetic emergencies. Pediatric Anesthesia. 2006;**16**(12):1302-1302

[152] Taylor M, Everett T, De Beer D, Mackinnon R. Managing emergencies in pediatric anesthesia (MEPA): Evolution of an international simulation training collaboration to improve the management of pediatric anesthetic emergencies: 10AP3-6. European Journal of Anaesthesiology. 2014;**31**:168-169

[153] Everett TC, MacKinnon R, de Beer D, Taylor M, Bould MD. Ten years of simulation-based training in pediatric anesthesia: The inception, evolution, and dissemination of the managing emergencies in pediatric anesthesia (MEPA) course. Paediatric Anaesthesia. 2017;**27**(10):984-990

[154] Advanced Life Support Group [Internet]. 2017. Available from: https://www.alsg.org

Section 5

Opioid Research

Chapter 11

Food-Derived Opioids: Production and the Effects of Opioids on Human Health

Sevda Arısoy, Işık Çoban and Özlem Üstün-Aytekin

Abstract

Traditional opioids have been used for the people who suffer from cancer, burns, surgery, HIV/AIDS, and other serious illness pains for years. However, numerous side effects like dizziness, apnea, physical dependence, tolerance, addiction, nausea, and vomiting push the researchers to look forward to the new opioid options. The opioid peptides which derived from foods provide significant advantages as the safe and natural alternative. The researchers reported that it is also promising a new functional food and nutraceutical. In this chapter, the type of food-derived opioids, their origins, possible receptors, their amino acid sequences, opioid effects, production techniques, and health benefits are reviewed.

Keywords: food opioids, exogenous opioid peptides, bioactive peptides

1. Introduction

Opioids have been acting on endogenous and exogenous opioidergic systems of the human. Endogenous opioids are generated in the human body. The system consists of mu (μ), delta (δ), kappa (κ), and nociception receptors (**Figure 1**) and their ligands (β-endorphins, enkephalins, dynorphins, and nociceptin/orphanin FQ) [1, 2]. The amino acid sequence of these opioids is almost the same as YGGF, except nociception/orphanin FQ [3].

Exogenous opioid peptides can bind act like endogenous. The most popular sample of exogenous opioids is morphine. It is a strong opioid isolated from plants and produced synthetically [3]. The chemical structure of morphine consists of a benzylisoquinoline alkaloid with two additional ring closures (**Figure 1**). Morphine, in both injectable and oral fast-acting formulations, can be used for acute and chronic pain and acts directly on the central nervous system (CNS). The most common application area is pain due to cancer, burns, surgery, HIV/AIDS, and other serious illnesses [4].

During the past two decades, morphine consumption reached almost record level 523 tons in 2013 followed by codeine and thebaine as 361 tons and 246 tons, respectively. The United States was the leader with 57.3% of global morphine consumption and followed by European countries (22.5%) and Canada (7.7%) [5].

Increasing of morphine and/or other opioid consumption has parallel increases in opioid overdoses. Because of the adverse effects of the exogenous opioids on human health such as dizziness, apnea, physical dependence, tolerance, nausea, vomiting, and addiction, interest in morphine-like food-derived

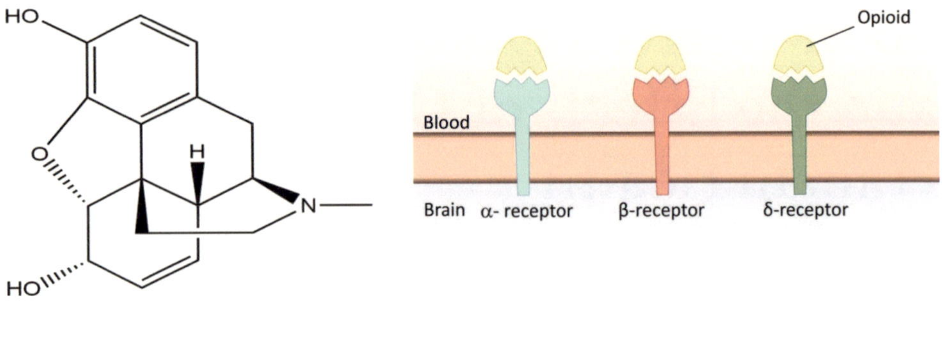

(a) (b)

Figure 1.
(a) Chemical structure of morphine, (b) The opioid receptors in human body.

Opioid peptide	Source	Amino acid sequence	Opioid receptor	Opioid effect	Reference
β-casomorphine-4	β-Casein/milk	YPFP	μ	Opioid agonist	[6, 7]
β-casomorphine-5	β-Casein/milk	YPFPG	μ	Opioid agonist	[6, 7]
β-casomorphine-6	β-Casein/milk	YPFPGP	μ	Opioid agonist	[6, 7]
β-casomorphine-7	β-Casein/milk	YPFPGPI	μ	Opioid agonist	[6, 7]
Lactoferroxin A	Lactoferrin/milk	YLGSGY	μ	Opioid antagonist	[8, 9–11]
Lactoferroxin B	Lactoferrin/milk	RYYGY	κ	Opioid antagonist	[8, 9–11]
Lactoferroxin C	Lactoferrin/milk	KYLGPGY	κ	Opioid antagonist	[8, 9–11]
α-Lactorphin	α-Lactalbumin/milk	YGLF	μ	Opioid agonist	[12, 13]
β-Lactorphin	β-Lactoglobulin/milk	YLLF	μ	Opioid agonist	[12, 13]
Casoxin A	κ-Casein/milk	YPSYGLN	μ	Opioid antagonist	[6, 14, 15]
Casoxin B	κ-Casein/milk	YPYY	μ	Opioid antagonist	[6, 14, 15]
Casoxin C	κ-Casein/milk	YIPIQYVLSR	μ	Opioid antagonist	[6, 14, 15]
Casoxin D	α-Casein/milk	YVPFPPF	μ	Opioid antagonist	[6, 14, 15]
Serorphin	Bovine serum protein	YGFQNA	δ	Opioid agonist	[16, 17]
Hermorphin	Hemoglobin	YPWT	μ	Opioid agonist	[16, 17]
Gluteomorphine A4	Wheat protein	GYYP	δ	Opioid agonist	[6, 18]
Gluteomorphine A5	Wheat protein	GYYPT	δ	Opioid agonist	[6, 18]
Gluteomorphine B4	Wheat protein	YGGW	δ	Opioid agonist	[6, 18]
Gluteomorphine B5	Wheat protein	YGGWL	δ	Opioid agonist	[6, 18]
Gluteomorphine C5	Wheat protein	YPISL	δ	Opioid agonist	[6, 18]
Gluteomorphine 7	Wheat protein	YPQPQPF	δ	Opioid agonist	[6, 18]
Soymorphine-5	Soy protein	YPFVV	μ	Opioid agonist	[19–21]

Opioid peptide	Source	Amino acid sequence	Opioid receptor	Opioid effect	Reference
Soymorphine-6	Soy protein	YPFVVN	μ	Opioid agonist	[19–21]
Soymorphine-7	Soy protein	YPFVVNA	μ	Opioid agonist	[19–21]
Rubiscolin-5	Spinach protein	YPLDL	δ	Opioid agonist	[22–24]
Rubiscolin-6	Spinach protein	YPLDLF	δ	—	[22–24]
Oryzatensin	Rice protein	GYPMYPLPR	μ	Opioid antagonist	[8, 25, 26]
Ovalulin	Ovalbumin/egg	YPLDLF	δ	—	[8, 9–11]

Table 1.
Food-derived opioid peptides, amino acid sequences, opioid receptors, opioid effects, and production method.

opioid peptides, exorphins, has been increased by researchers. Exorphins are generated from exogenous proteins, such as milk, meat, cereal, plant, or egg by enzymatic digestion [3, 8]. They across the blood-brain barrier, interact with opioid receptors, and stimulate analgesic activity and sedative effect on the nervous system. Most of the food-derived exorphins were tested for the opioid activity, and amino acid sequences were identified. The results showed that the exorphins generally have a tyrosine (Tyr; Y) residue at the amino terminal end (except α-casein opioids) (**Table 1**).

On the other hand, due to the lack of digestive enzymes in some people and their sensitivities on opioids, food-derived opioid peptide consumption might be involved in some important diseases. For example, the increase in β-casomorphin formation from β-caseins of either human or cow milk has a correlation with the sudden infant death (SID) syndrome [27, 28]. After the penetration of β-casomorphins into the infants' immature central nervous system, the respiratory center in the brain stem may be inhibited, resulting in breathing abnormality, hypercapnia, apnea, and mortality [29]. Moreover, in atopic eczema (a relapsing skin disease prevalent on infants' face, knees, and elbows), induced immune cells form β-casomorphin from breast milk β-caseins, resulting in histamine secretion that causes allergic skin reactions. The reason for this is the lack of DPPIV enzyme which is negatively correlated with the amount of β-casomorphin [30]. The DPPIV enzyme is also effective on autistic children on the treatment of some symptoms (e.g., insensitivity to pain, digestion problems, attention problems) which are caused by the effects of β-casomorphins and gluteomorphins [31]. β-casomorphins may also cause depression which is a significant risk factor for cardiac patient men [32].

2. Bioactive peptides and generation of the opioid peptides

Food proteins provide numerous important biologically active peptides. These peptides can be released by gastrointestinal digestive enzymes during digestion, ripening processes or fermentation with proteolytic starter culture and hydrolyzing with commercial protease derived from microorganisms or plants [6, 33]. Many recent articles have been focused on the effect of bioactive peptides on human health. Generally, these peptides are known as specific peptide fragments that have a positive effect on human body systems, functions, and conditions depending on their amino acid composition and sequence [7, 34]. Oral administration of the bioactive peptides may affect the nervous, cardiovascular, immune, and digestive system. Opioid peptides are one of the most studied bioactive peptides (**Figure 2**).

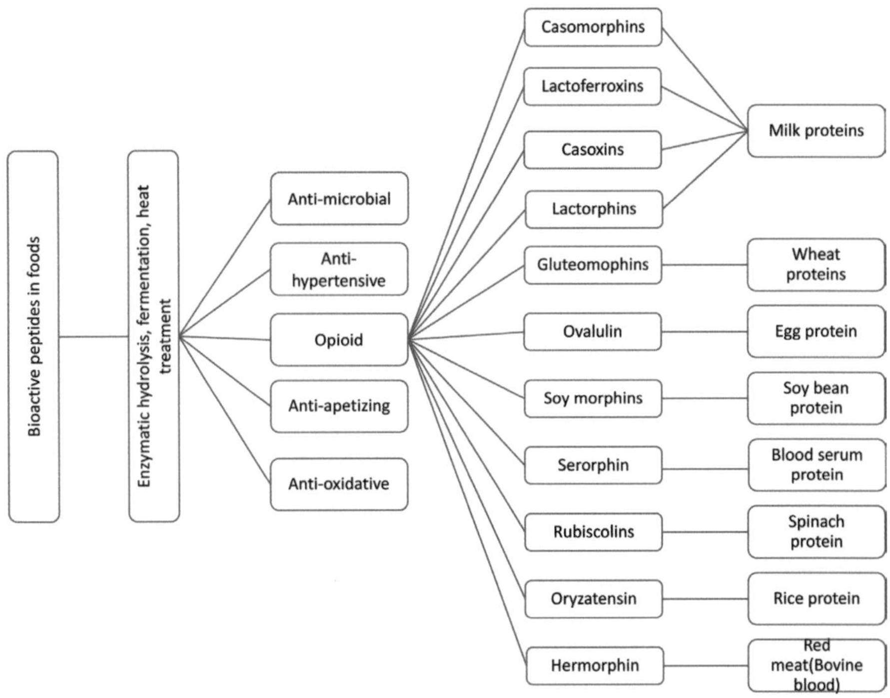

Figure 2.
Generation of bioactive peptides from foods and opioids.

3. Opioid peptides derived from animal protein

Because of the protein structures, milk proteins (80% casein; αS1-casein, αS2-casein, β-casein, and κ-casein and 20% whey protein; α-lactalbumin, β-lactoglobulin, serum albumin, immunoglobulins, and lactoferrins) have a great potential to occurrence of opioid peptides by fermentation, heat treatment, or enzymatic hydrolysis [35, 36]. Hydrolysis of these milk proteins lead to generate peptides that may have opioid activity. The milk-derived opioids have been named as β-casomorphins (β-casein), lactoferroxins (lactoferrin), casoxin (κ-casein, α -casein), α-lactorphin (α-lactalbumin), and β-lactophin (β-lactoglobulin) [9, 37]. β-casomorphins, the milk origin opioid peptides, were firstly detected in the infant's gastrointestinal system and blood plasma [10]. Then, the same structure was found in raw, processed sheep, buffalo, and human milk and fermented dairy products. The β-casomorphin group derived from β-casein consists of short-chain peptides such as β-casomorphin-4,-5,-6, and-7, and they act as opioid agonists on μ-type opioid receptors [9–11]. Researchers indicated that β-casomorphin is responsible for the calming effect of milk and stimulation of insulin and somatostatin release [12].

Lactoferrin is an iron-binding glycoprotein and known as a whey protein. It can be found not only in milk but also in secretion fluids such as tears, saliva, and synovial fluids. Lactoferrin is involved in many biological activities in human-like antimicrobial and anti-inflammatory effects and stimulating iron absorption [13]. After digestion, lactoferroxin A, B, and D forms are produced (**Table 1**). While lactoferroxins B and C act as an opioid antagonist to the κ-type receptor, lactoferroxin A acts opioid antagonists on μ-type opioid receptors. All lactoferroxin forms have weak opioid activities [8, 14–16].

α-lactorphin and β-lactorphin are derived from α-lactalbumin (bovine and human) and β-lactoglobulin (bovine), respectively. These two lactorphins are opioid agonist to the μ-type receptor; they inhibit the angiotensin-converting enzyme activity (ACE) and have been shown to have a smooth muscle contracting effect [17, 38].

All κ-casein fragments are known as casoxins that are produced by digestion of bovine casein with pepsin and trypsin. Casoxins A, B, and C were obtained from κ- casein by the enzymatic digestion, and casoxin D was produced from α-casein in bovine milk. Casoxins are the opioid antagonist to μ-type receptor-like lactoferrins, and casoxin C have the highest biological potency, and researchers reported that it can inhibit the ACE activity [9, 39, 40].

Other opioid peptides from animal sources are serorphin, historphin, valentorphin, kapporphin, hemorphin, and ovalulin. Serorphin has a δ-type opioid receptor ligand with agonist activity and generated from bovine serum proteins by digestion with pepsin. Historphin (YGFGG) and valentorphin (YGFIL) are structurally similar to the serorphin which are derived from histone H4 and carboxypeptidases A and B, respectively. An effective opioid on peristaltic movement, bladder spasm, and pain management, hemorphin is derived from digested hemoglobin, passes the blood-brain barrier, and acts as an opioid agonist to μ-type receptors [41, 42]. Researchers have reported that there is very limited knowledge about the last two opioid peptides: ovalulin and kapporphin. The origin of ovalulin is ovalbumin that is an egg protein and synthesized as a homolog of rubiscolin (spinach opioid) [43]. Kapporphin (YSFGG) is derived from immunoglobulin κ-chain [18].

4. Opioid peptides derived from plant/cereal protein

Among the possible opioids in plants, the major opioids are gluten exorphins (gluteomorphins, gliadorphins) that consist of a combination of gliadin and glutenin proteins and are found in some grains such as wheat, rye, barley, and oats. Studies have shown that gluteomorphins act as opioid agonists on δ-type opioid receptors and consist of gluteomorphin A4, A5, B4, B5, C, and 7. These are resistant to the intestinal and enterobacterial proteinases, cross the human intestinal epithelium, enter the bloodstream, and interfere with the central nervous system [9, 43–47]. Gluteomorphin A5 has been associated with antinociceptive effect and modulation of memory process and affects peripheral nervous system and central nervous system. Takahashi et al. [19] and Fanciulli et al. [44] revealed that gluteomorphin B5 induced prolactin secretion after peripheral injection in rats. Gluteomorphin C reduced anxiety and developed learning ability after consumption [9]. Casomorphins and gluteomorphins are associated with autism spectrum disorder because these opioid peptides found in the urine samples of autistic patients and removing casein and gluten proteins from autistic children's diet may improve learning abilities, concentration, attention and language problems, eye contact, and digestion problems [21, 31].

Soy protein is one of the widely used cereals in foods for gelation, emulsification, and viscosity [3]. Soymorphins are derived from the soybean β-conglycinin β-subunit by digestion with pancreatic elastase and leucine aminopeptidase and act as opioid agonists' anxiolytic-like activity on μ-type opioid receptors. The opioid activity of the soymorphin is twice than β-casomorphin. Soymorphin fractions consist of soymorphin-5, soymorphin-6, and soymorphin-7 had anxiolytic effects with oral administration at doses of 10–30 mg/kg in mice [23]. Oral administration of soymorphin suppresses food intake, especially soymorphin-7 which is more effective in suppressing food intake than soymorphin-5 and soymorphin-6 [24]. Soymorphins inhibit anxiety and overeating and are also effective on glucose and lipid metabolism. Soymorphin-5 associated with decreasing triglycerides both the plasma and liver in diabetic mice [25].

Rubiscolins are derived from spinach protein by digestion with pepsin. Rubiscolin-5 and rubiscolin-6 are opioid agonist to δ-type receptor. Oral administration at different doses of rubiscolin-6 may have an analgesic effect and anxiolytic effect and stimulate food intake and memory consolidation in mice [26, 48, 49].

Oryzatensin is derived from digestion of rice albumin with trypsin and acts as opioid antagonists on μ-type opioid receptors, and also oryzatensin has an affinity to C3a receptors and immunomodulating activities [8, 50, 51].

5. Production of food-derived exogenous opioid peptides

Although food sources do not exhibit opioid activity in their own right, the peptide products of the proteins of these foods can exhibit opioid activity. For the efficient production of opioids by using food proteins as substrate, three different production methods were mentioned: chemical digestion, enzymatic gastrointestinal or commercial hydrolysis, and microbial production.

5.1 Chemical digestion

On the purpose of improving protein digestion and peptide formation, acid hydrolysis is applied to food protein-rich substrate. For cheeses (e.g., Mozzarella), the profile of produced bioactive peptide might be affected from the type of acid used for hydrolysis [52]. Conventional conditions for acid hydrolysis (6 M HCl treatment at 110° C for more than 24 h) can cause the destruction of amino acids (e.g., tryptophan) [53]. On the other hand, in the food industry, alkali treatment is quite rarely applied for protein hydrolysis because of the loss of protein digestibility [52] and it can reduce arginine, cystine, serine, threonine, lysine, and/or isoleucine content and form unexpected amino acid residual forms such as lanthionine or lysinoalanine. Because of the difficulty of controlling chemical processes and yielding products with modified amino acids, the other treatment methods (enzymatic, fermentation) are preferred in bioactive peptide productions [53].

5.2 Enzymatic hydrolysis

A common way to produce opioid bioactive peptides is enzymatic hydrolysis, and the production of opioid peptides via enzymatic hydrolysis is mostly carried out by using microbial enzymes (e.g., thermolysin, alcalase) and gastrointestinal enzymes (e.g., trypsin, chymotrypsin, pepsin, and pancreatin) [54–56]. In some studies, an increase in opioid activity was reported by using a combination of gastrointestinal enzymes and microbial enzymes [54, 55]. Moreover, the components of these combinations are also significant in opioid types and concentrations. For example, food proteins are hydrolyzed by pepsin to produce opioids. Besides, pepsin-thermolysin combination produces gluten exorphins A5, B5, A4, and B4, while trypsin-chymotrypsin-pepsin hydrolysate forms gluten exorphin C [54, 55]. The pepsin-elastase hydrolysate, with its 250 μg/g concentration, has almost 5 times higher gluten exorphin A5 concentration than pepsin-thermolysin hydrolysate (40 μg/g) [57]. Soymorphin-4 and soymorphin-5 are released from soy protein by the activity of elastase and leucine aminopeptidase; however, soymorphin-6 is released by pepsin and pancreatic elastase activity [43]. Enzymatic hydrolysis is carried out by the following method regardless of the food protein used (**Figure 3**): preparation of raw material for enzymatic hydrolysis (size reduction, etc.), homogenization in buffer, temperature, and pH adjustment to the optimum values of the enzyme, and hydrolysis of food product by enzyme (ultrasonic-assisted hydrolysis

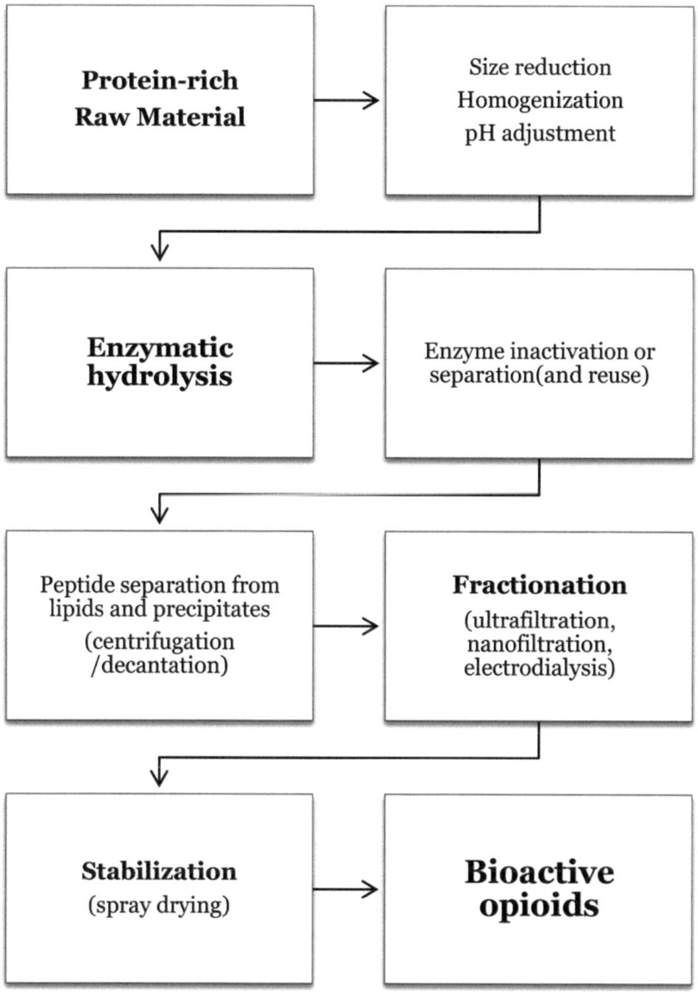

Figure 3.
Flow diagram to produce bioactive opioids.

for low molecular weight peptide production) [58, 59]. After inactivating or separating enzymes from hydrolysate, bioactive peptides are separated from the non-product residuals (e.g., lipids and precipitate) by centrifugation and decantation, subsequently fractionated (e.g., ultrafiltration, nanofiltration, electrodialysis), and then stabilized (e.g., spray drying) [60–62].

For producing desired peptides, using a proper enzyme and optimizing reaction conditions (e.g., time, pH, amount of the enzyme, temperature) are highly important [62]. For example, thermolysin enzyme obtained from *Bacillus thermoproteolyticus* has an optimum activation temperature range between 65 and 85°C and optimum pH between 5 and 8.5, while *Bacillus licheniformis* alcalase is active around 50°C and pH 8.

5.3 Microbial production

The use of protease-secreting microbial strains is an alternative method for chemical proteolysis and enzymatic hydrolysis for hydrolysis of food protein-rich substrates [63]. Enzymes secreted from microorganisms depending on the type of microbial production provide the secretion of opioids by hydrolyzing a protein-rich substrate [9]. The peptides produced during fermentation exhibit a high bioactivity and better opioid functions. For the fermentation of protein-rich sources to produce bioactive peptides, *Lactobacillus* is one of the most widely employed genera [9–26, 38–63]. Due to the use of lactic acid bacteria, protein-rich substrates become acidified because of lactic acid production. Lactic acid existence in the production media provides a microbiologically safe environment for production and extent shelf life of the opioid product because of the organic acid feature of lactic acid [63]. *Lactobacillus helveticus* L89 X-prolyl dipeptidyl aminopeptidase (Pep X)-deficient mutant strain was used for milk fermentation to produce β-casomorphin-4 [64].

Enzymatic proteolysis of *Lactobacillus* GG-fermented ultra-high temperature milk substrate by pepsin and trypsin resulted in the release of some opioid sequences (RYLGYLE, YPFP, YPFPGPIPNSL, YGLF) [65]. *L. delbrueckii* ssp. *bulgaricus* and *S. salivarius* ssp. *thermophilus* produce β-casomorphin precursors from fermented yogurt. But they cannot produce β-casomorphin because of an inability of these bacteria to hydrolyze β-casein to β-casomorphin. *Bacillus cereus* and *Pseudomonas aeruginosa* are also able to produce β-casomorphin from the fermentation of milk. *Kluyveromyces marxianus* var. *marxianus* can produce β-lactorphin from whey [9].

In addition, it is possible to produce opioid peptides from fungi fermentation. In Brie, Gouda, Gorgonzola, Cheddar, and Fontina cheeses, β-casomorphin was also detected in different concentrations.

To sum up, opioid peptides are promising new exogenous opioids because they are free from adverse effects on human health. Due to this feature, there is a growing interest to elucidate the function of food-derived opioid peptides in the human body. The production techniques of food-derived opioid peptides are mostly based on hydrolysis of food proteins by using commercial or/and gastrointestinal enzymes. Also, some of the researchers conclude that food-derived opioid peptides may be carefully considered as new nutraceutical candidates.

Conflict of interest

No potential conflict of interest was reported by the authors.

Author details

Sevda Arısoy[1], Işık Çoban[2] and Özlem Üstün-Aytekin[1*]

1 Faculty of Health Sciences, Department of Nutrition and Dietetics, University of Health Sciences, Istanbul, Turkey

2 Faculty of Engineering, Department of Bioengineering, İstanbul Medeniyet University, Istanbul, Turkey

*Address all correspondence to: ozlem.aytekin@sbu.edu.tr

References

[1] Teschemacher H. Opioid receptor ligands derived from food proteins. Current Pharmaceutical Design. 2003;**9**:1331-1344. DOI: 10.2174/1381612033454856

[2] Corder G, Castro DC, Bruchas MR, Scherrer G. Endogenous and exogenous opioids in pain. Annual Review of Neuroscience. 2018;**41**:453-473. DOI: 10.1146/annurev-neuro-080317-061522

[3] Stefanucci A, Mollica A, Macedonio G, Zengin G, Ahmed AA, Novellino E. Exogenous opioid peptides derived from food proteins and their possible uses as dietary supplements: A critical review. Food Reviews International. 2018;**34**:70-86. DOI: 10.1080/87559129.2016.1225220

[4] WHO. [Internet]. 2018. http://apps.who.int/iris/bitstream/handle/10665/274559/9789241514477-eng.pdf?ua=1 [Accessed: December 4, 2018]

[5] Comments on the Reported Statistics on Narcotic Drugs [Internet]. 2013. https://www.incb.org/documents/Narcotic-Drugs/Technical publications/2014/ND_TR_2014_2 Comments_EN.pdf [Accessed: December 4, 2018]

[6] Mann B, Athira S, Sharma R, Kumar R, Sarkar P. Bioactive peptides from whey proteins. In: Deeth HC, Bansal N, editors. Whey Proteins: From Milk to Medicine. Academic Press; 2019. pp. 519-547. DOI: 10.1016/B978-0-12-812124-5.00015-1

[7] Udenigwe CC, Aluko RE. Food protein-derived bioactive peptides: Production, processing, and potential health benefits. Journal of Food Science. 2012;**77**(1):R11-R24. DOI: 10.1111/j.1750-3841.2011.02455.x

[8] Yoshikawa M. Exorphins. In: Kastin AJ, editor. Handbook of Biologically Active Peptides. 2nd ed. London: Academic press; 2013. pp. 1570-1576

[9] Garg S, Nurgali K, Kumar Mishra V. Food proteins as source of opioid peptides—A review. Current Medicinal Chemistry. 2016;**23**:893-910. DOI: 10.2174/0929867323666160219115226

[10] Brantl V, Teschemacher H, Henschen A, Lottspeich F. Novel opioid peptides derived from casein (β-casomorphins). I. Isolation from bovine casein peptone. Hoppe-Seyler's Zeitschrift für Physiologische Chemie. 1979;**360**:1211-1224. DOI: 10.1515/bchm2.1979.360.2.1211

[11] Nguyen DD, Busetti F, Johnson SK, Solah VA. Degradation of β-casomorphins and identification of degradation products during yoghurt processing using liquid chromatography coupled with high resolution mass spectrometry. Foodservice Research International. 2018;**106**:98-104. DOI: 10.1016/j.foodres.2017.12.035

[12] Defilippi C, Gomez E, Charlin V, Silva C. Inhibition of small intestinal motility by casein: A role of beta casomorphins. Nutrition. 1995;**11**:751-754

[13] Suzuki YA, Kelleher SL, Yalda D, Wu L, Huang J, Huang N, et al. Expression, characterization, and biologic activity of recombinant human lactoferrin in rice. Journal of Pediatric Gastroenterology and Nutrition. 2003;**36**:190-199

[14] Teschemacher H, Koch G, Brantl V. Milk protein-derived opioid receptor ligands. Peptide Science. 1997;**43**:99-117

[15] Yildirım Z, Tokatlı M, Öncül N, Yildirım M. Laktoferrinin Biyolojik Aktivitesi. Academic Food Journal. 2011;(9):52-63

[16] Park YW, Nam MS. Bioactive peptides in milk and dairy products: A review. Korean Journal for Food Science of Animal Resources. 2015;**35**:831. DOI: 10.5851/kosfa.2015.35.6.831

[17] Antila P, Paakkari I, Järvinen A, Mattila MJ, Laukkanen M, Pihlanto-Leppälä A, et al. Opioid peptides derived from in-vitro proteolysis of bovine whey proteins. International Dairy Journal. 1991;**1**:215-229. DOI: 10.1016/0958-6946(91)90015-Z

[18] Tani F, Shiota A, Chiba H, Yoshikawa M. Serorphin, an opioid peptide derived from bovine. In: Β-Casomorphins and Related Peptides: Recent Developments. Kyoto; 1994. pp. 49-53

[19] Takahashi M, Fukunaga H, Kaneto H, Fukudome SI, Yoshikawa M. Behavioral and pharmacological studies on gluten exorphin A5, a newly isolated bioactive food protein fragment, in mice. The Japanese Journal of Pharmacology. 2000;**84**:259-265. DOI: 10.1254/jjp.84.259

[20] Fanciulli G, Dettori A, Fenude E, Demontis MP, Alberico E, Delitala G, et al. Intravenous administration of the food-derived opioid peptide gluten exorphin B5 stimulates prolactin secretion in rats. Pharmacological Research. 2003;**47**:53-58. DOI: 10.1016/S1043-6618(02)00267-0

[21] Zaky EA. Autism spectrum disorder (ASD): The past, the present, and the future. Journal of Child and Adolescent Behavior. 2017;**5**:1-4. DOI: 10.4172/2375-4494.1000e116

[22] Liu Z, Udenigwe CC. Role of food-derived opioid peptides in the central nervous and gastrointestinal systems. Journal of Food Biochemistry. 2018;**43**:e12629. DOI: 10.1111/jfbc.12629

[23] Ohinata K, Agui S, Yoshikawa M. Soymorphins, novel μ opioid peptides derived from soy β-conglycinin β-subunit, have anxiolytic activities. Bioscience, Biotechnology, and Biochemistry. 2007;**71**:2618-2621. DOI: 10.1271/bbb.70516

[24] Kaneko K, Iwasaki M, Yoshikawa M, Ohinata K. Orally administered soymorphins, soy-derived opioid peptides, suppress feeding and intestinal transit via gut μ1-receptor coupled to 5-HT1A, D2, and GABAB systems. American Journal of Physiology. Gastrointestinal and Liver Physiology. 2010;**299**:G799-G805. DOI: 10.1152/ajpgi.00081.2010

[25] Yamada Y, Muraki A, Oie M, Kanegawa N, Oda A, Sawashi Y, et al. Soymorphin-5, a soy-derived μ-opioid peptide, decreases glucose and triglyceride levels through activating adiponectin and PPARα systems in diabetic KKAy mice. American Journal of Physiology. Endocrinology and Metabolism. 2011;**302**:E433-E440. DOI: 10.1152/ajpendo.00161.2011

[26] Yang S, Kawamura Y, Yoshikawa M. Effect of rubiscolin, a δ opioid peptide derived from rubisco, on memory consolidation. Peptides. 2003;**24**:325-328. DOI: 10.1016/S0196-9781(03)00044-5

[27] Blair PS, Byard RW, Fleming PJ. Sudden unexpected death in infancy (SUDI): Suggested classification and applications to facilitate research activity. Forensic Science, Medicine, and Pathology. 2012;**8**:312-315. DOI: 10.1007/s12024-011-9294-x

[28] Sienkiewicz-Szłapka E, Jarmołowska B, Krawczuk S, Kostyra E, Kostyra H, Iwan M. Contents of agonistic and antagonistic opioid peptides in different cheese varieties. International Dairy Journal. 2009;**19**:258-263. DOI: 10.1016/j.idairyj.2008.10.011

[29] Sun Z, Cade R. Findings in normal rats following administration of gliadorphin-7 (GD-7). Peptides. 2003;**24**:321-323. DOI: 10.1016/S0196-9781(03)00043-3

[30] Jarmołowska B, Bielikowicz K, Iwan M, Sidor K, Kostyra E, Kaczmarski M. Serum activity of

dipeptidyl peptidase IV (DPPIV; EC 3.4. 14.5) in breast-fed infants with symptoms of allergy. Peptides. 2007;**28**:678-682. DOI: 10.1016/j.peptides.2006.11.014

[31] Arısoy S, Üstün-Aytekin Ö. Hydrolysis of food-derived opioids by dipeptidyl peptidase IV from *Lactococcus lactis* spp. *lactis*. Foodservice Research International. 2018;**111**:574-581. DOI: 10.1016/j.foodres.2018.05.068

[32] McLachlan CNS. β-Casein A1, ischaemic heart disease mortality, and other illnesses. Medical Hypotheses. 2001;**56**:262-272. DOI: 10.1054/mehy.2000.1265

[33] Korhonen H, Pihlanto A. Bioactive peptides: Production and functionality. International Dairy Journal. 2006;**16**:945-960. DOI: 10.1016/j.idairyj.2005.10.012

[34] Möller NP, Scholz-Ahrens KE, Roos N, Schrezenmeir J. Bioactive peptides and proteins from foods: Indication for health effects. European Journal of Nutrition. 2008;**47**(4):171-182. DOI: 10.1007/s00394-008-0710-2

[35] Mohanty DP, Mohapatra S, Misra S, Sahu PS. Milk derived bioactive peptides and their impact on human health—A review. Saudi Journal of Biological Sciences. 2016;**23**:577-583. DOI: 10.1016/j.sjbs.2015.06.005

[36] O'Callaghan TF, Sugrue I, Hill C, Ross RP, Stanton C. Nutritional aspects of raw milk: A beneficial or hazardous food choice. In: Nero LA, De Carvalho AF, editors. Raw Milk. London: Academic Press; 2019. pp. 127-148. DOI: 10.1016/C2016-0-00282-6

[37] Borad SG, Kumar A, Singh AK. Effect of processing on nutritive values of milk protein. Critical Reviews in Food Science and Nutrition. 2017;**57**:3690-3702. DOI: 10.1080/10408398.2016.1160361

[38] Nagpal R, Behare P, Rana R, Kumar A, Kumar M, Arora S, et al. Bioactive peptides derived from milk proteins and their health beneficial potentials: An update. Food & Function. 2011;**2**:18-27. DOI: 10.1039/C0FO00016G

[39] Xu RJ. Bioactive peptides in milk and their biological and health implications. Food Reviews International. 1998;**14**:1-16. DOI: 10.1080/87559129809541147

[40] Meisel H. Multifunctional peptides encrypted in milk proteins. BioFactors. 2004;**21**:55-61. DOI: 10.1002/biof.552210111

[41] Yoshikawa M, Chiba H. Biologically active peptides derived from food and blood proteins. In: Frontiers and New Horizons in Amino Acid Research. Kyoto: Elsevier Publishers; 1992. pp. 403-409

[42] Domenger D, Cudennec B, Kouach M, Touche V, Landry C, Lesage J, et al. Food-derived hemorphins cross intestinal and blood–brain barriers in vitro. Frontiers in Endocrinology. 2018;**9**:159. DOI: 10.3389/fendo.2018.00159

[43] Yoshikawa M. Bioactive peptides derived from natural proteins with respect to diversity of their receptors and physiological effects. Peptides. 2015;**72**:208-225. DOI: 10.1016/j.peptides.2015.07.013

[44] Vojdani A. The characterization of the repertoire of wheat antigens and peptides involved in the humoral immune responses in patients with gluten sensitivity and Crohn's disease. ISRN Allergy. 2011:1-12. DOI: 10.5402/2011/950104

[45] Czaja-Bulsa G. Non coeliac gluten sensitivity—A new disease with gluten intolerance. Clinical Nutrition. 2015;**34**:189-194

[46] Maggioni M, De Luca P, Arnaboldi F, Cornaghi L, Fiorilli A, Donetti E, et al.

CACO2/HT-29 coculture: An in vitro intestinal cell model to study nutrients-gut interaction. In: European Nutrition Conference (FENS): 2015 October 20-23. Karger. p. 223

[47] Pruimboom L, De Punder K. The opioid effects of gluten exorphins: Asymptomatic celiac disease. Journal of Health, Population, and Nutrition. 2015;**33**:24. DOI: 10.1186/s41043-015-0032-y

[48] Hirata H, Sonoda S, Agui S, Yoshida M, Ohinata K, Yoshikawa M. Rubiscolin-6, a δ opioid peptide derived from spinach rubisco, has anxiolytic effect via activating σ1 and dopamine D1 receptors. Peptides. 2007;**28**:1998-2003. DOI: 10.1016/j.peptides.2007.07.024

[49] Kaneko K, Lazarus M, Miyamoto C, Oishi Y, Nagata N, Yang S, et al. Orally administered rubiscolin-6, a δ opioid peptide derived from rubisco, stimulates food intake via leptomeningeal lipocalin-type prostaglandin D synthase in mice. Molecular Nutrition & Food Research. 2012;**56**:1315-1323. DOI: 10.1002/mnfr.201200155

[50] Agyei D, Danquah MK. Industrial-scale manufacturing of pharmaceutical-grade bioactive peptides. Biotechnology Advances. 2011;**29**:272-277. DOI: 10.1016/j.biotechadv.2011.01.001

[51] Takahashi M, Moriguchi S, Yoshikawa M, Sasaki R. Isolation and characterization of oryzatensin: A novel bioactive peptide with ileum-contracting and immunomodulating activities derived from rice albumin. Biochemistry and Molecular Biology International. 1994;**33**:1151-1158

[52] Kopf-Bolanz KA. Adjusting bioactive functions of dairy products via processing. In: Technological Approaches for Novel Applications in Dairy Processing. Rijeka: IntechOpen; 2017. DOI: 10.5772/intechopen.72927

[53] Tavano OL. Protein hydrolysis using proteases: An important tool for food biotechnology. Journal of Molecular Catalysis B: Enzymatic. 2013;**90**:1-11. DOI: 10.1016/j.molcatb.2013.01.011

[54] Fukudome SI, Yoshikawa M. Opioid peptides derived from wheat gluten: Their isolation and characterization. FEBS Letters. 1992;**296**:107-111. DOI: 10.1016/0014-5793(92)80414-C

[55] Fukudome SI, Yoshikawa M. Gluten exorphin C: A novel opioid peptide derived from wheat gluten. FEBS Letters. 1993;**316**:17-19. DOI: 10.1016/0014-5793(93)81727-H

[56] Pihlanto A. Bioactive peptides. In: Fuquay JW, Fox FP, PLH MS, editors. Encyclopedia of Dairy Sciences. Vol. 3. London: Academic Press; 2011. pp. 879-886

[57] Fukudome SI, Jinsmaa Y, Matsukawa T, Sasaki R, Yoshikawa M. Release of opioid peptides, gluten exorphins by the action of pancreatic elastase. FEBS Letters. 1997;**412**:475-479. DOI: 10.1016/S0014-5793(97)00829-6

[58] García-Moreno PJ, Pérez-Gálvez R, Guadix EM, Guadix A. Recent patents on the upgrading of fish by-products. Recent Patents on Chemical Engineering. 2010;**3**:149-162

[59] Kadam SU, Tiwari BK, Álvarez C, O'Donnell CP. Ultrasound applications for the extraction, identification and delivery of food proteins and bioactive peptides. Trends in Food Science and Technology. 2015;**46**:60-67. DOI: 10.1016/j.tifs.2015.07.012

[60] Abdul-Hamid A, Bakar J, Bee GH. Nutritional quality of spray dried protein hydrolysate from black tilapia (*Oreochromis mossambicus*). Food Chemistry. 2002;**78**(1):69-74. DOI: 10.1016/S0308-8146(01)00380-6

[61] Espejo-Carpio FJ, Guadix A, Guadix EM. Spray drying of goat milk protein hydrolysates with angiotensin converting enzyme inhibitory activity. Food and Bioprocess Technology. 2014;7(8):2388-2396. DOI: 10.1007/s11947-013-1230-5

[62] Kristinsson HG. In: Shahidi F, editor. Aquatic Food Protein Hydrolysates. Cambridge: Woodhead Publishing Limited; 2006. pp. 229-248

[63] Mora L, Reig M, Toldrá F. Bioactive peptides generated from meat industry by-products. Foodservice Research International. 2014;**65**:344-349. DOI: 10.1016/j.foodres.2014.09.014

[64] Matar C, Goulet J. β-Casomorphin 4 from milk fermented by a mutant of *Lactobacillus helveticus*. International Dairy Journal. 1996;**6**:383-397. DOI: 10.1016/0958-6946(95)00015-1

[65] Rokka T, Syväoja EL, Tuominen J, Korhonen HJ. Release of bioactive peptides by enzymatic proteolysis of *Lactobacillus* GG fermented UHT-milk. Milchwissenschaft. 1997;**52**:675-678